Anesthesia Care for Cancer Patients

Edited by

Bharathi Gourkanti, Irwin Gratz, William Marion, Rajiv Lingaraju & Grace Abramian

Department of Anesthesiology
Cooper Medical School of Rowan University
Cooper University Health Care
Camden, NJ, USA

Anesthesia Care for Cancer Patients

Editors: Bharathi Gourkanti, Irwin Gratz, William Marion, Rajiv Lingaraju & Grace Abramian

ISBN (Online): 979-8-89881-372-7

ISBN (Print): 979-8-89881-373-4

ISBN (Paperback): 979-8-89881-374-1

First published in 2025.

Bentham Science Publishers Pte. Ltd.
No. 9 Raffles Place
Office No. 26-01
Singapore 048619
Singapore
Email: subscriptions@benthamscience.net

BENTHAM SCIENCE

CONTENTS

FOREWORD

The field of oncoanesthesiology emerged in 2003 with a study investigating the effects of various anesthetic agents on tumor metastasis. Since this study, there have been numerous articles published describing the impact of various anesthetic techniques on natural killer cells, cytokines, T-lymphocytes, and cell apoptosis with the ultimate goal of discovering the preferred anesthetic technique when caring for the patient. This text emphasizes and addresses the importance of the perioperative care of the cancer patient. The anesthesia care these patients require is beyond the knowledge most anesthesia providers gained during their training; the vast body of literature available requires a clear, concise summary. The great news is that both goals are accomplished in this book.

The editors provide an outstanding summary of this emerging specialty, with chapters being written by leading experts. The uniformity in chapter presentation and minimal overlap are a testament to the efforts of the editors to provide a useful book on oncoanesthesiology that will provide new information for both novice and expert anesthesia providers. The inclusion of a chapter on the physiologic changes that occur in a patient with cancer is brilliant and unique. This book is a "must-read" for all who provide anesthesia to patients requiring surgery for cancer. Enjoy the read; You will be glad that you invested your time in reading this book.

Robert Gaiser
Professor of Anesthesiology
Yale School of Medicine
New Haven, Connecticut, USA

PREFACE

Why this Book?

Having experienced cancer in deeply personal ways—a family member who survived, another who succumbed, and the loss of dear friends—I have been closely involved in the journeys of those affected. Although I have been a practicing anesthesiologist for over 32 years, it had not fully occurred to me how integral anesthesia care is throughout the complex and often tumultuous course of a cancer patient's treatment.

Anesthesia does not cure cancer, but it is required at nearly every stage—from screening and diagnostic procedures to curative and palliative surgeries, as well as pain management. Following these personal experiences, I conducted an extensive literature review and found that while knowledge exists, it is scattered—presented in isolated journal articles, brief topics, or occasional textbook chapters. This realization became my motivation to create a single, comprehensive resource dedicated exclusively to anesthesia care for cancer patients.

Contributors to this Book

To ensure the breadth and depth of expertise, I invited board-certified anesthesiologists representing diverse subspecialties—including general anesthesia, pediatric anesthesia, cardiothoracic anesthesia, pain management, and critical care—to contribute. The team also included anesthesia residents, fellows, researchers, and even a few highly motivated medical students whose curiosity enriched the project. This collective expertise has enabled us to create a resource that we hope will serve as a comprehensive guide to anesthesia care for cancer patients. We believe it will be of value to anesthesia providers, residents, fellows in training, and medical students alike.

Contents of this Book

The book begins with an exploration of the role and importance of anesthesia in cancer treatment, followed by a review of the physiological changes caused by malignancy—knowledge essential for anesthetic planning. We summarize the complications of chemotherapy, radiation therapy, and immunotherapy, along with their anesthetic considerations. The potential effects of anesthesia on tumor metastasis are also discussed. Special chapters address anesthesia care for patients across different age groups with cancer.

We provide detailed guidance on perioperative management—spanning preoperative evaluation through postoperative care—for a wide range of oncologic surgeries, concluding with comprehensive sections on pain management and critical care in oncology.

Acknowledgements

My sincere thanks to Bentham Science Publishers for giving me the opportunity to write and publish this book. I am deeply grateful for the support of the Bentham Books team, particularly Dr. Obaid Sadiq, Manager, Bentham Books, and Fariya Zulfiqar, Manager, Bentham Books Publications, whose dedication made this work possible. My deepest gratitude goes to my co-editors and contributing authors for their countless hours of commitment to this project. I extend special thanks to Dr. Michael Mahrus and Brian McEniry, Clinical Research Coordinator, for their invaluable technical support.

Bharathi Gourkanti, Irwin Gratz, William Marion,
Rajiv Lingaraju & Grace Abramian
Department of Anesthesiology
Cooper Medical School of Rowan University
Cooper University Health Care
Camden, NJ, USA

List of Contributors

Aakash Patel	Department of Anesthesiology, Cooper Medical School of Rowan University, Cooper University Health Care, Camden, NJ, USA
Akhil Patel	Department of Anesthesiology, George Washington School of Medicine and Health Sciences, Washington, DC, USA
Amber Williams	Department of Anesthesiology, Cooper Medical School of Rowan University, Cooper University Health Care, Camden, NJ, USA
Bharathi Gourkanti	Department of Anesthesiology, Cooper Medical School of Rowan University, Cooper University Health Care, Camden, NJ, USA
Brian McEniry	Department of Anesthesiology, Cooper Medical School of Rowan University, Cooper University Health Care, Camden, NJ, USA
Colleen Naglee	Department of Anesthesiology, Cooper Medical School of Rowan University, Cooper University Health Care, Camden, NJ, USA
Christopher Potestio	Department of Anesthesiology, Cooper Medical School of Rowan University, Cooper University Health Care, Camden, NJ, USA
Chenxuan Zhou	Department of Anesthesiology and Perioperative Care, University of California, Irvine Medical Center, Orange, CA, USA
Crystal Adams	Department of Anesthesiology, George Washington School of Medicine and Health Sciences, Washington, DC, USA
Cathy Lee	Department of Anesthesiology, Cooper Medical School of Rowan University, Cooper University Health Care, Camden, NJ, USA
Dylan Windle-Puente	Mount Sinai Hospital, New York, USA
Eric You	Department of Anesthesiology, Cooper Medical School of Rowan University, Cooper University Health Care, Camden, NJ, USA
Flore Macenat Sulzynski	Temple University at Fox Chase Cancer Center, Philadelphia, PA, USA
Grace Abramian	Department of Anesthesiology, Cooper Medical School of Rowan University, Cooper University Health Care, Camden, USA
Irwin Gratz	Department of Anesthesiology, Cooper Medical School of Rowan University, Cooper University Health Care, Camden, NJ, USA
Ian Brotman	Department of Anesthesiology, Cooper Medical School of Rowan University, Cooper University Health Care, Camden, NJ, USA
Jason Vaz	Alberta Children's Hospital, Calgary, Alberta, Canada
Julie Mathew	Department of Anesthesiology, Cooper Medical School of Rowan University, Cooper University Health Care, Camden, NJ, USA
Kingsuk Ganguly	Department of Anesthesiology, Cooper Medical School of Rowan University, Cooper University Health Care, Camden, NJ, USA
Linh Le	Department of Anesthesiology and Perioperative Care, University of California, Irvine Medical Center, Orange, CA, USA

Michael Mahrous	Department of Anesthesiology, Cooper Medical School of Rowan University, Cooper University Health Care, Camden, NJ, USA
Michael Schwartz	Department of Anesthesiology and Perioperative Care, University of California, Irvine Medical Center, Orange, CA, USA
Madison Tanis	Department of Anesthesiology, Cooper Medical School of Rowan University, Cooper University Health Care, Camden, NJ, USA
Mia Ye	Department of Anesthesiology, George Washington School of Medicine and Health Sciences, Washington, DC, USA
Marcus Ryan Dal Nogare	Department of Anesthesiology, Cooper Medical School of Rowan University, Cooper University Health Care, Camden, NJ, USA
Mina Ghaly	Department of Anesthesiology, Cooper Medical School of Rowan University, Cooper University Health Care, Camden, NJ, USA
Nathalie Peiris	Nemours Children's Hospital, Wilmington, DE, USA
Osheen Abramian	Jefferson Einstein Montgomery Hospital, Thomas Jefferson University, Philadelphia, PA, USA
Rajiv Lingaraju	Department of Anesthesiology, Cooper Medical School of Rowan University, Cooper University Health Care, Camden, NJ, USA
Sophia Sinibaldi	Department of Anesthesiology, Cooper Medical School of Rowan University, Cooper University Health Care, Camden, NJ, USA
Siddhi Desai	Department of Anesthesiology, Cooper Medical School of Rowan University, Cooper University Health Care, Camden, NJ, USA
Shiu-Yi E Chen	Department of Anesthesiology, School of Medicine, UC Irvine, Irvine, CA 92617, USA
Taylor Tidwell	Department of Anesthesiology and Perioperative Care, University of California, Irvine Medical Center, Orange, CA, USA
William Marion	Department of Anesthesiology, Cooper Medical School of Rowan University, Cooper University Health Care, Camden, NJ, USA

CHAPTER 1

The Role of Anesthesia in Cancer Management

Irwin Gratz[1,*] and **Brian McEniry**[1]

[1] *Department of Anesthesiology, Cooper Medical School of Rowan University, Cooper University Health Care, Camden, NJ, USA*

Abstract: Cancer affects individuals across all age groups, with epidemiological data indicating a steady rise in the global cancer burden—a trend that closely parallels population growth and aging. As a substantial proportion of cancer patients will require surgical intervention during the course of their disease, this increasing incidence has led to a corresponding surge in demand for cancer-related surgical procedures worldwide. This chapter aims to contextualize the expanding role of oncoanesthesia within the framework of multidisciplinary cancer care, highlighting its influence not only on perioperative outcomes but also on long-term survivorship. To deliver optimal care, healthcare professionals involved in the perioperative management of oncology patients must possess a comprehensive understanding of evolving demographic trends, cancer epidemiology, tumor biology, and the perioperative implications of emerging oncologic therapies. As cancer care continues to evolve, anesthesiologists are increasingly recognized as integral contributors to improving both immediate and long-term outcomes in this growing patient population.

Keywords: Anesthesia, Cancer patients, GI tumors, Immunosuppression, Metastasis, NK cells, Oncoanesthesia, Perioperative management, Regional anesthesia, Total intravenous anesthesia (TIVA), Volatile anesthetics.

INTRODUCTION

Cancer: A Growing Global Health Crisis

Cancer remains one of the most formidable challenges in global public health, contributing significantly to both morbidity and mortality. By 2030, the number of new cancer cases is projected to exceed 22 million annually, underscoring the urgent need for advances in prevention, early detection, and treatment strategies [1]. With a rapidly aging global population and increasing incidence rates, cancer is on track to become the leading cause of death worldwide. Addressing this escalating crisis requires a multifaceted approach integrating research, public

* **Corresponding author Irwin Gratz:** Department of Anesthesiology, Cooper Medical School of Rowan University, Cooper University Health Care, Camden, NJ, USA; E-mail: gratz-irwin@cooperhealth.edu

Bharathi Gourkanti, Irwin Gratz, William Marion, Rajiv Lingaraju & Grace Abramian (Eds.)

health initiatives, healthcare policy reform, and specialized clinical care. Currently, cancer is responsible for nearly 10 million deaths annually, accounting for approximately one-sixth of all global deaths [1]. In 2022 alone, an estimated 20 million new cases and 9.7 million cancer-related deaths were reported worldwide [2]. Although cancer comprises a broad spectrum of diseases, a disproportionate burden arises from a few high-incidence malignancies, particularly breast, lung, colorectal, and prostate cancers [2]. Among these, gastrointestinal (GI) cancers, including colorectal, liver, gastric, esophageal, and pancreatic malignancies, are especially lethal, collectively responsible for approximately 34% of all global cancer-related deaths [2].

Despite significant progress in screening, adjuvant therapies, and surgical techniques [3], approximately 20% of patients undergoing curative-intent surgery will experience local or distant recurrence most commonly within the first three years postoperatively, with nearly 80% of recurrences occurring during this critical period [4]. These sobering statistics highlight the urgent need for innovative perioperative strategies to reduce recurrence rates and improve long-term, disease-free survival.

As cancer care becomes increasingly complex, the vast majority of patients will require anesthesia services at some point during their treatment or survivorship journey. This growing demand is further exacerbated by a global shortage of trained anesthesia providers [5, 6]. As cancer incidence continues to rise, the perioperative phase, particularly anesthetic management, has emerged as a crucial component of comprehensive oncologic care.

Global Disparities in Cancer Burden

Disparities in cancer care across the globe are shaped by variations in healthcare infrastructure, the Human Development Index (HDI), environmental exposures, and infection-related risks [2, 7]. High-HDI countries report higher cancer incidence but lower mortality, largely due to greater access to screening, timely diagnosis, and advanced treatments. Conversely, low-HDI countries are experiencing a growing burden in both incidence and mortality, a trend expected to accelerate in the coming decades.

Meanwhile, therapeutic advances, especially in high-income countries, have led to improved survival rates, contributing to a growing population of cancer survivors. These individuals often require anesthesia services for ongoing cancer-related procedures as well as unrelated surgeries throughout survivorship [8].

Anesthesia and Long-Term Cancer Outcomes

One of the most actively investigated areas in perioperative oncology is the potential influence of anesthetic technique on long-term cancer outcomes. While surgery remains the cornerstone of curative treatment for many solid tumors, metastasis is still the leading cause of cancer-related mortality. The perioperative period is characterized by physiological stressors that may inadvertently support tumor cell survival and dissemination. Micrometastases, which may persist or become dislodged during surgery despite optimal techniques, pose a significant risk for recurrence. Additionally, surgical stress can temporarily suppress immune function and trigger pro-inflammatory and pro-angiogenic pathways, creating a perioperative microenvironment conducive to recurrence and metastatic progression [9].

This book explores the connection of the global cancer burden with the evolving role of anesthesia and perioperative medicine. In particular, it examines how anesthetic techniques may influence cancer recurrence and long-term survival. Through this lens, we aim to emphasize the critical and expanding role of anesthesiologists as integral members of the multidisciplinary cancer care team actively contributing to improved oncologic outcomes worldwide.

The Expanding Scope of Oncoanesthesia

Oncoanesthesia, a specialized and increasingly vital field within cancer care, is a critical, yet often underrecognized, component of modern oncologic practice. Its role extends well beyond the administration of anesthesia, encompassing a broad range of perioperative responsibilities, including:

- Prehabilitation and patient optimization
- Advanced perioperative pain management
- Postoperative critical care
- Individualized, multidisciplinary strategies tailored to oncologic comorbidities

As cancer survival rates improve and the number of survivors increases, approximately 80% of cancer patients are expected to undergo one or more surgical procedures during the course of their treatment [2]. These procedures, ranging from curative resections to palliative surgeries, are becoming increasingly complex and often require significant perioperative planning and coordination.

Why Oncoanesthesia Matters

Modern cancer patients frequently present with a range of complex clinical challenges, such as:

- Poor nutritional status
- Immunosuppression
- Hematological abnormalities
- Organ dysfunction secondary to chemotherapy or radiotherapy

These complexities demand a nuanced, patient-centered approach to perioperative care. Oncoanesthesiologists play a vital role across the continuum of cancer care, not only during surgery but also in diagnostic procedures, treatment planning, survivorship, and end-of-life care.

Moreover, the need to closely coordinate surgical interventions with systemic therapies such as chemotherapy, immunotherapy, and radiation therapy underscores the importance of meticulous perioperative management. Prompt identification and treatment of complications are essential to prevent delays in adjuvant therapies, which, if postponed, may negatively impact oncologic outcomes [3, 4].

Multidisciplinary Integration and Sub-specialization in Cancer Care

Cancer care has increasingly shifted toward a multidisciplinary model, integrating multiple therapeutic modalities, including:

- Surgery
- Systemic Anticancer Therapy (SACT)
- Radiothcrapy
- Palliative Interventions

While surgical resection remains the most effective curative strategy for localized tumors, systemic and radiotherapeutic approaches are critical in reducing the risk of recurrence [5]. In metastatic disease, systemic therapies take precedence, with surgery serving a more selective, adjunctive role.

Within this evolving framework, the oncoanesthesiologist plays a vital role in ensuring that surgical interventions are safe, effective, and appropriately timed within the broader treatment plan [6]. Their expertise is increasingly important as patients undergo complex, multimodal care regimens.

The projected increase to 45 million cancer-related surgeries annually by 2030 underscores the urgent need for highly skilled anesthesia providers with specialized training in oncologic procedures.

Technical Demands and Innovations in Oncoanesthesia

Oncologic surgeries such as pancreaticoduodenectomy, esophagectomy, major head and neck resections, skull base procedures, thoracic surgeries, and complex genitourinary operations are classified as *supra-major procedures* due to their:

- Prolonged duration
- Significant blood loss
- Frequent need for massive transfusion protocols

These highly demanding surgeries require anesthesiologists with advanced expertise. The role of the oncoanesthesiologist includes proficiency in:

- Advanced airway management (*e.g.*, fiberoptic intubation, tracheostomy)
- Ultrasound-guided regional anesthesia and vascular access
- Invasive and non-invasive hemodynamic monitoring
- Perioperative critical care and pain management

In addition to complex surgeries, emerging cancer therapies present new physiological and anesthetic challenges. These include:

- Hyperthermic Intraperitoneal Chemotherapy (HIPEC)
- Pressurized Intraperitoneal Aerosol Chemotherapy (PIPAC)
- Isolated Limb Perfusion (ILP)
- Hyperthermic Intrathoracic Chemotherapy (HITHOC)

These modalities often involve extreme temperatures, pressure changes, and significant intravascular volume shifts, requiring highly precise and adaptable anesthetic management.

As cancer is projected to become the leading global cause of death, and with surgery playing a central role in both curative and palliative treatments, the importance of oncoanesthesiology has never been greater. Oncoanesthesiologists are crucial not only for improving short-term perioperative outcomes but also for enhancing long-term survival and quality of life.

To meet the complex needs of the growing global cancer population, anesthesiology must continue evolving through subspecialization, multidisciplinary collaboration, and the implementation of innovative perioperative strategies.

The Expanding Role of Oncoanesthesia

Oncoanesthesia extends well beyond the administration of anesthesia. It encompasses:

- Comprehensive pain management
- Postoperative care
- Personalized strategies tailored to the complex physiological and psychological needs of cancer patients

This field is becoming increasingly important, especially as the number of cancer survivors continues to grow, many of whom require multiple surgical interventions for either curative or palliative purposes. It is estimated that approximately 80% of cancer patients will undergo one or more surgeries during their disease [2]. Consequently, cancer-related procedures are expected to consume a growing share of surgical workload and healthcare resources.

Advancements in cancer treatments have significantly improved survival rates. As a result, an increasing number of patients now present with comorbidities and treatment-related complications, further highlighting the need for specialized anesthetic care to optimize surgical outcomes and quality of life.

Timing and Coordination in Cancer Surgery

Surgical intervention remains a cornerstone of cancer treatment, with many patients undergoing multiple procedures throughout their disease trajectory [2]. The timing of surgery is critical, as it must be coordinated to allow the early initiation of adjuvant therapies. Improved outcomes are closely linked to:

- Aggressive postoperative surveillance
- Prompt management of complications
- Effective strategies for managing cancer recurrence

These elements must align with systemic therapies to ensure optimal patient outcomes [3, 4].

A multidisciplinary approach is now the standard in cancer care. Increasingly, patients receive systemic anticancer therapy alongside surgical interventions. While surgery remains the most effective curative option for small, localized tumors, systemic therapies and radiotherapy are essential for minimizing recurrence risk [5]. In metastatic cases, systemic therapy is often the primary treatment modality. As cancer care evolves, the role of oncoanesthesiology within this framework is crucial to achieving the best possible outcomes [6].

Enhanced Recovery and RIOT: Optimizing Postoperative Care

The primary goal of perioperative anesthesia is to minimize hospital length of stay and facilitate enhanced recovery. Enhanced Recovery After Surgery (ERAS) protocols have demonstrated significant benefits, including:

- Reduced postoperative complications
- Shorter hospital stays
- Improved functional recovery

Originally introduced by Henrik Kehlet in 1997 for colorectal surgery [4], ERAS has since transformed traditional perioperative care [5 - 9].

Building on ERAS principles, the concept of Return to Intended Oncologic Treatment (RIOT) has emerged as a key metric in cancer surgery. RIOT emphasizes minimizing recovery time to enable earlier initiation of adjuvant therapies such as chemotherapy. First described in a 2014 observational study, RIOT showed a 10-day reduction in time to chemotherapy following liver resection [10].

Fluid Management in Major Oncologic Surgery

Fluid management plays a pivotal role in determining outcomes in major oncologic surgeries. These procedures regardless of tumor type are often prolonged and complex, with complications, such as:

- Impaired wound healing
- Postoperative ileus
- Pulmonary dysfunction
- Prolonged hospitalization

Excessive (liberal) fluid administration is associated with poorer postoperative outcomes. In response, intraoperative monitoring has advanced through minimally invasive technologies designed to predict fluid responsiveness and support precise fluid management. However, consistent evidence supporting their widespread routine use remains limited [8].

An increasingly valuable strategy is the use of:

- Goal-Directed Fluid Therapy (GDFT)
- Restrictive Fluid Therapy
- Zero-Balance Fluid Therapy

Among these, GDFT has shown promise. It enables individualized, real-time hemodynamic monitoring through assessment of fluid responsiveness using both dynamic and static parameters. This approach is especially beneficial in high-risk cancer surgeries associated with elevated morbidity and mortality [8].

Randomized controlled trials have demonstrated that GDFT can reduce complication rates in gastrointestinal and gynecological cancer surgeries, outperforming both liberal and restrictive strategies [9 - 11]. A systematic review and meta-analysis by Zhaosheng *et al.* further validated these findings [12], showing that intraoperative GDFT:

- Significantly reduced hospital length of stay
- Decreased postoperative complications
- Lowered unplanned hospital readmissions

These outcomes highlight GDFT's potential to enhance both short-term recovery and long-term resource efficiency in oncologic care.

Blood Management

As the complexity of cancer surgeries continues to increase, particularly those involving extensive dissection and anticipated blood loss exceeding 1,500 mL the use of packed red blood cells (pRBCs) remains a cornerstone of intraoperative hemorrhage management. While perioperative transfusions can be life-saving, mounting evidence indicates they may also have adverse oncologic consequences, largely attributed to immunomodulatory effects [13].

Transfusion-related immunosuppression has been linked to increased rates of tumor recurrence and decreased overall survival across a range of malignancies [14]. This has prompted ongoing investigation into the risks and benefits of blood transfusions in oncologic settings.

One landmark study addressing this issue is the ARCA-1 trial, an international, multicenter, prospective observational cohort study. Designed to evaluate the relationship between perioperative pRBC transfusion and outcomes following major cancer surgery, the study enrolled patients undergoing high-risk oncologic procedures. The vast majority of transfused patients received leukoreduced allogeneic pRBCs (76.6%) [15].

Although the study was terminated prematurely, its findings were striking: 1-year mortality was 19.7% in the transfused group compared to 6.5% among non-transfused patients. However, several limitations temper the interpretation of these results. The heterogeneity of included cancer types limited malignancy-specific conclusions. Moreover, patients requiring transfusion often had lower baseline hemoglobin, greater comorbidity burden, and higher frailty scores, which may have independently influenced outcomes.

These findings underscore the need for careful, individualized transfusion strategies in oncologic surgery. Where possible, efforts should focus on minimizing perioperative blood loss, optimizing preoperative hemoglobin levels, and adhering to evidence-based transfusion thresholds to balance the life-saving benefits of transfusion with potential long-term oncologic risks.

The underlying rationale for minimizing postoperative delays is that the earlier initiation of adjunctive therapy, such as chemotherapy or radiotherapy, may significantly improve survival outcomes. In contrast, delayed Return to Intended Oncologic Therapy (RIOT) has been associated with increased mortality, higher recurrence rates, and poorer overall oncologic outcomes [16, 17]. Multiple studies support this concept, demonstrating that both delays in and omission of adjuvant chemotherapy are correlated with worse overall survival [17]. A key hypothesis is that postponing systemic therapy allows residual microscopic disease to proliferate, particularly during the vulnerable postoperative period, when host immunity is suppressed and surveillance against tumor cells is compromised, especially following neoadjuvant treatments [18].

The perioperative period plays a critical role in influencing long-term cancer outcomes. During and after oncologic surgery, tumor cell dissemination may occur through several mechanisms, including mechanical manipulation, lymphatic spread, and hematogenous dissemination [18]. This window is characterized by heightened susceptibility to metastasis, driven in part by immune dysregulation and pro-inflammatory signaling cascades that promote angiogenesis, invasion, and tumor proliferation.

Despite curative-intent resection, up to one-third of patients will ultimately develop local or distant recurrence [19]. One contributing factor is the profound immunologic suppression induced by surgical stress and general anesthesia, particularly affecting natural killer (NK) cell activity and T-cell function, which may persist for up to one week postoperatively [20, 21]. This immune suppression creates a permissive microenvironment for residual tumor cells to survive, evade detection, and establish metastatic niches.

Additionally, perioperative practices such as the routine use of high inspired oxygen concentrations to prevent hypoxemia and optimize perfusion may have unintended oncologic consequences. At the cellular level, hyperoxia has been associated with enhanced tumor aggressiveness, increased oxidative stress, and upregulation of signaling pathways that may promote cancer progression and recurrence [22].

General anesthesia is the mainstay for the majority of tumor resections and is typically delivered using one of two principal modalities: inhalational anesthesia or total intravenous anesthesia (TIVA). Although widely practiced, the immunologic and oncologic effects of anesthesia are not yet fully understood, and the potential influence of anesthetic technique on long-term cancer outcomes remains an area of active investigation and ongoing debate [8 - 14].

Among inhalational agents, volatile anesthetics such as sevoflurane and isoflurane are commonly used for the maintenance of general anesthesia due to their predictable pharmacodynamics, ease of titration, and rapid onset and offset. However, emerging evidence suggests that these agents may exert proinflammatory effects, impair DNA repair mechanisms, inhibit natural killer (NK) cell function, and upregulate hypoxia-inducible factor-1α (HIF-1α), a transcription factor implicated in tumor progression and angiogenesis [23 - 28].

In contrast, TIVA involves the use of intravenous agents, most notably propofol, to maintain anesthesia without inhalational agents. TIVA regimens may include opioids, local anesthetics, dexmedetomidine, or ketamine, with propofol as the principal hypnotic agent. The choice of TIVA is often driven by clinical considerations such as reducing the incidence of postoperative nausea and vomiting (PONV) or enabling neuromonitoring during procedures where inhalational agents may interfere with somatosensory evoked potentials (SSEPs) or motor evoked potentials (MEPs) [29, 30].

Beyond these operational benefits, propofol has demonstrated several properties of potential relevance to oncologic outcomes. It exhibits free radical scavenging activity, reduces pulmonary complications in patients undergoing microvascular free flap reconstruction [31, 32], and may enhance postoperative pain control [33]. Furthermore, propofol has shown promise in reducing postoperative cognitive dysfunction, particularly in elderly patients with pre-existing mild cognitive impairment [34].

More recently, attention has been given to the anti-inflammatory and immunomodulatory effects of propofol, which may support tumor surveillance by preserving immune function in the vulnerable perioperative period [35]. These findings have sparked interest in TIVA as a potentially oncologically favorable anesthetic technique, though robust, prospective, randomized trials are still needed to confirm its impact on cancer recurrence and survival.

General anesthesia is the mainstay for the majority of tumor resections and is typically delivered using one of two principal modalities: inhalational anesthesia or total intravenous anesthesia (TIVA). Although widely practiced, the immunologic and oncologic effects of anesthesia are not yet fully understood, and the potential influence of anesthetic technique on long-term cancer outcomes remains an area of active investigation and ongoing debate [8 - 14].

Among inhalational agents, volatile anesthetics such as *sevoflurane* and *isoflurane* are commonly used for the maintenance of general anesthesia due to their predictable pharmacodynamics, ease of titration, and rapid onset and offset. However, emerging evidence suggests that these agents may exert proinflammatory effects, impair DNA repair mechanisms, inhibit natural killer (NK) cell function, and upregulate hypoxia-inducible factor-1α (HIF-1α), a transcription factor implicated in tumor progression and angiogenesis [23 - 28].

In contrast, TIVA involves the use of intravenous agents, most notably propofol, to maintain anesthesia without inhalational agents. TIVA regimens may include opioids, local anesthetics, dexmedetomidine, or ketamine, with propofol as the principal hypnotic agent. The choice of TIVA is often driven by clinical considerations such as reducing the incidence of postoperative nausea and vomiting (PONV) or enabling neuromonitoring during procedures where inhalational agents may interfere with somatosensory evoked potentials (SSEPs) or motor evoked potentials (MEPs) [29, 30].

Beyond these operational benefits, propofol has demonstrated several properties of potential relevance to oncologic outcomes. It exhibits free radical scavenging activity, reduces pulmonary complications in patients undergoing microvascular free flap reconstruction [31, 32], and may enhance postoperative pain control [33]. Furthermore, propofol has shown promise in reducing postoperative cognitive dysfunction, particularly in elderly patients with pre-existing mild cognitive impairment [34].

More recently, attention has focused on the anti-inflammatory and immunomodulatory effects of propofol, which may support tumor surveillance by preserving immune function in the vulnerable perioperative period [35]. These findings have sparked interest in TIVA as a potentially oncologically favorable anesthetic technique, though robust, prospective, randomized trials are still needed to confirm its impact on cancer recurrence and survival.

Despite the theoretical and preliminary clinical advantages of specific anesthetic techniques, large-scale data remain inconclusive. A population-based study using the Swedish National Registry, which evaluated patients with stage I–III colorectal cancer, found no significant difference in overall or disease-free survival between those who received inhalational anesthesia and those who received propofol-based total intravenous anesthesia (TIVA) [36]. Similar outcomes were reported in large observational studies by Makito *et al.* and Hasselager *et al.*, both of which failed to demonstrate a survival benefit favoring one anesthetic technique over another [37, 38].

However, the limitations inherent to observational designs, including selection bias, residual confounding, and lack of tumor-specific stratification, may obscure meaningful differences. Furthermore, the biologic heterogeneity of tumors may contribute to inconsistent findings across studies.

Supporting this notion, a randomized controlled trial by Kwon *et al.* examined a homogeneous cohort of 536 patients undergoing elective hepatectomy for hepatocellular carcinoma. Participants were randomized to receive either TIVA with propofol or inhalational anesthesia with sevoflurane. Notably, the propofol group exhibited significantly improved overall survival and lower recurrence rates in subgroup analysis [39].

These findings emphasize the need for tumor-specific investigations and rigorously designed, prospective randomized controlled trials to determine the true impact of anesthetic technique on long-term oncologic outcomes. Until such data are available, anesthetic choice should be guided by individual patient characteristics, surgical context, and institutional protocols, while remaining cognizant of the evolving evidence base.

Nutrition

While surgery remains a cornerstone of cancer treatment, preoperative malnutrition is a significant and often underrecognized risk factor for adverse postoperative outcomes. Among the various markers of nutritional status, hypoalbuminemia is one.

Even in its mild form, it has been identified as an independent predictor of both morbidity and mortality [40]. A large-scale study by Hu *et al.* using data from 30,676 colorectal cancer patients in the American College of Surgeons National Surgical Quality Improvement Program (ACS-NSQIP) revealed that mild hypoalbuminemia (serum albumin levels of 30–35 g/L) was significantly associated with increased postoperative mortality, as well as complications including deep vein thrombosis, pulmonary embolism, surgical site infection, pneumonia, septic shock, and prolonged hospitalization [40].

These findings underscore the critical importance of preoperative nutritional assessment and optimization, particularly with regard to serum albumin levels, in reducing perioperative risk and improving surgical outcomes [41].

Malnutrition is especially prevalent among patients with gastrointestinal (GI) and head and neck cancers (HNC), two populations particularly vulnerable due to both tumor-related and treatment-related factors. In GI cancers, diminished appetite, mechanical obstruction, and malabsorption contribute to malnutrition, with prevalence rates ranging from 20% to over 70%, depending on tumor type and stage [42]. Similarly, patients with HNC often experience dysphagia, mucositis, and altered anatomy secondary to the tumor or its treatment, severely impairing oral intake and nutritional status [43].

Malnutrition in these populations compromises immune function, delays wound healing, and increases susceptibility to postoperative infections and other complications. Additionally, the catabolic stress of major cancer surgery, when superimposed on preexisting sarcopenia and nutritional deficits, further exacerbates immune dysregulation and contributes to a heightened risk of infectious and systemic complications [44].

Optimizing nutritional status through early assessment and targeted intervention should be a routine component of preoperative planning for cancer patients, particularly those undergoing complex surgical procedures. Multidisciplinary collaboration, including dietitians, surgeons, oncologists, and anesthesiologists, is essential to mitigate risk and enhance recovery.

FUTURE DIRECTIONS IN ONCOANESTHESIA

The future of cancer care will not rely solely on novel therapeutics or advanced surgical techniques, but increasingly on the integration and optimization of perioperative elements, a domain where oncoanesthesiologists are uniquely positioned to lead. Emerging innovations such as AI-guided anesthetic planning, precision fluid and hemodynamic management, and personalized enhanced recovery protocols informed by tumor biology and patient-specific genomic profiles are poised to transform perioperative care into a more predictive, preventative, and individualized practice.

This evolving paradigm highlights the imperative for anesthesiologists to be proactive members of the multidisciplinary oncology team, influencing not only intraoperative safety but also long-term cancer control, survivorship, and quality of life. As perioperative medicine advances, oncoanesthesia will be central to bridging the gap between surgical intervention and sustained oncologic outcomes, positioning anesthesiologists at the forefront of modern cancer care.

CONCLUSION

As cancer incidence rises globally, the perioperative period, particularly anesthetic management, is increasingly recognized as a key factor in patient outcomes. Oncoanesthesiologists now play a vital role beyond the operating room, contributing to preoperative preparation, intraoperative care, and postoperative recovery. Evidence linking anesthesia practices to immune function, recurrence, and survival underscores the need for personalized, evidence-based strategies. In this evolving landscape, oncoanesthesia is a critical component of multidisciplinary cancer care. Improving long-term outcomes will require continued research, specialized training, and greater integration of perioperative medicine into the broader cancer treatment paradigm.

REFERENCES

[1] Divatia JV, Thota RS, Garg TR, Ramkiran S. Onco-anaesthesiology as an emerging sub-speciality domain: Need of the hour! Indian J Anaesth 2020; 64(1): 69-71.
[http://dx.doi.org/10.4103/ija.IJA_838_19] [PMID: 32001913]

[2] Bray F, Laversanne M, Sung H, *et al.* Global cancer statistics 2022: GLOBOCAN estimates of incidence and mortality worldwide for 36 cancers in 185 countries. CA Cancer J Clin 2024; 74(3): 229-63.
[http://dx.doi.org/10.3322/caac.21834] [PMID: 38572751]

[3] Schellenberg M, Abudayyeh S, Ahmed A, Elsayed A. Recurrence patterns and risk factors in stage I–III colorectal cancer after curative surgery: A competing risk analysis. BMC Gastroenterol 2022; 22: 161.
[http://dx.doi.org/10.1186/s12876-022-02161-9] [PMID: 35241002]

[4] Ryu S, An S, Park M, Youn S, Chun H. Postoperative recurrence patterns and risk factors in colorectal cancer: A retrospective cohort study. Cancers (Basel) 2023; 15(24): 5791. Available from: https://www.mdpi.com/2072-6694/15/24/579110.3390/cancers15245791
[PMID: 38136337]

[5] Wildgaard K, Petersen RH, Hansen HJ, *et al.* Anesthesia and surgical considerations in the care of the cancer patient. CA Cancer J Clin 2021; 71(3): 217-35.

[6] Law TJ, Lipnick MS, Morriss W, Gelb AW, Mellin-Olsen J, Filipescu D, Rowles J, Rod P, Khan F, Yazbeck P, Zoumenou E, Ibarra P, Ranatunga K, Bulamba F; Collaborators. The Global Anesthesia Workforce Survey: Updates and Trends in the Anesthesia Workforce. Anesth Analg. 2024 Jul 1; 139(1): 15-24.
[http://dx.doi.org/10.1213/ANE.0000000000006836] [PMID: 38470828]

[7] Sung H, Ferlay J, Siegel RL, *et al.* Global cancer statistics 2020: GLOBOCAN estimates of incidence and mortality worldwide for 36 cancers in 185 countries. CA Cancer J Clin 2021; 71(3): 209-49.
[http://dx.doi.org/10.3322/caac.21660] [PMID: 33538338]

[8] Ljungqvist O, Scott M, Fearon KC. Enhanced recovery after surgery: A review. JAMA Surg 2017; 152(3): 292-8.
[http://dx.doi.org/10.1001/jamasurg.2016.4952] [PMID: 28097305]

[9] Srinivasa S, Taylor MH, Singh PP, *et al.* Goal-directed therapy in major cancer surgery: A meta-analysis of randomized controlled trials. Br J Anaesth 2013; 111(4): 561-73.
[PMID: 23293274]

[10] Miller KD, Nogueira L, Devasia T, *et al.* Cancer treatment and survivorship statistics, 2022. CA Cancer J Clin 2022; 72(5): 409-36.
[http://dx.doi.org/10.3322/caac.21731] [PMID: 35736631]

[11] Yildiz GO, Hergunsel GO, Sertcakacilar G, Akyol D, Karakaş S, Cukurova Z. Perioperative goal-directed fluid management using noninvasive hemodynamic monitoring in gynecologic oncology. Braz J Anesthesiol 2022; 72(3): 322-30.
[http://dx.doi.org/10.1016/j.bjane.2021.12.012]

[12] Zhaosheng H, Xuelian L, Zhen H, *et al.* Effect of goal-directed fluid therapy on postoperative outcomes: A systematic review and meta-analysis of randomized controlled trials. Int J Surg 2023; 110: 123-31.
[http://dx.doi.org/10.1016/j.ijsu.2023.123131]

[13] Gupta R, Patel K, Yi WS, *et al.* Perioperative blood transfusion adversely affects cancer-specific survival in patients with non–small cell lung cancer. Ann Thorac Surg 2020; 110(6): 1742-9.
[http://dx.doi.org/10.1016/j.athoracsur.2020.03.042]

[14] Cata JP, Guerra-Londono JJ, Ramirez MF, *et al.* The association between perioperative red blood cell transfusions and 1-year mortality after major cancer surgery: An international multicenter observational study. Anesth Analg 2025; 140(4): 782-94.
[http://dx.doi.org/10.1213/ANE.0000000000007236] [PMID: 39504267]

[15] Cata J, Ramirez M, Forget P, *et al.* International multicentre observational study to evaluate the association between perioperative red blood cell transfusions and 1-year mortality after major cancer surgery (ARCA-1): study design, statistical analysis plan and study protocol. BMJ Open 2021; 11(3): e043453.
[http://dx.doi.org/10.1136/bmjopen-2020-043453] [PMID: 33737431]

[16] Aloia TA, Zimmitti G, Conrad C, *et al.* Return to intended oncologic treatment (RIOT): A novel metric for evaluating the quality of oncologic surgery. J Surg Oncol 2014; 110(8): 1071-7.
[http://dx.doi.org/10.1002/jso.23729]

[17] Grass F, Slankamenac K, Pache B, *et al.* Impact of time to adjuvant chemotherapy on survival after colorectal cancer resection: A population-based study. Int J Cancer 2020; 146(6): 1501-8.
[http://dx.doi.org/10.1002/ijc.32418]

[18] Biagi JJ, Raphael MJ, Mackillop WJ, Kong W, King WD, Booth CM. Association between time to initiation of adjuvant chemotherapy and survival in colorectal cancer: a systematic review and meta-analysis. JAMA 2011; 305(22): 2335-42.
[http://dx.doi.org/10.1001/jama.2011.749] [PMID: 21642686]

[19] Hiller JG, Perry NJ, Poulogiannis G, *et al.* Perioperative immunomodulation in cancer surgery: New therapeutic opportunities. Cancer J 2018; 24(3): 146-53.
[http://dx.doi.org/10.1097/PPO.0000000000000319]

[20] Nguyen XD, Horn A, Fischer D, *et al.* Suppressive effects of deep balanced anesthesia on cellular immunity and protein expression: a randomized-controlled pilot study. BMC Anesthesiol 2025; 25(1): 129.
[http://dx.doi.org/10.1186/s12871-025-02980-9] [PMID: 40097954]

[21] Ristescu AI, Tiron CE, Dricu A, Dudea D, Niculescu A. Perioperative immunomodulation and cancer recurrence: Current concepts and therapeutic perspectives. Biomedicines 2021; 9(8): 874.

[http://dx.doi.org/10.3390/biomedicines9080874] [PMID: 34440079]

[22] Ristescu AI, Tiron CE, Tiron A, Grigoras I. Exploring hyperoxia effects in cancer—from perioperative clinical data to potential molecular mechanisms. Biomedicines 2021; 9(9): 1213. [http://dx.doi.org/10.3390/biomedicines9091213] [PMID: 34572400]

[23] Li JM, Shao JL, Zeng WJ, Liang RB. General/epidural anesthesia in combination preserves NK cell activity and affects cytokine response in cervical carcinoma patients undergoing radical resection: a cohort prospective study. Eur J Gynaecol Oncol 2015; 36(6): 703-7. [PMID: 26775356]

[24] Welden B, Gates G, Mallari R, Garrett N. Effects of anesthetics and analgesics on natural killer cell activity. AANA J 2009; 77(4): 287-92. [PMID: 19731847]

[25] Kutza J, Gratz I, Afshar M, Murasko DM. The effects of general anesthesia and surgery on basal and interferon stimulated natural killer cell activity of humans. Anesth Analg 1997; 85(4): 918-23. [http://dx.doi.org/10.1213/00000539-199710000-00037] [PMID: 9322480]

[26] Wu Y, Yin M, Xia W, Dou B, Liu X, Sun R. Enhancing NK cell antitumor activity with natural compounds: Research advances and molecular mechanisms. Phytother Res 2025; 39(5): 1905-29. [http://dx.doi.org/10.1002/ptr.8456] [PMID: 39931789]

[27] Tarazona R, Lopez-Sejas N, Guerrero B, *et al.* Current progress in NK cell biology and NK cell-based cancer immunotherapy. Cancer Immunol Immunother 2020; 69(5): 879-99. [http://dx.doi.org/10.1007/s00262-020-02532-9] [PMID: 32130453]

[28] Greppi M, De Franco F, Obino V, *et al.* NK cell receptors in anti-tumor and healthy tissue protection: Mechanisms and therapeutic advances. Immunol Lett 2024; 270: 106932. [http://dx.doi.org/10.1016/j.imlet.2024.106932] [PMID: 39303993]

[29] Apfel CC, Korttila K, Abdalla M, *et al.* A factorial trial of six interventions for the prevention of postoperative nausea and vomiting. N Engl J Med 2004; 350(24): 2441-51. [http://dx.doi.org/10.1056/NEJMoa032196] [PMID: 15190136]

[30] Sloan TB. Anesthetic effects on electrophysiologic recordings. J Clin Neurophysiol 1998; 15(3): 217-26. [http://dx.doi.org/10.1097/00004691-199805000-00005] [PMID: 9681559]

[31] Yu B, Kirsch JR, Bloch KD, *et al.* Propofol activates eNOS and is a scavenger of reactive oxygen species. Anesthesiology 2002; 96(3): 523-8. [http://dx.doi.org/10.1097/00000542-200203000-00012] [PMID: 11873021]

[32] Seruya M, Venturi ML, Patel KM, *et al.* Propofol-based total intravenous anesthesia decreases pulmonary complications in patients undergoing head and neck free flap reconstruction. Ann Plast Surg 2013; 70(5): 555-60. [http://dx.doi.org/10.1097/SAP.0b013e31823b6c77]

[33] Cheng SS, Yeh J, Flood P. Anesthesia matters: patients anesthetized with propofol have less postoperative pain than those anesthetized with isoflurane. Anesth Analg 2008; 106(1): 264-9. [http://dx.doi.org/10.1213/01.ane.0000287653.77372.d9] [PMID: 18165589]

[34] Wu L, Sun D, Tan Y, *et al.* Comparison of propofol and sevoflurane anesthesia on postoperative cognitive dysfunction in elderly cancer patients with mild cognitive impairment: A randomized controlled trial. J Clin Anesth 2020; 62: 109716. [http://dx.doi.org/10.1016/j.jclinane.2020.109716]

[35] Kochiyama T, Li X, Nakayama H, *et al.* Effect of propofol on the production of inflammatory cytokines by human polarized macrophages. Mediators Inflamm 2019; 2019: 1-13. [http://dx.doi.org/10.1155/2019/1919538] [PMID: 31007601]

[36] Enlund A, Nikberg M, Berglund A, Östberg E, Enlund M. Total intravenous or inhalational volatile anaesthesia and survival after colorectal cancer surgery: a Swedish national registry study. Anaesthesia

2025; 80(4): 386-94.
[http://dx.doi.org/10.1111/anae.16495] [PMID: 39676618]

[37] Makito K, Matsui H, Fushimi K, Yasunaga H. Volatile versus total intravenous anesthesia for cancer prognosis in patients having digestive cancer surgery. Anesthesiology 2020; 133(4): 764-73.
[http://dx.doi.org/10.1097/ALN.0000000000003440] [PMID: 32930730]

[38] Hasselager RP, Hallas J, Gögenur I. Inhalational versus total intravenous anesthesia and recurrence after colorectal cancer surgery: A propensity score matched Danish registry-based study. BMC Anesthesiol 2021; 21(1): 33.
[http://dx.doi.org/10.1186/s12871-021-01433-6] [PMID: 33530942]

[39] Kwon JH, Kim J, Yeo H, *et al.* Recurrence-free survival after hepatectomy using propofol-based total intravenous anaesthesia and sevoflurane-based inhalational anaesthesia: a randomised controlled study. Anaesthesia 2025; 80(4): 366-77.
[http://dx.doi.org/10.1111/anae.16488] [PMID: 39776101]

[40] Zhong JX, Kang K, Shu XL. Effect of nutritional support on clinical outcomes in perioperative malnourished patients: a meta-analysis. Asia Pac J Clin Nutr 2015; 24(3): 367-78.
[PMID: 26420176]

[41] Hu WH, Cajas-Monson LC, Eisenstein S, Parry L, Cosman B, Ramamoorthy S. Preoperative serum albumin levels predict 30-day postoperative mortality and morbidity in colorectal cancer surgery patients: A population-based cohort study. Clin Nutr 2020; 39(2): 676-83.
[http://dx.doi.org/10.1016/j.clnu.2019.02.021]

[42] Arends J, Baracos V, Bertz H, *et al.* ESPEN expert group recommendations for action against cancer-related malnutrition. Clin Nutr 2017; 36(5): 1187-96.
[http://dx.doi.org/10.1016/j.clnu.2017.06.017] [PMID: 28689670]

[43] Cook F, Rodriguez JM, McCaul LK. Malnutrition, nutrition support and dietary intervention: the role of the dietitian supporting patients with head and neck cancer. Br Dent J 2022; 233(9): 757-64.
[http://dx.doi.org/10.1038/s41415-022-5107-8] [PMID: 36369557]

[44] Chapek MA, Martindale RG. Nutrition in cancer therapy: Overview for the cancer patient. JPEN J Parenter Enteral Nutr 2021; 45(S2) (Suppl. 2): 33-40.
[http://dx.doi.org/10.1002/jpen.2259] [PMID: 34459006]

CHAPTER 2

Physiological Changes during Malignancy and its Anesthetic Considerations

Shiu-Yi E. Chen[1,*] and **Chenxuan Zhou**[2]

[1] *Department of Anesthesiology, School of Medicine, UC Irvine, Irvine, CA 92617, United States*

[2] *Department of Anesthesiology and Perioperative Care, University of California, Irvine Medical Center, Orange, CA, USA*

Abstract: The perioperative management of cancer patients is complex due to cancer-related physiological alterations and treatment-induced toxicities, requiring tailored anesthetic strategies. Malignancies and therapies like chemotherapy and radiation cause multisystem organ dysfunction, impacting cardiovascular, pulmonary, gastrointestinal, hepatic, renal, and hematologic systems. Surgical stress responses, including catecholamine release and immunosuppression, may promote metastasis. Anesthetic choices, such as total intravenous anesthesia (TIVA) and regional techniques, may mitigate immunosuppression and reduce recurrence risks compared to volatile agents. Preoperative evaluation must address organ-specific toxicities, such as anthracycline-induced cardiotoxicity, bleomycin-associated pulmonary damage, and platinum-based nephrotoxicity. Intraoperative management involves advanced hemodynamic monitoring, lung-protective ventilation, and coagulation management. Postoperative care focuses on early mobilization, multimodal analgesia, and the prevention of complications. Special considerations include tumor lysis syndrome, endocrine paraneoplastic syndromes, and neurotoxicity from chemotherapy. A multidisciplinary approach integrating oncologists, surgeons, and anesthesiologists is essential to optimize outcomes. Prospective studies are needed to validate the impact of anesthetic techniques on long-term oncologic results.

Keywords: Neurotoxicity, Organ dysfunction, Paraneoplastic syndromes, Perioperative management, Pulmonary toxicity, Regional anesthesia, Renal dysfunction, Surgical stress response, Total intravenous anesthesia (TIVA), Tumor lysis syndrome, Volatile anesthetics.

[*] **Corresponding author Shiu-Yi E. Chen:** Department of Anesthesiology, School of Medicine, UC Irvine, Irvine, CA 92617, United States; E-mail: shiuyic@hs.uci.edu

INTRODUCTION

The perioperative management of cancer patients presents unique challenges for anesthesiologists, stemming from both the pathophysiological alterations induced by malignancies and the complexities introduced by various cancer treatments. A comprehensive understanding of these factors is essential to optimize anesthetic care and improve patient outcomes.

Cancer and its treatments can lead to significant physiological changes affecting multiple organ systems. For instance, certain chemotherapeutic agents are known to cause organ-specific toxicities: bleomycin is associated with pulmonary damage, anthracyclines with cardiotoxicity, and platinum-based compounds with nephrotoxicity. Additionally, many chemotherapy agents can impair liver function and cause gastrointestinal disturbances.

Surgical interventions, while often necessary for cancer treatment, can inadvertently promote tumor metastasis and recurrence. The physiological stress response to surgery, characterized by the release of catecholamines, growth factors, and prostaglandins, may suppress immune function and create a microenvironment conducive to cancer cell dissemination. Local tissue injury during surgery further exacerbates this by inducing inflammation and releasing cytokines, such as interleukin-6 and prostaglandin E_2, which can inhibit natural killer cell activity.

Anesthetic management plays a pivotal role in modulating these perioperative factors. Retrospective data suggest that the choice of anesthetic agents and techniques can influence cancer outcomes. For example, regional anesthesia and the use of total-intravenous anesthesia (TIVA) for general anesthesia have been associated with reduced perioperative immunosuppression, potentially decreasing the risk of cancer recurrence. Conversely, volatile anesthetic agents may have immunosuppressive effects that could promote tumor progression. These are encouraging data that motivate future prospective research to evaluate the potential benefits for cancer recurrence prevention and TIVA-based anesthesia in cancer surgery.

Effective pain management is another critical consideration in the anesthetic care of cancer patients. Uncontrolled pain can lead to chronic pain syndromes and negatively impact the quality of life. Therefore, anesthesiologists must employ multimodal analgesia strategies tailored to the individual patient's needs, balancing effective pain control with minimal side effects.

As an introduction, the anesthetic care of cancer patients requires a nuanced understanding of the disease's impact on physiology, the effects of various treatments, and the implications of anesthetic choices on cancer progression and patient well-being. A multidisciplinary approach, involving close collaboration with oncologists and surgeons, is essential to navigate these complexities and provide optimal perioperative care [1].

CARDIOVASCULAR CHANGES DURING MALIGNANCY-ASSOCIATED ANESTHETIC CONSIDERATIONS

Cardiovascular Changes Induced by Malignancy

Cancer and its treatments profoundly impact the cardiovascular system, presenting challenges to anesthetic management. Malignancies, directly and indirectly, influence cardiac function through tumor-related cytokine release, paraneoplastic syndromes, and tumor invasion of cardiovascular structures. Additionally, the systemic inflammatory response associated with cancer can exacerbate endothelial dysfunction, pro-coagulant states, and myocardial strain.

Chemotherapy-Induced Cardiotoxicity

Certain chemotherapeutic agents are well-known for their cardiotoxic potential. Anthracyclines, for example, are associated with dose-dependent cardiomyopathy and heart failure due to oxidative stress and mitochondrial dysfunction. Similarly, trastuzumab, a monoclonal antibody targeting HER2, disrupts cardiomyocyte survival pathways, leading to reversible cardiac dysfunction. Platinum-based agents and vascular endothelial growth factor (VEGF) inhibitors contribute to hypertension, ischemia, and left ventricular dysfunction by inducing endothelial damage and impairing nitric oxide production [2 - 4].

The clinical manifestations of cardiotoxicity vary depending on the timing and extent of myocardial injury. Acute toxicity occurs immediately after treatment and manifests as ECG changes, QT prolongation, and various arrhythmias, with rare cases of ventricular fibrillation leading to sudden death. Subacute toxicity may cause acute left ventricular failure, pericarditis, or pericarditis-myocarditis syndrome, particularly in children, while elderly patients with preexisting heart disease may develop transient CHF. Chronic cardiotoxicity, primarily dose-dependent, often leads to cardiomyopathy, cardiomegaly, and progressive CHF, with the risk increasing significantly beyond 550 mg/m^2 of doxorubicin, for instance. Late-onset cardiotoxicity can emerge years after treatment, with previously asymptomatic patients developing heart failure and arrhythmias, potentially due to subclinical myocardial injury that impairs cardiac growth and function over time [2].

Preoperative Cardiac Evaluation

Preoperative cardiac evaluation in cancer patients aims to identify pre-existing cardiovascular diseases, assess the risk of cancer therapy-related cardiotoxicity (*e.g.*, from anthracyclines, HER2-targeted therapies, radiation, or immune checkpoint inhibitors), and determine functional capacity and hemodynamic stability for surgery. This involves clinical assessment, ECG, cardiac biomarkers, and imaging (*e.g.*, echocardiography or cardiac MRI) to stratify risk and guide perioperative management, ensuring patient safety and optimizing outcomes. Key components of evaluation and risk stratification should include:

- **Clinical Assessment:** Evaluate symptoms, cancer therapy history, and cardiovascular risk (*e.g.*, RCRI score).
- **ECG & Biomarkers:** Detect arrhythmias, myocardial injury (troponin, B-type natriuretic peptide), and electrolyte imbalances.
- **Cardiac Imaging:** Use echocardiography (left ventricular ejection fraction, global longitudinal strain) for baseline function, MRI for fibrosis/inflammation, and coronary CT for ischemia in high-risk cases.
- **Risk Stratification & Management:** Optimize medications, monitor high-risk patients, and tailor perioperative care to minimize cardiac complications.

Based on the preoperative cardiac evaluation results, cancer patients undergoing preoperative cardiac evaluation are stratified into three risk categories. Low-risk patients with a normal cardiovascular profile can proceed with surgery under standard monitoring. Moderate-risk patients with mild LV dysfunction or controlled CAD may require optimization of heart failure therapy, including beta-blockers, ACE inhibitors, or statins if indicated. High-risk patients with severe LV dysfunction or recent cardiac events should undergo further cardiology consultation, potential surgery delay for cardiac optimization, or consideration of alternative cancer treatment strategies to minimize perioperative complications [5].

Intraoperative Monitoring

Intraoperative cardiac monitoring in cancer patients with chemotherapy-induced cardiotoxicity requires a risk-stratified approach to minimize complications. Standard monitoring includes continuous electrocardiography (ECG), pulse oximetry, end-tidal CO_2, and non-invasive blood pressure measurement. In high-risk patients, invasive monitoring with an arterial line, central venous pressure, or pulmonary artery catheterization may be necessary.

Cardiac biomarkers (troponin, BNP) and electrolyte monitoring (potassium, magnesium) help detect myocardial injury and prevent arrhythmias. Intraoperative transesophageal echocardiography (TEE) provides real-time assessment of ventricular function and volume status in hemodynamically unstable patients. These tools enable real-time assessment of cardiac function, facilitating the early detection of myocardial ischemia or dysfunction.

Anesthetic considerations play a crucial role in these patients. It is important to avoid anesthetic agents that may exacerbate myocardial depression and maintain normovolemia to prevent sudden blood pressure fluctuations. Propofol, with its vasodilatory properties, should be used cautiously in patients with limited cardiac reserve. Volatile anesthetics may provide cardioprotective effects but can exacerbate hypotension in hypovolemic patients. In a patient with optimized coagulation status, regional anesthesia may be advantageous in minimizing systemic hemodynamic changes. Vasoactive medications should be used judiciously, with careful titration of vasopressors and inotropes to optimize perfusion while avoiding excessive myocardial oxygen demand in patients with compromised cardiac function. Overall, a tailored, multimodal approach optimizes intraoperative stability and improves perioperative outcomes [5, 6].

Postoperative Considerations

Postoperative care must focus on optimizing cardiac function, preventing complications, and early recognition and treatment of cardiac diseases. Management in cancer patients with pre-existing or therapy-induced cardiac dysfunction requires continuous hemodynamic monitoring, including electrocardiography, pulse oximetry, and blood pressure assessment, to detect arrhythmias, hypotension, or ischemic changes. Cardiac biomarkers such as troponin and brain natriuretic peptide should be measured in high-risk patients to assess myocardial injury and heart failure risk, while electrolyte imbalances must be corrected to prevent arrhythmias.

Optimized fluid management and early mobilization are essential to prevent volume overload and thromboembolic events, with diuretics or vasoactive agents used as needed to maintain hemodynamic stability. Patients with prior chemotherapy-related cardiotoxicity should continue or initiate guideline-directed medical therapy, including beta-blockers and angiotensin-converting enzyme inhibitors, to support myocardial recovery. Enhanced recovery protocols, emphasizing early mobilization and multimodal analgesia, can help mitigate the cardiovascular stress of surgery and promote better outcomes.

Long-term cardiac surveillance with serial echocardiography and biomarker assessments is recommended, particularly in those previously treated with anthracyclines or human epidermal growth factor receptor 2-targeted therapies. A multidisciplinary approach, integrating cardiology, oncology, and perioperative medicine, is essential for individualized postoperative care and optimal cardiovascular and oncologic outcomes [5, 6].

The interplay between cancer, its treatments, and the cardiovascular system necessitates a meticulous and multidisciplinary approach to anesthetic care. Understanding the pathophysiological changes induced by malignancy and chemotherapy, coupled with tailored perioperative management strategies, is essential for optimizing outcomes in this high-risk population.

PULMONARY CHANGES DURING MALIGNANCY AND ANESTHETIC CONSIDERATIONS

Tumor Invasion and Mass Effect

Tumor invasion and mass effect refer to the structural and functional consequences of a malignant growth within or near the lungs. As tumors expand, they can compress or invade adjacent structures, leading to a variety of pulmonary complications. Large or centrally located tumors may cause partial or complete airway obstruction, resulting in atelectasis, post-obstructive pneumonia, or respiratory distress. Tumor invasion into major blood vessels, such as the pulmonary artery or superior vena cava, can lead to life-threatening complications, including pulmonary embolism, hemoptysis, or superior vena cava syndrome.

Additionally, tumors extending into the pleura often cause malignant pleural effusions, leading to dyspnea and impaired lung expansion. Nerve involvement is another concern; invasion of the recurrent laryngeal nerve may result in vocal cord paralysis and hoarseness, while phrenic nerve involvement can cause diaphragmatic paralysis and reduced lung function. In cases where large tumors compress the mediastinum, patients may experience dysphagia from esophageal compression, airway compromise due to tracheal involvement, or even cardiac tamponade if the heart is affected [7, 8].

Chemotherapy and Radiation-Induced Pulmonary Toxicity

Pulmonary toxicity from chemotherapy and radiation is a major concern in cancer treatment, as these therapies can lead to acute and chronic lung injury. Chemotherapy-induced pulmonary injury can present as early or late-onset disease [7].

Early-onset chemotherapy-induced pulmonary injury includes inflammatory interstitial pneumonitis, a hypersensitivity-like reaction seen with agents such as methotrexate, bleomycin, and paclitaxel. Patients with this condition often develop dyspnea, dry cough, and low-grade fever. Another complication, noncardiogenic pulmonary edema, occurs due to increased vascular permeability and is associated with drugs like cytosine arabinoside, interleukin-2, and all-tran--retinoic acid. Additionally, capillary leak syndrome, seen with interleukin-2 and gemcitabine, can cause pulmonary edema and hypoxemia, requiring aggressive management.

Late-onset chemotherapy-induced pulmonary injury primarily manifests as pulmonary fibrosis, commonly caused by bleomycin, busulfan, and carmustine. This condition is often progressive and irreversible, leading to significant respiratory impairment. Another late-onset complication is bronchiolitis obliterans with organizing pneumonia (BOOP), which has been associated with bleomycin and methotrexate. Patients with BOOP may present with patchy alveolar infiltrates and worsening respiratory function over time [7, 8].

Radiation therapy also causes lung injury, with effects typically confined to the irradiated field. Acute radiation pneumonitis develops within 2 to 3 months after radiation therapy and presents with dyspnea, cough, fever, and hypoxemia. Imaging usually reveals ground-glass opacities and alveolar infiltrates in the affected area. Treatment includes corticosteroids and supportive care. Chronic radiation fibrosis, which appears 6 to 12 months post-treatment, is characterized by progressive scarring, volume loss, and reduced lung compliance. Imaging findings often show reticulations and traction bronchiectasis, while pulmonary function tests indicate a restrictive pattern with decreased diffusing capacity [7, 8].

Anesthetic Considerations and Management

Preoperative Pulmonary Evaluation

A thorough preoperative pulmonary evaluation is critical for patients with cancer-related or therapy-induced pulmonary changes. The assessment should always include:

- **History and physical examination:** Identifying symptoms like dyspnea, chronic cough, or exercise intolerance can help assess the severity of pulmonary compromise.

- **Pulmonary function tests (PFTs):** These are used to assess restrictive, obstructive, or diffusion impairments. Measurement of diffusion capacity (DLCO) is particularly useful for detecting early fibrosis [9].
- **Imaging studies:** Chest X-rays or CT scans can identify structural abnormalities such as tumor mass effects, pleural effusions, fibrosis, or signs of pneumonitis.
- **Advanced diagnostics:** Cardiopulmonary exercise testing or arterial blood gas analysis may be needed for patients with borderline pulmonary function [9].

Intraoperative Management

Ventilation Strategies & Monitoring

Intraoperative anesthetic management requires tailored strategies to accommodate compromised pulmonary function to prevent further injury.

- **Lung-protective ventilation:** Low tidal volumes (6–8 mL/kg ideal body weight) and permissive hypercapnia minimize ventilator-induced lung injury.
- **Positive end-expiratory pressure (PEEP):** Careful titration of PEEP prevents atelectasis while avoiding hemodynamic compromise, particularly in patients with right heart dysfunction.
- **Monitoring:** Continuous pulse oximetry and capnography help assess oxygenation and ventilation. Advanced tools like electrical impedance tomography can provide real-time insights into lung recruitment and ventilation-perfusion matching.

Anesthetic Agent Selection

The selection of anesthetic agents also requires special consideration to optimize oxygenation, ventilation, and maintain hemodynamic stability.

- **Volatile anesthetics:** Isoflurane and sevoflurane provide bronchodilation, making them beneficial for patients with airway obstruction.
- **Intravenous agents:** Propofol and dexmedetomidine offer hemodynamic stability and are preferred in patients with limited respiratory reserve.
- **Oxygen management:** In patients with bleomycin-induced pulmonary toxicity, high inspired oxygen fractions ($FiO2 > 30\%$) should be avoided to reduce the risk of oxygen toxicity [10].
- **Fluid management:** Restrictive fluid strategies are essential to prevent pulmonary edema, particularly in patients with chemotherapy-induced vascular permeability changes.

- **Patient positioning:** Patients with large pleural effusions may require modified lateral positioning to optimize ventilation and prevent lung compression [7, 10 - 12].

Postoperative Considerations

Postoperative care is crucial to prevent respiratory complications such as pneumonia, acute respiratory distress syndrome (ARDS), and exacerbations of preexisting pulmonary conditions. The plan should include utilization of non-invasive ventilation support, mobility, and pain management.

- **Early mobilization:** Helps reduce atelectasis and the risk of venous thromboembolism.
- **Optimal pain management:** Regional anesthesia techniques, such as thoracic epidurals, can improve postoperative respiratory function by minimizing opioid use.
- **Noninvasive ventilation (NIV) and high-flow nasal cannula (HFNC):** These modalities can support oxygenation and prevent intubation in patients with borderline respiratory function [11, 12].

In conclusion, the management of pulmonary changes during malignancy demands a multidisciplinary approach to address the intricate interplay between tumor-related effects, therapy-induced toxicity, and anesthetic implications. A comprehensive understanding of these factors, coupled with meticulous preoperative assessment and individualized intraoperative strategies, is vital for optimizing outcomes in this high-risk patient population.

GASTROINTESTINAL CHANGES DURING MALIGNANCY AND ANESTHETIC CONSIDERATIONS

Malignancies often induce significant gastrointestinal (GI) alterations, which may affect various aspects of anesthetic management. These changes include alterations in gastrointestinal motility, such as gastroparesis and obstruction, which can occur due to either tumor-related mechanical effects or systemic factors. Chemotherapy-induced nausea and vomiting (CINV) is another critical aspect of GI changes, significantly impacting patients' quality of life and perioperative care. Furthermore, malignancy and its treatment can impair liver function, leading to metabolic disturbances, coagulopathies, and altered drug metabolism [13].

Gastrointestinal Motility: Gastroparesis and Obstruction

Gastrointestinal motility disorders, including gastroparesis and obstruction, are common in malignancy. These conditions may arise from direct tumor invasion, compression of the gastrointestinal tract, consequences of medical or surgical intervention, or autonomic dysfunction. Gastroparesis, characterized by delayed gastric emptying without mechanical obstruction, leads to symptoms such as nausea, vomiting, and bloating. Similarly, obstruction, whether mechanical or functional (pseudo-obstruction), can result in acute or chronic symptoms that may complicate anesthetic planning. These motility disorders necessitate a tailored approach to perioperative management to reduce the risk of aspiration and optimize nutritional status [13].

Chemotherapy-Induced Nausea and Vomiting (CINV)

CINV is a prevalent side effect of chemotherapy, often categorized into acute, delayed, anticipatory, or breakthrough types. The pathophysiology involves complex interactions between central and peripheral pathways, particularly the chemoreceptor trigger zone and the gastrointestinal tract. Despite the use of antiemetics, nausea remains difficult to control, especially delayed nausea, which occurs more than 24 hours post-chemotherapy. Effective management of CINV is essential to improve patient comfort and enhance quality of life. Various pharmacological agents, such as serotonin antagonists, neurokinin-1 receptor antagonists, and corticosteroids, play a key role in its prevention and treatment. Non-pharmacologic approaches, such as ginger supplementation and acupressure, have also shown promise in reducing nausea when used alongside standard therapies. Research suggests that preemptive treatment before chemotherapy improves nausea control, highlighting the need for further innovations in managing CINV [14].

Impaired Liver Function

Liver dysfunction in cancer patients can result from primary or metastatic liver disease, chemotherapy, or paraneoplastic syndromes. Impaired hepatic function affects the synthesis of proteins, metabolism of drugs, and coagulation pathways. These changes not only complicate anesthetic management, particularly with drugs metabolized by the liver, but also impact surgical outcomes, increasing the risk of postoperative complications such as infections and prolonged recovery. Additionally, liver dysfunction may lead to portal hypertension, ascites, and an increased risk of bleeding, requiring comprehensive preoperative evaluation and intraoperative vigilance. Prognostic models, such as the Child-Turcotte-Pugh score and Model for End-Stage Liver Disease score, can help guide perioperative decision-making and risk stratification. Further discussion on hepatic implications in cancer patients will be covered in the next section dedicated to liver changes [15].

Anesthetic Considerations in Patients with GI Changes

Anesthetic management of patients with gastrointestinal changes necessitates a thorough understanding of the underlying pathophysiology and tailored perioperative strategies. Preoperative assessment should include evaluation of gastrointestinal motility, liver function, chemotherapy- or radiotherapy-induced toxicities, and nutritional status. Intraoperatively, strategies to minimize aspiration risk, optimize hemodynamic stability, and account for altered drug metabolism are paramount. Patients who have received chemotherapy require careful monitoring for pulmonary fibrosis (from bleomycin), cardiotoxicity (from anthracyclines), and nephrotoxicity (from platinum-based agents). Postoperatively, attention to pain management, early mobilization, and gastrointestinal function recovery is crucial. Advanced techniques, including total intravenous anesthesia and regional anesthesia, may offer advantages in specific cases, reducing the risk of postoperative nausea and vomiting while also minimizing perioperative immunosuppression, which may impact cancer recurrence.

In conclusion, gastrointestinal changes during malignancy present unique challenges to anesthetic management. A multidisciplinary approach involving oncologists, gastroenterologists, and anesthesiologists is essential to optimize patient care and outcomes by addressing both perioperative risks and long-term oncologic considerations [16, 17].

LIVER CHANGES DURING MALIGNANCY AND ANESTHETIC CONSIDERATIONS

Coagulopathy in Cancer

Coagulopathy is a common manifestation in patients with liver involvement during malignancy. The liver is central to the synthesis of coagulation factors, and its impairment leads to reduced levels of clotting proteins, increased bleeding tendencies, and thrombocytopenia. In malignancy, coagulopathy is often further compounded by the hypercoagulable state associated with cancer, as tumor cells release prothrombotic factors, which can trigger disseminated intravascular coagulation in severe cases. Additionally, chemotherapy, particularly agents such as asparaginase, can exacerbate coagulopathy by inducing thrombocytopenia and disrupting coagulation pathways. Liver metastases, hepatocellular carcinoma, or chemotherapy-induced hepatic injury can worsen clotting abnormalities.

The diagnostic workup includes prolonged prothrombin time, increased international normalized ratio, and reduced fibrinogen levels, often reflecting impaired liver function and ongoing coagulation disturbances. Platelet dysfunction may also occur due to splenomegaly from portal hypertension. Treatment focuses on managing the underlying malignancy, correcting coagulation deficits with fresh frozen plasma, vitamin K, or cryoprecipitate, and carefully balancing anticoagulation therapy in cases where thrombosis and bleeding risks coexist [16 - 18].

Impaired Liver Function

Liver dysfunction in malignancy can result from primary liver tumors, metastases, or systemic effects of cancer therapy. The liver's role in detoxification, metabolism, and protein synthesis is compromised, leading to hyperbilirubinemia, hypoalbuminemia, and impaired drug metabolism. Additionally, underlying cirrhosis, often present in gastrointestinal malignancies, further exacerbates hepatic impairment, increasing the risk of complications such as portal hypertension and coagulopathy. Tumor burden or chemotherapy-induced hepatotoxicity may also accelerate liver fibrosis or cirrhosis.

Patients with impaired liver function may present with jaundice, ascites, encephalopathy, and susceptibility to infections. The severity of liver dysfunction is commonly assessed using scoring systems like the Child-Turcotte-Pugh (CTP) and Model for End-Stage Liver Disease (MELD) scores, which help guide treatment decisions and predict surgical risk. Liver function tests, including serum transaminases, bilirubin levels, and albumin levels, are critical for assessing hepatic reserve. Imaging and liver biopsy may be necessary to evaluate structural changes.

Management strategies include preoperative optimization, individualized anesthetic planning, and postoperative monitoring to minimize complications. Dose adjustments of hepatotoxic medications are crucial, while minimally invasive treatments, such as endoscopic mucosal resection (EMR) and endoscopic submucosal dissection (ESD), may be preferred over major surgeries to reduce morbidity. For symptomatic management, diuretics can be used for ascites, and ammonia-lowering agents like lactulose are effective for hepatic encephalopathy [15].

Anesthetic Considerations in Patients with Hepatic Changes

Anesthetic management in cancer patients with liver dysfunction requires careful consideration due to altered drug metabolism, coagulopathy, and fluid-electrolyte imbalances.

Preoperative Assessment

A comprehensive evaluation of liver function should include prothrombin time/international normalized ratio, liver enzymes, bilirubin, albumin levels, and coagulation studies. Additionally, imaging such as ultrasound, CT, or MRI may be needed to assess the extent of liver involvement. Risk stratification using the Child-Turcotte-Pugh or Model for End-Stage Liver Disease scores can help predict perioperative morbidity and mortality. Correction of coagulopathy with vitamin K, fresh frozen plasma, or prothrombin complex concentrate should be individualized, and electrolyte imbalances such as hyponatremia should be addressed preoperatively.

Intraoperative Management

- **Anesthetic Agents:** Many anesthetic agents are metabolized by the liver, necessitating cautious selection. Propofol and etomidate are preferred due to their extrahepatic metabolism, with propofol also offering advantages in reducing perioperative immunosuppression. Volatile anesthetics like isoflurane and sevoflurane are generally well-tolerated, but halothane should be strictly avoided due to its association with immune-mediated hepatotoxicity.
- **Neuromuscular Blockers:** Cisatracurium and atracurium are the agents of choice, as they undergo Hofmann elimination, independent of liver metabolism. Rocuronium and vecuronium require dose adjustment due to prolonged duration of action in hepatic dysfunction.
- **Analgesics:** Opioids should be used judiciously, as impaired hepatic metabolism can lead to prolonged sedation and respiratory depression. Morphine should be avoided due to its active metabolite accumulation, while fentanyl and remifentanil are preferred due to their shorter half-lives and predictable metabolism.

Coagulopathy Management

Coagulopathy in liver disease is complex, involving both prothrombotic and hemorrhagic risks. Transfusions of fresh frozen plasma (FFP), cryoprecipitate, or platelets should be administered based on clinical needs rather than routine correction of lab values. Thromboelastography (TEG) or rotational thromboelastometry (ROTEM) should be used to guide targeted coagulation therapy rather than relying solely on PT/INR values.

Hemodynamic Stability

Maintaining hepatic perfusion is critical, as patients with liver dysfunction often have a hyperdynamic circulation with low systemic vascular resistance.

Hypotension should be aggressively managed to prevent hepatic ischemia. Vasopressors such as norepinephrine are preferred over phenylephrine due to better preservation of hepatic blood flow.

Fluid Management

Judicious fluid management is essential to avoid exacerbating ascites, portal hypertension, or fluid overload. Colloid administration, particularly albumin infusions, can be beneficial in maintaining oncotic pressure and preventing intravascular hypovolemia. Excessive crystalloid use should be avoided due to the risk of worsening edema and pulmonary congestion.

Postoperative Care

Postoperative monitoring is critical, as patients are at increased risk of bleeding, infections, hepatic encephalopathy, and delayed drug clearance. Multimodal pain management strategies should be prioritized to reduce opioid use. Regional anesthesia, such as epidural or transversus abdominis plane (TAP) blocks, may help minimize systemic drug exposure but must be used cautiously in the presence of coagulopathy [18, 19].

Hepatic changes during malignancy, including coagulopathy and impaired liver function, significantly impact perioperative care. Comprehensive preoperative assessment, tailored anesthetic strategies, and meticulous intraoperative and postoperative management are crucial for optimizing outcomes. Collaboration between anesthesiologists, oncologists, and hepatologists ensures a multidisciplinary approach to these complex patients.

HEMATOLOGIC CHANGES DURING MALIGNANCY AND ANESTHETIC CONSIDERATIONS

Hematologic changes are a frequent consequence of malignancy and its treatment, profoundly impacting anesthetic management. These alterations include anemia, leukocytosis, immunosuppression, thrombocytopenia, and coagulopathy, all of which pose unique perioperative challenges.

Anemia

Anemia is a common complication in cancer patients, arising from tumor-induced chronic inflammation, nutritional deficiencies, bone marrow suppression, and blood loss, with chemotherapy and radiotherapy further exacerbating erythropoiesis impairment. It disrupts iron metabolism, leading to either absolute or functional iron deficiency, and contributes to increased perioperative transfusion rates, cardiovascular strain, pulmonary complications, and cognitive dysfunction. Reduced oxygen delivery impairs wound healing and heightens surgical risks. Management strategies include preoperative iron supplementation, erythropoiesis-stimulating agents, and restrictive transfusion strategies to minimize immunomodulation, thromboembolic events, and infection risks. Anesthesiologists must balance optimizing hemoglobin levels with minimizing transfusion-related complications to improve surgical outcomes [20 - 25].

Leukocytosis and Immunosuppression

Leukocytosis in cancer patients may result from tumor-induced cytokine production, bone marrow stimulation, or paraneoplastic syndromes, potentially masking underlying infections or bone marrow dysfunction. Conversely, immunosuppression arises from malignancy itself, chemotherapy, or radiotherapy, increasing susceptibility to infections, delayed wound healing, and sepsis. Anesthetic management requires stringent infection control, timely antibiotic prophylaxis, and close monitoring of leukocyte counts and immune function. Perioperative considerations include optimizing immune status, assessing for occult infections, and managing hemodynamic instability in septic patients with cautious fluid resuscitation and vasopressor support. Additionally, the immunomodulatory effects of anesthetic agents, particularly volatile anesthetics and opioids, should be considered to minimize further immune suppression and improve perioperative outcomes [24, 25].

Thrombocytopenia and Coagulopathy

Thrombocytopenia in cancer patients is often multifactorial, arising from bone marrow suppression, tumor invasion, or chemotherapy-induced toxicity, and significantly increases the risk of perioperative bleeding. Malignancy-associated coagulopathy, including disseminated intravascular coagulation (DIC) and a hypercoagulable state, further complicates surgical management by predisposing patients to both thrombotic and hemorrhagic events. This necessitates a nuanced approach to anticoagulation and hemostasis, balancing the risks of clot formation and excessive bleeding. Preoperative evaluation should include platelet counts, coagulation profiles, and assessment for underlying prothrombotic conditions. Correction strategies may involve platelet transfusions, clotting factor replacement, or antifibrinolytic agents when appropriate. Anesthetic considerations include minimizing invasive procedures, avoiding neuraxial techniques in severe thrombocytopenia, and optimizing intraoperative coagulation monitoring to reduce complications and improve surgical outcomes [26, 27].

Anesthetic Considerations in Patients with Hematologic Changes

In summary, effective anesthetic management of patients with hematologic changes requires a comprehensive preoperative evaluation and individualized perioperative strategies. Anemia necessitates careful assessment of cardiovascular and respiratory function to optimize oxygen delivery. For patients with leukocytosis or immunosuppression, stringent aseptic techniques and infection prophylaxis are critical. Thrombocytopenia and coagulopathy demand meticulous attention to bleeding risks, necessitating the use of minimally invasive techniques and hemostatic agents where applicable. Advanced intraoperative monitoring, including thromboelastography, may aid in real-time assessment of coagulation status.

In conclusion, hematologic changes during malignancy pose significant anesthetic challenges. A multidisciplinary approach, involving oncologists, hematologists, and anesthesiologists, is vital to ensure optimal patient outcomes.

CENTRAL NERVOUS SYSTEM (CNS) CHANGES DURING MALIGNANCY AND ANESTHETIC CONSIDERATIONS

Tumor Mass Effect in the Central and Peripheral Nervous Systems

Malignancies involving the central (CNS) and peripheral nervous system (PNS) can cause significant structural and functional disruptions, leading to severe neurological consequences. CNS tumors exert mass effects, resulting in increased intracranial pressure (ICP), brain edema, hydrocephalus, and compression of critical neural structures, manifesting as headaches, altered mental status, seizures, and focal neurological deficits. Tumors affecting the PNS can cause nerve compression, leading to neuropathic pain, motor weakness, and sensory deficits. Compression of vital structures such as the brainstem or spinal cord can result in life-threatening complications, including respiratory failure and autonomic dysfunction. Metastases to the CNS, commonly from lung cancer, breast cancer, and melanoma, further exacerbate neurological impairment by disrupting the blood-brain barrier, promoting inflammatory responses, and increasing peritumoral edema. Anesthetic management focuses on preserving cerebral perfusion, mitigating ICP fluctuations, and optimizing neuromuscular function. Preoperative imaging, corticosteroids for edema reduction, seizure prophylaxis, and careful selection of anesthetic agents are crucial to minimizing perioperative risks and ensuring optimal neurological outcomes [28, 29].

Cancer Treatment-Related Peripheral and Central Toxicity

Cancer treatments such as chemotherapy and radiation therapy can cause significant neurotoxicity affecting both the central nervous system (CNS) and peripheral nervous system (PNS). Chemotherapy-induced peripheral neuropathy (CIPN) is a common complication, characterized by numbness, tingling, burning pain, and motor deficits that impair quality of life and may necessitate dose reductions or treatment discontinuation. Agents frequently implicated in CIPN include platinum-based compounds, taxanes, and vinca alkaloids, which induce neuronal damage through oxidative stress, mitochondrial dysfunction, and microtubule disruption. Central neurotoxicity manifests as cognitive impairment ("chemo brain"), encephalopathy, seizures, and radiation-induced necrosis or leukoencephalopathy, often exacerbated by cumulative treatment effects and blood-brain barrier disruption. Radiation therapy can further contribute to neuroinflammation, white matter injury, and long-term cognitive decline. Management strategies focus on dose modifications, symptomatic relief with neuropathic pain agents, and supportive interventions such as physical therapy and cognitive rehabilitation to optimize functional outcomes [28, 29].

Anesthetic Considerations in Patients with Cancer-related CNS and PNS Changes

Patients with CNS and PNS changes due to malignancy require meticulous anesthetic planning to mitigate risks and optimize perioperative outcomes. Preoperative evaluation should assess for increased intracranial pressure (ICP), airway compromise due to mass effect, and existing neurological deficits. Imaging studies, such as MRI or CT scans, provide crucial information regarding tumor location, size, and associated complications, guiding anesthetic management. For patients with elevated ICP, induction and maintenance should focus on preventing further pressure increases - propofol is often preferred for its neuroprotective effects and ability to reduce cerebral metabolic demand. Avoiding hypercapnia, maintaining adequate oxygenation, and minimizing fluctuations in blood pressure are essential to prevent cerebral ischemia and edema. Neuromuscular monitoring is particularly important in patients with chemotherapy-induced peripheral neuropathy (CIPN) or pre-existing neuromuscular deficits, as they may have prolonged responses to neuromuscular blocking agents, requiring cautious dosing and reversal.

Intraoperative management may involve the use of corticosteroids to reduce cerebral edema, anticonvulsants for seizure prophylaxis, and hemodynamic monitoring to manage autonomic instability, which is common in patients with extensive nerve involvement. For patients with PNS involvement, meticulous positioning is critical to prevent exacerbation of neuropathic pain and avoid nerve compression injuries. Additionally, opioid dosing should be carefully titrated, as patients with CNS or PNS pathology may exhibit altered pain sensitivity, necessitating a multimodal analgesic approach. Postoperative care should focus on early detection and management of neurological complications, such as new deficits, seizures, or worsening cerebral edema. Given the complexity of these cases, a multidisciplinary approach involving anesthesiologists, neurologists, oncologists, and surgeons is essential to ensure comprehensive and individualized perioperative management [30, 31].

RENAL CHANGES DURING MALIGNANCY AND ANESTHETIC CONSIDERATIONS

Tumor Lysis Syndrome (TLS)

Tumor lysis syndrome (TLS) is a life-threatening metabolic complication commonly seen in patients with rapidly proliferating malignancies such as leukemia and lymphoma. TLS occurs when tumor cells lyse spontaneously or in response to cytotoxic therapy, releasing intracellular contents into the bloodstream. The release of potassium, phosphate, nucleic acids, and calcium leads to a cascade of metabolic derangements, including hyperkalemia, hyperphosphatemia, hyperuricemia, and hypocalcemia. These imbalances can result in acute kidney injury (AKI), cardiac arrhythmias, seizures, and, if untreated, death.

Renal injury in TLS is primarily caused by uric acid and calcium phosphate crystal deposition within the renal tubules, resulting in obstructive nephropathy. The onset of TLS is typically within 12–72 hours of initiating chemotherapy or radiation, but it can also occur spontaneously. Risk factors for TLS include a large tumor burden, high cell turnover rates, preexisting renal impairment, and dehydration. Prophylaxis involves aggressive hydration, allopurinol, and the use of urate oxidase (rasburicase) in high-risk patients to prevent hyperuricemia. Dialysis may be required in severe cases of AKI or refractory metabolic disturbances [32, 33].

Anesthetic Considerations in Patients with Renal Changes

Preoperative assessment is critical, especially for patients with high-grade hematologic malignancies, and should include evaluation of renal function, electrolyte levels, and hydration status. Aggressive intravenous hydration is essential to maintain renal perfusion and promote the excretion of uric acid and phosphate. Continuous monitoring of potassium, calcium, phosphate, and uric acid levels is necessary to prevent arrhythmias and other complications. Urine alkalinization with sodium bicarbonate may be used cautiously to increase uric acid solubility, though it risks worsening hypocalcemia. Hypouricemic agents like allopurinol or rasburicase are key for managing hyperuricemia, with rasburicase being particularly effective. In severe cases with acute kidney injury, renal replacement therapy, such as hemodialysis, may be required. Anesthetists must also avoid nephrotoxic drugs and contrast agents to protect renal function. Early recognition and proactive management are vital to improving patient outcomes [32 - 34].

Intraoperative Management

Anesthetic Agents

The selection of anesthetic agents should prioritize renal safety, avoiding those with potential nephrotoxicity or significant renal clearance. Inhalational agents such as sevoflurane, while generally well-tolerated, can produce compound A, a nephrotoxic metabolite, particularly in low-flow anesthesia settings, so their use should be cautious. Intravenous agents like propofol and dexmedetomidine are preferred due to their minimal renal metabolism and hemodynamic stability. Non-depolarizing neuromuscular blockers that rely on renal clearance, such as vecuronium and pancuronium, should be avoided or used with dose adjustments, while cisatracurium, which undergoes Hofmann elimination, is a safer alternative [34 - 36].

Fluid Management

Maintaining euvolemia is crucial for renal perfusion and reducing the risk of acute kidney injury. Balanced crystalloids (*e.g.*, lactated Ringer's or Plasma-Lyte) are preferred over normal saline, as chloride-rich solutions can contribute to hyperchloremic metabolic acidosis and renal vasoconstriction. Colloids (*e.g.*, hydroxyethyl starch) should be avoided due to their association with worsening renal outcomes. Urine output monitoring is essential, but diuretics like furosemide should be used cautiously, primarily in fluid-overloaded patients, to avoid worsening intravascular depletion and electrolyte disturbances [34 - 36].

Electrolyte Monitoring

Patients with tumor lysis syndrome (TLS) are at high risk for hyperkalemia, hyperphosphatemia, hypocalcemia, and metabolic acidosis, which can cause life-threatening arrhythmias and neuromuscular dysfunction. Continuous intraoperative electrolyte monitoring is critical, and hyperkalemia should be managed with calcium gluconate (for cardiac stabilization), insulin with glucose (to shift potassium intracellularly), sodium bicarbonate (if acidotic), and loop diuretics or dialysis if severe [34 - 36].

Hemodynamic Stability

Maintaining stable hemodynamics is paramount for preventing renal hypoperfusion and ischemic injury. Hypotension exacerbates renal ischemia, leading to AKI, so fluid resuscitation should be balanced with vasopressor support if needed. Norepinephrine is the preferred vasopressor due to its ability to sustain mean arterial pressure without excessive vasoconstriction of renal vasculature, while dopamine is generally not recommended due to its lack of renal protective effects in critically ill patients and higher risks for tachycardia and dysrhythmia at moderate to high doses. Continuous arterial blood pressure monitoring is recommended for high-risk patients to guide real-time hemodynamic management [35, 36].

Postoperative Considerations

Postoperative monitoring of renal function is critical, particularly in high-risk patients. Pain management strategies should prioritize non-nephrotoxic medications, avoiding NSAIDs when possible due to their potential to impair renal function. Early recognition and treatment of complications, such as fluid overload or electrolyte imbalances, are essential to improving outcomes. Dialysis support may be needed for patients with severe renal impairment [34 - 36].

Renal changes associated with malignancy, particularly TLS, pose significant perioperative challenges. Early recognition and management of metabolic derangements, along with careful selection of anesthetic agents and meticulous intraoperative monitoring, are crucial for optimizing outcomes in these patients. A multidisciplinary approach involving oncologists, nephrologists, and anesthesiologists is key to providing comprehensive care.

ENDOCRINE CHANGES DURING MALIGNANCY AND ANESTHETIC CONSIDERATIONS

Introduction

Endocrine changes during malignancy can significantly impact patient care, particularly in the perioperative setting. These changes may result from the direct effects of tumors, paraneoplastic syndromes, or cancer treatments, and they often involve the hypothalamic-pituitary axis, adrenal glands, thyroid, and parathyroid glands. For example, pituitary tumors can lead to conditions like acromegaly or Cushing's disease, while adrenal tumors may cause hypercortisolism or hyperaldosteronism. Thyroid and parathyroid tumors can result in hyperthyroidism or hypercalcemia, respectively. These endocrine disturbances can complicate anesthesia by affecting airway management, cardiovascular stability, electrolyte balance, and glucose regulation [37].

Carcinoid Tumors

Carcinoid tumors are neuroendocrine tumors originating from enterochromaffin cells, commonly found in the gastrointestinal tract and lungs. These tumors secrete serotonin, histamine, bradykinin, and other vasoactive substances, leading to carcinoid syndrome, which is characterized by flushing, diarrhea, bronchospasm, and carcinoid heart disease. The risk of carcinoid crisis, a life-threatening perioperative complication, poses significant anesthetic challenges [38 - 40].

Perioperative Concerns

- Carcinoid Crisis Risk: Triggered by surgical stress, tumor manipulation, or anesthetic agents, leading to severe hypotension, hypertension, arrhythmias, and bronchospasm.
- Carcinoid Heart Disease: Fibrotic changes in the right-sided heart valves due to prolonged exposure to serotonin, leading to tricuspid regurgitation and pulmonary stenosis, which can result in heart failure and perioperative hemodynamic instability.
- Unpredictable Physiologic Changes: Patients may exhibit uncontrolled vasoactive hormone release, causing hemodynamic instability refractory to conventional inotropes and vasopressors [38 - 40].

Management

- **Preoperative Optimization**
    - Somatostatin Analog Therapy: Preoperative administration of octreotide helps suppress hormone secretion and reduce crisis risk. However, recent studies suggest prophylactic octreotide does not significantly reduce intraoperative carcinoid crisis incidence, raising the need for individualized therapy [39].
    - Cardiac Evaluation: Patients with suspected carcinoid heart disease should undergo echocardiography and NT-proBNP testing to assess cardiac function and valve pathology [40].
    - Electrolyte and Volume Status: Chronic diarrhea can lead to hypovolemia, hypokalemia, and niacin deficiency (pellagra), requiring correction before surgery [40]

- **Intraoperative Management**
  - Anesthetic Drug Selection:
    - Avoid histamine-releasing agents (*e.g.*, morphine, atracurium) and catecholamine-releasing drugs (*e.g.*, ephedrine, ketamine) that may exacerbate vasoactive hormone release.
    - Preferred agents include propofol for induction and remifentanil or dexmedetomidine for analgesia due to their stable hemodynamic profile.
    - Non-depolarizing neuromuscular blockers like rocuronium or cisatracurium are preferred to minimize cardiovascular instability.
  - Hemodynamic Stability:
    - Maintain adequate intravascular volume with balanced crystalloids; avoid rapid fluid shifts.
    - Norepinephrine is the preferred vasopressor if needed, as it provides stable vasoconstriction without triggering carcinoid hormone release.
  - Carcinoid Crisis Management:
    - Bolus octreotide (50-500 mcg) and infusion (50-200 mcg/hr) should be readily available for intraoperative crisis treatment.
    - Treat bronchospasm with nebulized beta-2 agonists (*e.g.*, albuterol) rather than epinephrine to prevent worsening hormone release.
    - Continuous arterial blood pressure monitoring is recommended for real-time hemodynamic assessment [39, 40].
- **Postoperative Considerations**
  - **Continue somatostatin analogs** to prevent delayed carcinoid symptoms.
  - **Monitor for rebound hypotension, arrhythmias, and respiratory complications** in a step-down unit or an intensive care unit, depending on patients' needs.
  - **Assess for post-op cardiac decompensation** in patients with pre-existing carcinoid heart disease [38, 40].

Thyroid Disorders

Thyroid dysfunction in cancer patients may be primary (*e.g.*, thyroid cancer) or secondary to treatments like radiation or immunotherapy [41, 42].

- **Hyperthyroidism:** Increased thyroid hormone levels can lead to thyrotoxicosis with tachycardia, hypertension, and arrhythmias.
- **Hypothyroidism:** Associated with bradycardia, hypothermia, and impaired drug metabolism.

Management

- **Preoperative:** Normalize thyroid function with antithyroid drugs, beta-blockers, or thyroid hormone replacement. Assess airway for thyroid enlargement or tracheal deviation.
- **Intraoperative:** Avoid sympathetic stimulation in hyperthyroid patients. Hypothyroid patients may require reduced doses of sedatives and opioids.
- **Postoperative:** Monitor for thyroid storm or myxedema coma, rare but life-threatening complications.

Adrenal Tumors

Adrenal tumors encompass a spectrum of functional and non-functional lesions, with pheochromocytomas being the most clinically significant due to their excessive catecholamine secretion, leading to episodic hypertension, tachycardia, diaphoresis, and headaches. Other adrenal tumors, such as adrenocortical carcinomas (ACC), may produce excess cortisol or androgens, contributing to Cushing's syndrome or virilization. Proper preoperative, intraoperative, and postoperative management is essential to prevent complications such as hypertensive crises, hemodynamic instability, and metabolic disturbances [43].

Management

- **Preoperative:** Alpha-adrenergic blockade (*e.g.*, phenoxybenzamine) to normalize blood pressure and volume status. Beta-blockade may be used to control tachycardia. Patients with ACC and cortisol excess should receive preoperative steroid replacement therapy to prevent adrenal insufficiency postoperatively.
- **Intraoperative:** Anesthetic considerations include avoiding catecholamine-releasing agents such as ketamine and ephedrine, maintaining hemodynamic stability with short-acting vasodilators (*e.g.*, nitroprusside, nicardipine) for hypertension, and using vasopressors (*e.g.*, norepinephrine, vasopressin) judiciously for post-resection hypotension. Continuous invasive monitoring *via* arterial lines and central venous catheters is essential for real-time blood pressure and volume assessment.
- **Postoperative:** patients require frequent monitoring of hemodynamics, glucose, and electrolytes to detect delayed complications such as hypotension or adrenal insufficiency. A multidisciplinary approach involving anesthesiologists, endocrinologists, and surgeons is crucial for optimizing outcomes in these [43].

Pituitary Tumors

Pituitary tumors can cause hormonal excess (*e.g.*, Cushing's disease, acromegaly) or deficiency (*e.g.*, panhypopituitarism). These tumors may also cause mass effect symptoms such as headache and visual disturbances [44 - 47].

Management

- **Preoperative:** Assess endocrine function and correct hormonal imbalances. Perform MRI to evaluate tumor size and extension.
  - **Intraoperative:** Intraoperative considerations include avoiding agents that increase intracranial pressure, careful airway management in acromegaly patients with difficult intubation, and maintaining hemodynamic stability, particularly in patients with cardiovascular complications from hormonal excess. Hormone replacement therapy may be required for endocrine deficiencies, and patients undergoing transsphenoidal surgery should be monitored for cerebrospinal fluid (CSF) leaks.
  - **Postoperative:** Careful observation for diabetes insipidus and syndrome of inappropriate antidiuretic hormone (SIADH) is critical, as both conditions can cause severe electrolyte imbalances and hemodynamic instability. A multidisciplinary approach, involving anesthesiologists, endocrinologists, and neurosurgeons, is essential for optimizing outcomes [45 - 47].

Parathyroid Tumors

Parathyroid adenomas or carcinomas may cause primary hyperparathyroidism with hypercalcemia, leading to nephrolithiasis, bone pain, and neurocognitive dysfunction [48, 49].

Management

- **Preoperative:** Correct hypercalcemia with intravenous fluids, bisphosphonates, or calcitonin.
- **Intraoperative:** Monitor calcium levels and avoid hyperventilation, which exacerbates hypocalcemia.
- **Postoperative:** Watch for hypocalcemia (*e.g.*, Chvostek's and Trousseau's signs) due to "hungry bone syndrome."

Anesthetic Considerations in Cancer Patients with Endocrine Changes

Cancer patients with endocrine alterations pose unique challenges for anesthetic management. Key considerations include:

1. **Preoperative:** Comprehensive evaluation of endocrine function and tumor-related complications. Optimize hormonal and metabolic status before surgery.
2. **Intraoperative:** Tailor anesthetic agents based on the endocrine pathology. Maintain hemodynamic stability, avoid exacerbating endocrine crises, and manage electrolyte disturbances.
3. **Postoperative:** Close monitoring for delayed complications like adrenal insufficiency, thyroid storm, or calcium imbalances.

Endocrine changes during malignancy require meticulous perioperative assessment and management. Anesthetic care must be individualized to address the specific endocrine pathology, ensure patient safety, and optimize surgical outcomes. Multidisciplinary collaboration between anesthesiologists, endocrinologists, and oncologists is critical for success.

ROLE OF REGIONAL ANESTHESIA IN MALIGNANCY AND ANESTHETIC CONSIDERATIONS IN CANCER PATIENTS

Introduction

Regional anesthesia plays a significant role in the perioperative management of patients with malignancy. By targeting specific nerves or nerve groups, regional techniques offer pain control, reduce the need for systemic opioids, and may influence oncologic outcomes by modulating immune and inflammatory responses. This chapter discusses the mechanisms, potential benefits, and anesthetic considerations of regional anesthesia in cancer patients.

Mechanisms of Regional Anesthesia in Cancer Management

Regional anesthesia works by blocking afferent nerve signals from the site of surgery to the central nervous system. By reducing the neuroendocrine stress response and lowering circulating catecholamines, regional anesthesia can potentially improve the immune environment, which is critical for patients undergoing oncologic surgery.

Additionally, regional anesthesia minimizes the need for volatile anesthetics and opioids, which have been shown in some studies to suppress natural killer (NK) cell function, a key component in tumor immunosurveillance. Emerging evidence suggests that techniques such as epidurals and peripheral nerve blocks may play a role in mitigating metastatic spread, although further research is needed to confirm these effects [50].

Benefits of Regional Anesthesia in Cancer Patients

Pain Control

Regional anesthesia provides superior analgesia compared to systemic opioid use, particularly in surgeries with significant postoperative pain, such as breast, thoracic, or abdominal cancer surgeries. Techniques like thoracic epidurals or paravertebral blocks can significantly reduce pain scores and enhance patient recovery.

Reduced Opioid Consumption

By providing localized pain relief, regional anesthesia reduces the need for systemic opioids, thereby minimizing opioid-related side effects such as nausea, vomiting, ileus, and sedation. This can enhance recovery and reduce the length of hospital stay.

Immunomodulatory Effects

Regional techniques may influence the immune response favorably by limiting the perioperative stress response. A reduction in the use of systemic anesthetics and opioids may help preserve NK cell activity and improve the host's ability to combat micro-metastases.

Potential Impact on Recurrence and Survival

Studies have suggested a possible link between regional anesthesia and improved long-term cancer outcomes. Although the data are not definitive, regional anesthesia may reduce tumor recurrence by limiting perioperative immune suppression and systemic inflammatory responses.

Anesthetic Considerations in Cancer Patients Using Regional Techniques

Patient Selection

Regional anesthesia is not suitable for all patients. Coagulopathy, often seen in patients with malignancy due to liver dysfunction, disseminated intravascular coagulation (DIC), or the effects of chemotherapy, may contraindicate neuraxial techniques due to the increased risk of bleeding. Patients with tumor involvement of the nervous system may require modified block techniques due to anatomical alterations.

Medication Considerations

Many cancer patients are on anticoagulants or antiplatelet medications, necessitating careful planning to minimize the risk of hematoma. Additionally, certain chemotherapy agents may increase the risk of neurotoxicity, which could interact with local anesthetics.

Perioperative Challenges

- **Neurotoxicity**: Chemotherapy-induced peripheral neuropathy can complicate the placement of regional blocks or exacerbate pre-existing neurologic symptoms.
- **Tumor Involvement**: Patients with malignancies affecting the spine or nervous system may have altered anatomy, complicating regional anesthesia techniques.
- **Immunosuppression**: Cancer patients are often immunosuppressed, either due to the disease itself or its treatment. This increases the risk of infection, requiring strict aseptic techniques during block placement.

Monitoring and Follow-Up

Continuous monitoring of regional anesthesia effects is critical, especially in cancer patients with complex comorbidities. Postoperative follow-up ensures timely identification of complications, such as hematoma, infection, or prolonged block duration [50].

CONCLUSION AND FUTURE DIRECTIONS

While studies highlight the potential benefits of regional anesthesia in oncologic surgery, more robust, large-scale, randomized controlled trials are needed to determine its definitive impact on cancer outcomes. Current research focuses on identifying which patient populations benefit most and understanding the molecular mechanisms through which regional anesthesia may influence tumor biology.

Regional anesthesia is a valuable tool in the anesthetic management of cancer patients, offering significant benefits in pain control, reduced opioid requirements, and potential improvements in oncologic outcomes. However, careful patient selection and an understanding of the unique challenges posed by malignancy are essential. As the field evolves, integrating regional techniques into multimodal anesthesia plans will likely remain a cornerstone of personalized perioperative care in cancer patients.

REFERENCES

[1] Keane E, Nestor C. Implications of anaesthesia on cancer surgery. Anaesthesia Tutorial of the Week. 2022 Dec 20; 487: 1-6. Available from: https://resources.wfsahq.org/wp-content/uploads/atow-487-00.pdf

[2] Gehdoo RP. Anticancer Chemotherapy and it's Anaesthetic Implications (Current Concepts). Indian J Anaesth 2009; 53(1): 18-29. [PMID: 20640073]

[3] Tu Y, Zhou S, Wang H, *et al.* Neoadjuvant chemotherapy and perioperative cardiotoxicity. Vol. 3, Journal of Anesthesia and Translational Medicine. Elsevier BV; 2024. p. 171–80. [http://dx.doi.org/10.1016/j.jatmed.2024.11.003]

[4] Curigliano G, Lenihan D, Fradley M, *et al.* Management of cardiac disease in cancer patients throughout oncological treatment: ESMO consensus recommendations. Ann Oncol 2020; 31(2): 171-90. [http://dx.doi.org/10.1016/j.annonc.2019.10.023] [PMID: 31959335]

[5] Scalia IG, Gheyath B, Tamarappoo BK, Moudgil R, Otton J, Pereyra M, *et al.* Chemotherapy Related Cardiotoxicity Evaluation—A Contemporary Review with a Focus on Cardiac Imaging. Vol. 13, Journal of Clinical Medicine. MDPI AG; 2024. p. 3714. [http://dx.doi.org/10.3390/jcm13133714]

[6] Dent SF, Moore H, Raval P, Alder L, Guha A. How to Manage and Monitor Cardiac Dysfunction in Patients With Metastatic HER2-Positive Breast Cancer. Vol. 4, JACC: CardioOncology. Elsevier BV; 2022. p. 404–8. [http://dx.doi.org/10.1016/j.jaccao.2022.06.002]

[7] Dhamija E, Meena P, Ramalingam V, Sahoo R, Rastogi S, Thulkar S. Chemotherapy-induced pulmonary complications in cancer: Significance of clinicoradiological correlation. Vol. 30, Indian Journal of Radiology and Imaging. Georg Thieme Verlag KG; 2020. p. 20–6. [http://dx.doi.org/10.4103/ijri.IJRI_178_19]

[8] Malhotra V, Perry MC. Radiation-induced and chemotherapy-induced pulmonary injury. Vol. 13, Current Opinion in Oncology. Ovid Technologies (Wolters Kluwer Health); 2001. p. 242–8. [http://dx.doi.org/10.1097/00001622-200107000-00006]

[9] Win T, Jackson A, Sharples L, *et al.* Relationship between pulmonary function and lung cancer surgical outcome. Vol. 25, European Respiratory Journal. European Respiratory Society (ERS); 2005. p. 594–9. [http://dx.doi.org/10.1183/09031936.05.00077504]

[10] Huh J, Hwang W. The Role of Anesthetic Management in Lung Cancer Recurrence and Metastasis: A Comprehensive Review. Vol. 13, Journal of Clinical Medicine. MDPI AG; 2024. p. 6681. [http://dx.doi.org/10.3390/jcm13226681]

[11] Wang J, Liu L, Song Y, Jiao J, Zhong Y. Current Understanding on Perioperative Management in Lung Cancer: Implications for Anesthetic Considerations. Drug Des Devel Ther 2021; 15: 835-42. [http://dx.doi.org/10.2147/DDDT.S297200] [PMID: 33658765]

[12] Lederman D, Easwar J, Feldman J, Shapiro V. Anesthetic considerations for lung resection: preoperative assessment, intraoperative challenges and postoperative analgesia. Ann Transl Med 2019; 7(15): 356. [http://dx.doi.org/10.21037/atm.2019.03.67] [PMID: 31516902]

[13] Shafi MA. Gastrointestinal Motility Issues in Cancer Patients. Curr Gastroenterol Rep 2019; 21(12): 69. [http://dx.doi.org/10.1007/s11894-019-0738-x] [PMID: 31823129]

[14] Ryan JL. Treatment of Chemotherapy-induced Nausea in Cancer Patients. Vol. 06, European Oncology & Haematology. Touch Medical Media, Ltd.; 2010. p. 14.

[http://dx.doi.org/10.17925/EOH.2010.06.02.14]

[15] Xiang Z, Li Y, Zhu C, *et al.* Gastrointestinal Cancers and Liver Cirrhosis: Implications on Treatments and Prognosis. Vol. 11, Frontiers in Oncology. Frontiers Media SA; 2021. [http://dx.doi.org/10.3389/fonc.2021.766069]

[16] Kiamanesh D, Rumley J, Moitra VK. Monitoring and managing hepatic disease in anaesthesia. Vol. 111, British Journal of Anaesthesia. Elsevier BV; 2013. p. i50–61. [http://dx.doi.org/10.1093/bja/aet378]

[17] Gudaitytė J, Dvylys D, Šimeliūnaitė I. Anaesthetic challenges in cancer patients: current therapies and pain management. Vol. 24, Acta medica Lituanica. Vilnius University Press; 2017. p. 121–7. [http://dx.doi.org/10.6001/actamedica.v24i2.3493]

[18] Brentjens TE, Chadha R. Anesthesia for the Patient with Concomitant Hepatic and Renal Impairment. Vol. 34, Anesthesiology Clinics. Elsevier BV; 2016. p. 645–58. [http://dx.doi.org/10.1016/j.anclin.2016.06.002]

[19] Bedewy A, El-Kassas M. Anesthesia in patients with chronic liver disease: An updated review. Vol. 47, Clinics and Research in Hepatology and Gastroenterology. Elsevier BV; 2023. p. 102205. [http://dx.doi.org/10.1016/j.clinre.2023.102205]

[20] Patel MS, Carson JL. Anemia in the Preoperative Patient. Vol. 93, Medical Clinics of North America. Elsevier BV; 2009. p. 1095–104. [http://dx.doi.org/10.1016/j.mcna.2009.05.007]

[21] Weber RS, Jabbour N, Martin RCG II. Anemia and transfusions in patients undergoing surgery for cancer. Ann Surg Oncol 2008; 15(1): 34-45. [http://dx.doi.org/10.1245/s10434-007-9502-9] [PMID: 17943390]

[22] Liu X, Qiu H, Huang Y, *et al.* Impact of preoperative anemia on outcomes in patients undergoing curative resection for gastric cancer: a single□institution retrospective analysis of 2163 Chinese patients. Vol. 7, Cancer Medicine. Wiley; 2018. p. 360–9. [http://dx.doi.org/10.1002/cam4.1309]

[23] Busti F, Marchi G, Ugolini S, Castagna A, Girelli D. Anemia and Iron Deficiency in Cancer Patients: Role of Iron Replacement Therapy. Vol. 11, Pharmaceuticals. MDPI AG; 2018. p. 94. [http://dx.doi.org/10.3390/ph11040094]

[24] Taylor M, Abah U, Hayes T, Eadington T, Smith M, Shackcloth M, *et al.* Preoperative Anemia is Associated With Worse Long-Term Survival After Lung Cancer Resection: A Multicenter Cohort Study of 5,029 Patients. Vol. 36, Journal of Cardiothoracic and Vascular Anesthesia. Elsevier BV; 2022. p. 1373–9. [http://dx.doi.org/10.1053/j.jvca.2021.08.029]

[25] Pan K, Pang S, Robinson M, Goede D, Meenrajan S. A review of perioperative anemia: A modifiable and not so benign risk factor. Vol. 11, Journal of Family Medicine and Primary Care. Medknow; 2022. p. 5004–9. [http://dx.doi.org/10.4103/jfmpc.jfmpc_2209_21]

[26] Kasuga I, Makino S, Kiyokawa H, Katoh H, Ebihara Y, Ohyashiki K. Tumor-related leukocytosis is linked with poor prognosis in patients with lung carcinoma. Vol. 92, Cancer. Wiley; 2001. p. 2399–405. [http://dx.doi.org/10.1002/1097-0142(20011101]

[27] Bezu L, Akçal Öksüz D, Bell M, *et al.* Perioperative Immunosuppressive Factors during Cancer Surgery: An Updated Review. Vol. 16, Cancers. MDPI AG; 2024. p. 2304. [http://dx.doi.org/10.3390/cancers16132304]

[28] Deshpande SP, Henderson RA, Ajith AU, Zimrin AB, Williams B. Cancer-Related Coagulopathy and Perioperative Considerations. Anesthesia & Analgesia. Ovid Technologies (Wolters Kluwer Health); 2024.

[http://dx.doi.org/10.1213/ANE.0000000000007286]

[29] Khorana AA. Cancer and coagulation. Vol. 87, American Journal of Hematology. Wiley; 2012. [http://dx.doi.org/10.1002/ajh.23143]

[30] Mendez JS, DeAngelis LM. Metastatic Complications of Cancer Involving the Central and Peripheral Nervous Systems. Vol. 36, Neurologic Clinics. Elsevier BV; 2018. p. 579–98. [http://dx.doi.org/10.1016/j.ncl.2018.04.011]

[31] Le TT, Oudin MJ. Understanding and modeling nerve–cancer interactions. Vol. 16, Disease Models & Mechanisms. The Company of Biologists; 2023. [http://dx.doi.org/10.1242/dmm.049729]

[32] Kvolik S, Glavas-Obrovac L, Sakic K, Margaretic D, Karner I. Anaesthetic implications of anticancer chemotherapy. Vol. 20, European Journal of Anaesthesiology. Ovid Technologies (Wolters Kluwer Health); 2005. p. 859–71. [http://dx.doi.org/10.1017/S026502150300139X]

[33] Adeyinka A, Kaur A, Bashir K. Tumor lysis syndrome. Treasure Island (FL): StatPearls Publishing; 2025 Jan– [updated 2024 Oct 5; cited 2025 Feb 17]. Available from: https://www.ncbi.nlm.nih.gov/books/NBK518985/

[34] Mahfooz K, Sohail H, Gvajaia A, *et al.* Rasburicase in treating tumor lysis syndrome: An umbrella review. Vol. 1, Cancer Pathogenesis and Therapy. Elsevier BV; 2023. p. 262–71. [http://dx.doi.org/10.1016/j.cpt.2023.07.001]

[35] Domi R, Huti G, Sula H, *et al.* From Pre-Existing Renal Failure to Perioperative Renal Protection: The Anesthesiologist's Dilemmas. Vol. 6, Anesthesiology and Pain Medicine. Brieflands; 2016. [http://dx.doi.org/10.5812/aapm.32386]

[36] Motayagheni N, Phan S, Eshraghi C, Nozari A, Atala A. A Review of Anesthetic Effects on Renal Function: Potential Organ Protection. Vol. 46, American Journal of Nephrology. S. Karger AG; 2017. p. 380–9. [http://dx.doi.org/10.1159/000482014]

[37] Dougherty TB, Cronau LH Jr. Anesthetic implications for surgical patients with endocrine tumors. Int Anesthesiol Clin 1998; 36(3): 31-44. [http://dx.doi.org/10.1097/00004311-199803630-00006] [PMID: 10812414]

[38] Powell B, Al Mukhtar A, Mills GH. Carcinoid: the disease and its implications for anaesthesia. Vol. 11, Continuing Education in Anaesthesia Critical Care & Pain. Elsevier BV; 2011. p. 9–13. [http://dx.doi.org/10.1093/bjaceaccp/mkq045]

[39] Xu A, Suz P, Reljic T, *et al.* Perioperative Carcinoid Crisis: A Systematic Review and Meta-Analysis. Cancers (Basel) 2022; 14(12): 2966. [http://dx.doi.org/10.3390/cancers14122966] [PMID: 35740631]

[40] Kaltsas G, Caplin M, Davies P, *et al.* ENETS Consensus Guidelines for the Standards of Care in Neuroendocrine Tumors: Pre- and Perioperative Therapy in Patients with Neuroendocrine Tumors. Neuroendocrinology 2017; 105(3): 245-54. [http://dx.doi.org/10.1159/000461583] [PMID: 28253514]

[41] Bajwa SJ, Sehgal V. Anesthesia and thyroid surgery: The never ending challenges. Indian J Endocrinol Metab 2013; 17(2): 228-34. [http://dx.doi.org/10.4103/2230-8210.109671] [PMID: 23776893]

[42] Bacuzzi A, Dionigi G, Del Bosco A, *et al.* Anaesthesia for thyroid surgery: Perioperative management. Vol. 6, International Journal of Surgery. Ovid Technologies (Wolters Kluwer Health); 2008. p. S82–5. [http://dx.doi.org/10.1016/j.ijsu.2008.12.013]

[43] Else T, Kim AC, Sabolch A, Raymond VM, Kandathil A, Caoili EM, *et al.* Adrenocortical Carcinoma. Vol. 35, Endocrine Reviews. The Endocrine Society; 2013. p. 282–326. [http://dx.doi.org/10.1210/er.2013-1029]

[44] Xu L, Khaddour K, Chen J, Rich KM, Perrin RJ, Campian JL. Pituitary carcinoma: Two case reports and review of literature. Vol. 11, World Journal of Clinical Oncology. Baishideng Publishing Group Inc.; 2020. p. 91–102.
[http://dx.doi.org/10.5306/wjco.v11.i2.91]

[45] Bajwa SJS, Bajwa S. Anesthesia and Intensive care implications for pituitary surgery: Recent trends and advancements. Vol. 15, Indian Journal of Endocrinology and Metabolism. Medknow; 2011. p. 224.
[http://dx.doi.org/10.4103/2230-8210.84872]

[46] Saini V, Malhotra SK, Sharma K. Pituitary Surgery and Anesthetic Management: An Update. Vol. 5, World Journal of Endocrine Surgery. Jaypee Brothers Medical Publishing; 2013. p. 1–5.
[http://dx.doi.org/10.5005/jp-journals-10002-1114]

[47] Smith M, Hirsch NP. Pituitary disease and anaesthesia. Vol. 85, British Journal of Anaesthesia. Elsevier BV; 2000. p. 3–14.
[http://dx.doi.org/10.1093/bja/85.1.3]

[48] Bajwa SJ, Sehgal V. Anesthetic management of primary hyperparathyroidism: A role rarely noticed and appreciated so far. Vol. 17, Indian Journal of Endocrinology and Metabolism. Medknow; 2013. p. 235.
[http://dx.doi.org/10.4103/2230-8210.109679]

[49] Sasidharan P, Johnston IG. Parathyroid Physiology & Anaesthesia. 2022 [cited 2025 Feb 17]. Available from: https://resources.wfsahq.org/atotw/parathyroid-physiology-anaesthesia-anaesthe-ia-tutorial-of-the-week-142/

[50] Bhuyan S, Bhuyan D, Rahane S. Optimizing Regional Anesthesia for Cancer Patients: A Comprehensive Review of Current Practices and Future Directions. Cureus 2024; 16(9): e69315. [http://dx.doi.org/10.7759/cureus.69315] [PMID: 39398679]

CHAPTER 3

Chemotherapy: Complications and Anesthetic Considerations

Christopher Potestio[1,*], **Sophia Sinibaldi**[1] and **Madison Tanis**[1]

[1] *Department of Anesthesiology, Cooper Medical School of Rowan University, Cooper University Health Care, Camden, NJ, USA*

Abstract: This chapter explores the relationship between chemotherapy and anesthesia, highlighting the challenges faced in perioperative management of cancer patients. As chemotherapy remains a cornerstone of modern oncologic therapy, its systemic toxicities—including cardiotoxicity, neurotoxicity, hepatotoxicity, nephrotoxicity, and myelosuppression—present unique anesthetic considerations. The chapter systematically reviews major chemotherapeutic drug classes, including alkylating agents, antimetabolites, plant alkaloids, anti-tumor antibiotics, hormonal therapies, and biological response modifiers, alongside their mechanisms, indications, and adverse effects. Common malignancies, such as breast, colorectal, brain, and lung cancers—are discussed in detail to demonstrate how chemotherapy impacts anesthesia choices and perioperative planning. Strategies such as regional anesthesia, preoperative organ function assessment, and individualized anesthetic approaches are emphasized to mitigate risk. The chapter underscores the importance of multidisciplinary collaboration between oncologists, anesthesiologists, and surgeons to optimize outcomes and safety in the evolving field of oncologic surgery.

Keywords: Chemotherapy, Glioblastoma, Lung cancer, Alkylating agents, Anthracyclines, Regional anesthesia, Chemotherapy-induced complications, Anesthetic risk stratification, Oncologic anesthesia.

INTRODUCTION

Cancer is the leading cause of long-term mortality following surgery. Even after a "curative" surgery with complete resection, postoperative cancer returns in up to one-third of patients [1]. As such, many patients who undergo surgery as a means of treating cancer will receive chemotherapy and radiation as indicated to help maximize survival. As cancer care incorporates these multimodal treatment strat-

* **Corresponding author Christopher Potestio:** Department of Anesthesiology, Cooper Medical School of Rowan University, Cooper University Health Care, Camden, NJ, USA; E-mail: potestio-christopher@cooperhealth.edu

Bharathi Gourkanti, Irwin Gratz, William Marion, Rajiv Lingaraju & Grace Abramian (Eds.)

egies, understanding the pharmacological and physiological interactions between anesthetic agents and chemotherapeutic drugs has become critically important for optimizing patient outcomes and minimizing perioperative risks.

Chemotherapeutic agents, while essential in managing malignancies, are often associated with systemic toxicities that can significantly influence anesthetic management. For instance, cardiotoxicity from anthracyclines, pulmonary complications from bleomycin, and neurotoxicity from agents like vincristine present unique challenges during anesthesia. Recognizing and anticipating these complications is vital for tailoring perioperative care to individual patient needs.

In addition to direct systemic toxicities, chemotherapy-induced immunosuppression and hematologic disturbances, such as thrombocytopenia and neutropenia, impact preoperative planning and intraoperative vigilance. Perioperative management of the cancer patient mandates a multidisciplinary approach involving oncologists, anesthesiologists, and surgeons to ensure cohesive and informed care. Through case discussions and evidence-based recommendations, the chapter serves as a practical guide for clinicians navigating the perioperative management of cancer patients undergoing anesthesia. Focus on patient safety, individualized care, and interdisciplinary collaboration highlights the evolving demands of modern oncologic anesthesia.

DEFINITIONS

Chemotherapy is described as the use of any drug to target neoplastic cells by targeting mechanisms used by cells that rapidly divide, such as DNA replication, RNA synthesis, and protein synthesis. In doing so, chemotherapeutic drugs can target benign, healthy cells, thereby causing common side effects such as nausea, vomiting, hair loss, diarrhea, fatigue, and easy bruising and bleeding.

The roles of chemotherapy can be curative, palliative, adjuvant, and neoadjuvant. The goal of curative chemotherapy is to achieve complete remission, while the goal of palliative chemotherapy is to relieve symptoms. Adjuvant chemotherapy's goal is to destroy any remaining neoplastic cells and prevent recurrence or relapse. Neoadjuvant chemotherapy is given before surgery or radiation therapy to shrink or prevent the growth of the tumor.

There are numerous types of cancers that respond to chemotherapy, such as leukemias, lymphomas, bone cancer, endometrial cancer, testicular cancer, breast cancer, *etc*., but advanced-stage solid tumors remain more difficult to treat with chemotherapeutic drugs [2]. Solid tumors are difficult to treat with chemotherapy, likely due to a combination of factors, including the presence of a hypoxic and acidic tumor microenvironment and overall tumor heterogeneity.

The overarching strategy of chemotherapeutic agents is to target cell division. Chemotherapies can act in a number of ways, including alkylation, nitrosoureas, antimetabolites, plant alkaloids and natural products, anti-tumor antibiotics, hormonal agents, and biological response modifiers.

MAJOR CLASSES OF CHEMOTHERAPY, COMMON INDICATIONS, SIDE EFFECTS

Alkylating Agents

Alkylating agents are drugs or chemicals that form electrophilic intermediates that bind to the N7 nitrogen of two adjacent guanine nucleotides, causing crosslinking between DNA strands and inhibiting DNA replication or transcription [3]. In the 1940s, these agents were the first non-hormonal drugs to be used in cancer treatment. Nitrogen mustards are commonly used alkylating agents; these agents typically contain a nitrogen group with two chloroethyl groups that act as electrophiles in the alkylation process. SN1 is the first type of alkylating agent [4]. SN1 agents act directly on biological molecules. This is in contrast to SN2 alkylating agents, which create a reactive intermediate. Common alkylating drugs are cyclophosphamide, ifosfamide, chlorambucil, mechlorethamine, and melphalan [3]. Cyclophosphamide is an SN2 alkylating agent that is converted into an active metabolite by cytochrome P450 enzymes and is typically used to treat non-Hodgkin lymphomas, breast, lung, and ovarian cancer. In a randomized trial, a combination treatment of cyclophosphamide, fluorouracil, and epirubicin (CEF) was compared to a combination of cyclophosphamide, methotrexate, and fluorouracil (CMF). Ten-year overall survival rates for CEF and CMF were 62% and 58%, respectively, suggesting a benefit from combination therapies with cyclophosphamide [5]. Ifosfamide is another SN2 agent used to treat sarcomas and testicular cancer. In a meta-analysis, ifosfamide used as preoperative chemotherapy was associated with an increased rate of limb salvage in patients with osteosarcomas of the limbs with an odds ratio of 4.06 ($p<0.001$). Chlorambucil is an SN1 agent used to treat Chronic lymphocytic leukemia or non-Hodgkin lymphoma, while mechlorethamine is an SN1 agent used for Hodgkin and non-Hodgkin lymphoma. In a randomized controlled clinical trial, the event-free survival rate of patients with mucosa-associated lymphoid tissue lymphoma treated with rituximab alone was 50%, but it increased to 68% when combined with chlorambucil [5]. Melphalan is an SN1 primarily used for multiple myeloma, breast, and ovarian cancer. In a randomized clinical trial, melphalan in a drug regimen with bortezomib, daratumumab, and prednisone increased the 18-month progression-free survival of patients with multiple myeloma to 71.6% [6].

Overall, indications for alkylating agents are hematological malignancies, breast, ovarian, uterine, and lung cancer, Hodgkin lymphoma, multiple myeloma, and sarcomas. Common side effects of alkylating agents are hematopoietic toxicity, nausea, vomiting, gastrointestinal damage, pulmonary damage, renal toxicity, antidiuresis, hypersensitivity reactions, alopecia, and immunosuppression [3].

Nitrosoureas

Nitrosoureas are lipophilic alkylating and carbamoylating agents used in chemotherapy that have a nitroso functional group and a urea functional group [4]. Their mechanism of action includes the formation of reactive intermediates, followed by crosslinking of DNA [2]. Examples include carmustine, lomustine, and streptozocin, which can be given orally or intravenously. Because of their lipophilicity, these agents can pass through the blood-brain barrier, creating "cerebrospinal fluid concentrations that are 30% of plasma concentrations" [2]. This allows nitrosoureas to be useful in cancers such as glioblastomas, Hodgkin and non-Hodgkin lymphomas, and pancreatic islet cell tumors [4]. Therefore, nitrosourea agents are often indicated for targeting rapid DNA replication in areas protected by the blood-brain barrier, including glioblastomas. They are also indicated in metastatic Hodgkin and non-Hodgkin lymphomas and metastatic pancreatic islet cell tumors.

Carmustine and lomustine can be used for brain tumors such as astrocytomas, while streptozocin is used for pancreatic islet cell tumors [2]. In a systematic review and meta-analysis of randomized controlled trials, patients with glioblastoma had a 15% higher chance of progression-free survival and overall survival than those not treated with carmustine [7]. In patients with anaplastic oligodendrogliomas, there was an increased overall survival when treated with procarbazine, lomustine, and vincristine (PCV) with radiotherapy (42.3 months) as opposed to radiotherapy alone (30.6) [8]. In another randomized clinical trial, patients with advanced islet cell carcinoma treated with chlorozotocin achieved a 30% regression rate, while treatment with doxorubicin and streptozocin showed a 69% regression rate [9]. The side effects of nitrosurea agents are demyelination resulting in neuropathy, decreased cardiac output, pulmonary fibrosis, hepatocyte necrosis, jaundice, and bone marrow toxicity. Hepatotoxicity is found in 26% of patients treated with nitrosourea analogs [4].

Anti-metabolites

Folic Acid Analog

Anti-metabolites are chemotherapeutic agents that block enzymes involved in DNA synthesis [2]. This can be done by mimicking purines and pyrimidines, incorporating into DNA or RNA, and inhibiting replication or transcription. Anti-metabolites can also cause double-strand breaks. Because they block DNA replication, anti-metabolites are effective mostly in the S-phase of the cell cycle, where the cell is replicating its DNA. Methotrexate is a commonly used anti-metabolite drug that can be used as an immunosuppressant, as well as in cancer treatment. Methotrexate is a folic acid analog that enters cells and prevents the creation of tetrahydrofolate, which is used for thymidine and purine synthesis [2]. Methotrexate has a large volume of distribution but does not cross the blood-brain barrier.

Pemetrexed is another analog of folic acid. Methotrexate is given orally or intravenously, while pemetrexed is only given intravenously [2]. Indications for methotrexate include childhood leukemia, trophoblastic tumors, breast cancer, and osteosarcomas. In a randomized phase III trial, methotrexate, vinblastine, and cisplatin (CMV) were used as a combined neoadjuvant for patients with muscle-invasive urothelial cancer of the bladder, where it was found to have a 16% reduction in the risk of death, which corresponded to a 10-year survival compared to those who did not have the CMV neoadjuvant [10]. Indications for pemetrexed are non-small cell lung cancer and mesothelioma. In a phase three trial, the combination of pemetrexed with cisplatin had a response rate of 41.3% compared to the response rate of 16.7% from cisplatin alone in the treatment of malignant pleural mesothelioma [11]. Common side effects include myelosuppression, oral ulceration, and hepatotoxicity.

Pyrimidine Analog

Fluorouracil is another commonly used anti-metabolite that blocks thymidylate synthetase, which converts deoxyuridine monophosphate to deoxythymidine monophosphate. Fluorouracil is considered a pyrimidine analog. Fluorouracil has two active metabolites. The first, 5-fluorodeoxyuridine monophosphate, blocks thymidylate synthetase, while the second, 5-fluorodeoxyuridine triphosphate, incorporates itself and blocks RNA function. Fluorouracil is commonly used for gastric, pancreatic, breast, and colorectal cancers [2]. Another everyday use for fluorouracil is topically to treat actinic keratoses. In a randomized control trial, patients with advanced esophagogastric cancer were treated with either a combination regimen of epirubicin, cisplatin, and protracted venous infusion fluorouracil (5-FU), doxorubicin, and methotrexate (FAMTX). It was reported that the two-year survival rate of those treated with ECF was 14%, while the survival rate for FAMTX was 5% [12].

Cytarabine is another pyrimidine anti-metabolite used as an analog of cytosine, allowing it to block DNA polymerase. Cytarabine is indicated in breast cancer as well as colorectal cancer. In a randomized control trial, systemic therapy combined with intrathecal liposomal cytarabine showed a median overall survival of 7.3 months compared to 4.0 months in the systemic therapy only group [13]. Common side effects of pyrimidine analogs include myelosuppression, oral ulceration, and gastric ulceration.

Purine Analog

Two common purine analogs include mercaptopurine and thioguanine, which are analogs of hypoxanthine and guanine. Mercaptopurine creates active thioguanine nucleotide metabolites, which block adenylosuccinate synthetase, inosine monophosphate dehydrogenase, and glutamine phosphoribosyl aminotransferase [5]. Mercaptopurine can be used along with methotrexate to prolong remission in patients with acute lymphocytic leukemia. In a randomized, double-blind clinical trial, patients with acute leukemia were assigned to either 6-mercaptopurine or a placebo, and it was shown that patients in the 6-mercaptopurine group had a median survival of 54 weeks, while those in the placebo group had a median survival of 44 weeks. In this trial, there was also a statistically significant increase in remission time for those treated with 6-mercaptopurine [14]. Thioguanine is commonly used for acute myeloid leukemia. In a phase II clinical trial, the effects of the combination of low-dose cytarabine and thioguanine in elderly patients with acute myeloid leukemia were examined. It was shown that those newly diagnosed with AML had a 74% response rate, and those with refractory disease had a 25% response rate. Both of these responses show a beneficial outcome in the use of thioguanine and low-dose cytarabine [15]. Fludarabine and cladribine are two purine anti-metabolites that cause DNA chain termination [2]. Fludarabine is indicated in chronic lymphocytic leukemia. In patients with previously untreated B-cell chronic lymphocytic leukemia, there was an 80.2% response rate when treated with fludarabine. In addition, there were 12.3% complete remission and 67.9% partial remission [16].

Common side effects of anti-metabolites are myelosuppression, oral ulceration, hepatotoxicity, nausea, and vomiting [2]. Tumor lysis syndrome can be caused by mercaptopurine and thioguanine, when used in combination with allopurinol, a xanthine oxidase inhibitor. Specific adverse effects of cladribine are muscle weakness, black stools, blood in urine, fever, and chills [12].

Plant Alkaloids and Natural Products

Plant alkaloids are typically characterized as mitotic and topoisomerase inhibitors. Colchicine is a common mitotic inhibitor that acts by inhibiting B-tubulin polymerization in microtubules. This blocks chromosomal arrangement along the metaphase plate and anaphase. This also affects mitochondrial associations with microtubules and cellular content transportation. Colchicine is indicated as a neoadjuvant for inflammation. Colchicine is derived from autumn crocus, *Colchicum autumnale*, or the glory lily, *Gloriosa superba* [3]. Taxol is another anti-microtubule agent and is also known as paclitaxel. Paclitaxel is derived from the Pacific yew tree, *Taxus brevifolia*, and it works by binding and stabilizing microtubules, causing clumping and decreased microtubule function. Paclitaxel has many indications, including breast, gastric, ovarian, bladder, lung, prostate, and esophageal cancer, as well as melanoma [3]. In a randomized phase III trial, patients with triple-negative breast cancer were treated with either cyclophosphamide, epirubicin, docetaxel, and fluorouracil (CEF-T) or Paclitaxel plus carboplatin (PCb). This study found that those treated with PCb had a statistically significantly greater five-year disease-free survival [86.5%] than those treated with CEF-T (80.3%) [17].

Vinca alkaloids are another group of alkaloids derived from *Catharanthus roseus* [2]. Two vinca alkaloids, vinblastine and vincristine, are used in chemotherapy. Their structure consists of two multi-ringed nuclei with an indole and a dihydroindole nucleus. These agents also disrupt polymerization and assembly of microtubules. Indications for vinca alkaloids are acute leukemia, Hodgkin and non-Hodgkin lymphoma, gliomas, sarcomas, breast, lung, and testicular cancer. In the VINILO trial, vinblastine showed a longer progression-free survival (15 months) compared to the combination therapy of vinblastine plus nilotinib (8 months) for children and young adults diagnosed with low-grade gliomas [18]. Side effects of plant alkaloids are nausea, vomiting, gastrointestinal bleeding, fatigue, arrhythmias, and teratogenicity [3].

An example of a topoisomerase inhibitor is camptothecin (CPT). CPT was originally found in the bark of the *Camptotheca acuminata* tree. CPT acts by targeting topoisomerase I, thereby halting DNA replication, as the DNA supercoil cannot be relaxed [4]. This eventually causes apoptosis of the cell. Camptothecin is indicated in ovarian, colon, lung, and breast cancer. Side effects of topoisomerase inhibitors include mouth sores, diarrhea, anemia, hair loss, and decreased immune response [4]. In a phase II trial with Belotecan, a camptothecin derivative, patients with SCLC had a 42.9% overall response rate and a median overall survival of 11.9 months and 10.5 months for chemotherapy-naïve and chemotherapy-sensitive patients [19]. Podophyllotoxins are a group of microtubule-inhibiting agents derived from mandrake and mayapple plants [2]. Two main podophyllotoxins are etoposide and teniposide. Both are topoisomerase inhibitors as well as microtubule inhibitors. Etoposide is used to treat testicular cancer, lung cancer, and non-Hodgkin lymphoma. Teniposide is only used to treat acute leukemias. Side effects of podophyllotoxins are nausea, vomiting, alopecia, and myelosuppression [2].

Anti-tumor Antibiotics

Anti-tumor antibiotics are biopharmaceuticals derived from various bacteria or fungi. These agents act by interfering with cellular DNA or protein synthesis. This can be done by generating free radicals, inhibiting topoisomerase, and cross-linking DNA. The anthracycline drugs, bleomycin and dactinomycin, are a major group of anti-tumor antibiotics.

Anthracycline drugs include doxorubicin, daunorubicin, and mitomycin, which are all obtained from the *Streptomyces* species [2]. These drugs contain quinone and hydroquinone groups, which form free radicals, disrupting cellular functions. Anthracyclines cause a double-strand break in DNA by blocking topoisomerase II, along with the creation of hydroxyl radicals. These drugs typically have long half-lives and large volumes of distribution, but do not cross the blood-brain barrier. Doxorubicin is indicated for breast, bladder, and ovarian cancer. Acute myeloid leukemia is an indication for daunorubicin and idarubicin. Common side effects of anthracyclines are cardiotoxicity, nausea, vomiting, and myelosuppression. In a randomized controlled trial, patients with metastatic breast cancer were either treated with doxorubicin, bisantrene, or mitoxantrone. Patients treated with doxorubicin had a 28% response rate, compared to 13% and 14% for bisantrene and mitoxantrone, respectively. Patients in the doxorubicin group had a median survival of 315 days compared to 290 days in the bisantrene group, and 177 days in the mitoxantrone-treated group [20].

Bleomycin is another type of antitumor antibiotic that originates from *Streptomyces verticillus*. The mechanism of action of bleomycin is by the creation of free radicals and mainly acts on the G2 phase of the cell cycle, preventing mitosis from occurring. Bleomycin is largely used for solid tumors but is also useful for non-Hodgkin lymphoma and testicular cancer. Side effects of bleomycin are pulmonary fibrosis and severe inflammation of the mucus membrane [2]. Pulmonary fibrosis can be particularly debilitating. In a randomized control trial, patients with pathologic Stage I-IE and II-IIE non-Hodgkin lymphoma with diffuse histology, were treated with either a combination of cyclophosphamide, vincristine, and prednisone (CVP) or bleomycin, adriamycin, cyclophosphamide, vincristine, and prednisone (BACOP). Patients treated with BACOP had a 5-year progression-free survival of 78% compared to those treated with CVP (62%) [21].

A third major anti-tumor antibiotic is dactinomycin, which acts by intercalating DNA [22]. Dactinomycin is derived from *Streptomyces parvulvus*. Dactinomycin is typically indicated for the treatment of trophoblastic tumors and pediatric tumors. Common side effects of dactinomycin include alopecia, anemia, nausea, mouth ulcers, easy bruising, and easy bleeding. In a randomized phase III trial, methotrexate was compared to dactinomycin in the treatment of those with low-risk gestational trophoblastic neoplasia. The results showed that dactinomycin had a statistically significant overall response rate, 73%, compared to those treated with methotrexate, who had a 58% response rate [22].

Hormonal Agents

Major hormonal agents used for chemotherapy include estrogen antagonists, androgen antagonists, 5α-reductase inhibitors, gonadotropin-releasing hormone agonists, and corticosteroids. These agents act by blocking of hormone agonist binding, activating receptors, or inhibiting hormone production *via* competitive and noncompetitive mechanisms.

Examples of estrogen antagonists are tamoxifen and fulvestrant. Tamoxifen and toremifene are selective estrogen receptor modulators, acting on estrogen receptors as both agonists and antagonists, depending on the tissue. Tamoxifen and toremifene both inhibit HER2 and other growth factors involved in breast cancer and are indicated in metastatic breast cancer. Side effects of tamoxifen and toremifene include nausea, vomiting, and menstrual abnormalities. In a randomized controlled trial, patients who received tamoxifen as postoperative therapy had significantly longer disease-free survival compared to those treated with a placebo (83% vs 77%) in the treatment of node-negative breast cancer and estrogen-positive tumors [23].

Fulvestrant is a selective estrogen receptor degrader, which works by binding a monomer of the estrogen receptor, preventing dimerization and causing receptor degradation by a proteasome. Fulvestrant is indicated in tamoxifen-resistant breast cancer and metastatic breast cancer. Side effects include headache, nausea, diarrhea, fatigue, bone pain, and rashes. In a phase I/II trial, fulvestrant showed a clinical benefit rate of 69% in patients with tamoxifen-resistant advanced breast cancer [24].

Androgen antagonists include flutamide, bicalutamide, enzalutamide, and nilutamide, which are competitive inhibitors of testosterone for the androgen receptor. These drugs, along with gonadotropin-releasing hormone, are indicated for prostate cancer. Side effects include osteoporosis, sexual dysfunction, anemia, fatigue, and depression. In a randomized controlled trial, patients with prostate cancer received radiation therapy along with either bicalutamide or a placebo. The study demonstrated a statistically significant difference in overall survival rates for those treated with bicalutamide (76.3%) compared to those treated with placebo (71.3%) in the treatment of prostate cancer [25].

5α-Reductase Inhibitors include finasteride and dutasteride, which decrease dihydrotestosterone in target tissues such as the prostate gland. These agents are indicated in benign prostatic hyperplasia. Side effects include sexual dysfunction, anxiety, and depression.

Gonadotropin-releasing hormone agonists act by binding to pituitary cells and decreasing the release of luteinizing hormone and follicle-stimulating hormone. An example of a GnRH agonist is Leuprolide, which is indicated in metastatic prostate cancer. Side effects include fatigue, weight gain, osteoporosis, and metabolic abnormalities. In a randomized clinical trial, patients with advanced prostate cancer, prostatic carcinoma, were either treated with leuprolide and flutamide or leuprolide and placebo. Patients who received leuprolide in the combination regimen experienced an increase in progression-free survival to 16.5 months, compared to 13.0 months in the placebo group. There was also an increase in overall survival for those treated with combination therapy. Both regimens demonstrate the efficacy of leuprolide in the treatment of prostatic carcinoma [26].

Corticosteroids are another very common hormonal agent used for chemotherapy. Corticosteroids act by inducing apoptosis, tumor antigen release, and immune-mediated reactions. Examples of corticosteroids are prednisone and dexamethasone, which are both indicated in lymphocytic leukemias, lymphomas, and multiple myeloma. Side effects of corticosteroids include weight gain, osteoporosis, glycemic abnormalities, delayed wound healing, and indigestion [27]. In a clinical trial comparing a combination treatment of gemcitabine, cisplatin, prednisone, and thalidomide (GDPT] to cyclophosphamide, doxorubican, vincristine, and prednisone (CHOP] in the treatment of newly diagnosed peripheral T-cell lymphoma, it was reported that those in the GDPT group had a higher complete remission rate, 52%, and overall response rate, 67%, compared to those in the CHOP group with a 33% complete remission rate and 49% overall response rate. Both treatment regimens show the efficacy of using prednisone in combination treatments for newly diagnosed peripheral T-cell lymphoma [28]. In another trial comparing the efficacy of prednisone and dexamethasone, there was found to be no statistically significant difference between the regimens when treating acute lymphoblastic leukemia or lymphoblastic lymphoma [29].

Biological Response Modifiers

Biological response modifiers are agents that regulate the body's immune response to cancer cells. This can be achieved by stimulating the immune system, targeting cancer cells, and modulating cell growth. Vaccines, cytokines, and antibodies can all be used as biological response modifiers and immunotherapy. T helper 2 cells stimulate antibody production and facilitate the production of cytokines, such as interleukins and interferons, for immunotherapy. IL-2 specifically is indicated in renal cell carcinoma and metastatic melanoma. Examples of biological response modifiers are pembrolizumab and nivolumab for melanoma, renal cell cancer, non-squamous lung cancer, lymphoma, and gastrointestinal cancers. Biological response modifiers can cause fever, chills, muscle aches, loss of appetite, nausea, vomiting, diarrhea, and rashes. In patients with non-small-cell lung cancer, it was found that those treated with pembrolizumab had a 5-year survival of 16.6-21.9% compared to 8.5-10.1% with a combination of carboplatin and paclitaxel or pemetrexed [30]. Additionally, in a phase III trial for resected stage IIB/C melanoma, nivolumab was found to significantly improve recurrence-free survival by 42% compared to placebo when used as adjuvant therapy [31].

Steroids in Chemotherapy

Corticosteroids have a broad range of uses in chemotherapy, including the treatment of cancers such as leukemias, lymphomas, and multiple melanomas. They can also be used to treat the side effects of chemotherapy and help with immunotherapy.

Corticosteroids reduce the expression of genes encoding for cytokines, prostaglandins, and eicosanoids, therefore decreasing inflammation [27]. Their immunosuppressive effect is mostly linked to decreasing cytokines such as IL1β, TNF, IFNγ, and IL6 and increasing T regulatory cells, which secrete IL10 and TGFβ. They also decrease leukocyte recruitment to sites of inflammation, decreasing damage caused by chronic inflammation. This reduction in inflammation and the immune response can alleviate side effects such as nausea and vomiting.

Some common corticosteroids used in chemotherapy are prednisone and dexamethasone, which are indicated for acute lymphoblastic leukemia, non-Hodgkin lymphomas, and multiple myelomas. Glucocorticoids are also commonly used as adjuvants for cancer treatment in solid tumors and combination therapy. Some of these include dexamethasone, prednisolone, and betamethasone, and they are commonly indicated in breast cancer and prostate cancer. They can also ameliorate chemotherapy-induced toxicity.

The immunosuppressive effects of steroids decrease the tumor-surveillance of our immune system by inducing the expression of immune checkpoint inhibitors, PD1, TIM3, LAG3, and TGIT, which can lead to tumor growth associated with high doses and extended use of corticosteroids [27]. Baseline steroid doses of greater than 50 mg prednisone equivalents were associated with poor median overall survival in advanced melanoma on anti-PD-1 therapy compared to those with a lower dose of 0-49 mg of prednisone equivalents [32]. It is recommended that the lowest effective dose be used for patients, and they should be followed up regularly. Overall, steroids in chemotherapy make a significant impact on the quality of life and ease the side effects of cancer treatment. In a randomized, double-blind study, dexamethasone was found to decrease gastrointestinal side effects of chemotherapy by 26% compared to placebo in patients being treated for breast cancer [33].

Table **1** reviews the common classes of chemotherapeutic agents, their indications, and common side effects.

Table 1. Common chemotherapeutic agents.

Drug	Indications	Common Side effects
Alkylating Agents		
Cyclophosphamide	Non-Hodgkin lymphomas, breast, lung, and ovarian cancer	Nausea, vomiting, alopecia, mouth sores, hepatotoxicity, and damage to the digestive tract.
Ifosfamide	sarcomas and testicular cancer	Nausea, vomiting, alopecia, mouth sores, hepatotoxicity, and damage to the digestive tract.
Chlorambucil	CLL or non-Hodgkin lymphoma	Diarrhea, seizures, vomiting, and hypersensitivity reactions.
Melphalan	Multiple myeloma, breast, and ovarian cancer	Mouth ulcer, nausea, diarrhea, and rash.
Nitrosoureas		
Carmustine	Brain tumors	Nausea, tiredness, loss of appetite, decreased platelet count, and blurred vision.
Lomustine	Brain tumors	Alopecia, mouth ulcer, vomiting, blurred vision, and confusion.
Streptozocin	Pancreatic islet cell tumors	Bruising, bleeding, chills, nausea, and liver toxicity.
Anti-metabolites		
Folic Acid analogs: Methotrexate and Pemetrexed	Childhood leukemia, trophoblastic tumors, breast cancer, osteosarcomas, non-small cell lung cancer, and mesothelioma.	Myelosuppression, oral ulceration, and hepatotoxicity.

(Table 1) cont.....

Drug	Indications	Common Side effects
Pyrimidine Analogs: Fluorouracil and Cytarabine	Gastric, pancreatic, breast, colorectal cancers, actinic keratoses, breast and colorectal cancer.	Myelosuppression, oral ulceration, and gastric ulceration.
Purine Analogs: Mercaptopurine and thioguanine	Acute lymphocytic leukemia and acute myeloid leukemia.	Myelosuppression, oral ulceration, hepatotoxicity, nausea, and vomiting.
Fludarabine	Chronic lymphocytic leukemia	Nausea, fatigue, and muscle pain.
Cladribine	Chronic lymphocytic leukemia	Muscle weakness, black stools, blood in urine, fever, and chills.
Plant alkaloids and natural products		
Paclitaxel and colchicine	Breast, ovarian, bladder, lung, prostate, melanoma, and esophageal cancer	Nausea, vomiting, gastrointestinal bleeding, fatigue, arrhythmias, and teratogenicity.
vinblastine and vincristine	Acute leukemia, Hodgkin and non-Hodgkin lymphoma, sarcomas, breast, lung, and testicular cancer	Nausea, vomiting, gastrointestinal bleeding, fatigue, arrhythmias, and teratogenicity.
camptothecin	Ovarian, colon, lung, and breast cancer	Mouth sores, diarrhea, anemia, hair loss, and decreased immune response.
Podophyllotoxins	Treat testicular cancer, lung cancer, non-Hodgkin lymphoma, and acute leukemias.	Nausea, vomiting, alopecia, and myelosuppression
Antitumor antibiotics		
Anthracycline drugs	Breast, bladder, ovarian cancer, and acute myeloid leukemia.	Cardiotoxicity, nausea, vomiting, and myelosuppression.
Bleomycin	Solid tumors, non-Hodgkin lymphoma, and testicular cancer	Pulmonary and mucous membrane reactions.
Dactinomycin	Trophoblastic tumors or pediatric tumors	Alopecia, anemia, nausea, mouth ulcers, easy bruising, and easy bleeding
Hormonal Agents		
Estrogen antagonists	Metastatic breast cancer	Nausea, vomiting, menstrual abnormalities, headache, diarrhea, fatigue, bone pain, and rashes.
Androgen antagonists	Prostate cancer	Osteoporosis, sexual dysfunction, anemia, fatigue, and depression.
5α-Reductase Inhibitors	Benign prostatic hyperplasia	Sexual dysfunction, anxiety, and depression.

(Table 1) cont.....

Drug	Indications	Common Side effects
Gonadotropin-Releasing Hormone Agonists	Metastatic prostate cancer	Fatigue, weight gain, osteoporosis, and metabolic abnormalities.
Corticosteroids	Lymphocytic leukemias, lymphomas, and multiple myeloma	Weight gain, osteoporosis, glycemic abnormalities, delayed wound healing, and indigestion.
Biological Response Modifier		
Interleukin-2	Renal cell carcinoma and metastatic melanoma.	Fever, chills, muscle aches, loss of appetite, nausea, vomiting, diarrhea, and rashes.
Pembrolizumab and nivolumab	Melanoma, renal cell cancer, non-squamous lung cancer, lymphoma, and gastrointestinal cancers.	Fever, chills, muscle aches, loss of appetite, nausea, vomiting, diarrhea, and rashes

ANESTHETIC CONSIDERATIONS FOR PATIENTS UNDERGOING CHEMOTHERAPY

Depending on the type of cancer, treatment may take many forms. Operative management is a cornerstone of many oncologic treatment plans. This can frequently follow the administration of chemotherapy. Neoadjuvant chemotherapy's primary role is to decrease tumor burden in order to increase the chance of complete resection of the cancerous tissue.

The selection of thc modc of ancsthesia best suited for a patient who has undergone chemotherapy treatment may be influenced by the patient's overall state of health and by each individual's chemotherapy course. Chemotherapy is a broad term encompassing the classes of powerful medications used to destroy cancerous cells in the body. Because of their inherent toxicity, many chemotherapy drugs can damage healthy tissue as well.

As discussed above, classes such as alkylating agents can cause mucosal degradation as well as pulmonary and hepatic fibrosis. Anthracyclines can cause profound cardiac toxicities, even years after the last administration of the medication [34]. Additionally, most chemotherapy treatments cause myelosuppression, which can complicate a patient's postoperative course. For example, a patient who has received treatment with an agent causing pulmonary fibrosis, utilizing a regional anesthetic approach, when applicable, may allow for decreased ICU stays as well as decreased time with a chest tube [35].

Patients who have undergone chemotherapy treatment with doxorubicin or other anthracycline agents who have developed cardiomyopathy following treatment may have similar anesthetic considerations as patients with low-output heart failure. Specifically, young cancer survivors are at the highest risk of developing cardiotoxicity even years following chemotherapy administration [36]. A severely decreased cardiac output can lead to a significant increase in mortality due to increased risk of arrhythmia and myocardial infarction in the postoperative period. Patients are also likely to experience acute exacerbation in heart failure in the perioperative period, leading to longer hospital stays [35].

Breast Cancer

Neoadjuvant chemotherapy is frequently used in breast cancer treatment to reduce tumor size and facilitate surgical intervention. The most commonly utilized regimens include anthracyclines (*e.g.*, doxorubicin, epirubicin) and taxanes (*e.g.*, paclitaxel, docetaxel), both of which have significant systemic effects that must be considered when planning anesthetic management. These agents can impact cardiovascular function, immune response, hematologic status, and postoperative recovery, which can influence the choice of anesthetic technique for surgeries such as mastectomy, lumpectomy, or reconstructive procedures.

Anthracyclines are known for their potential to cause cardiotoxicity and cardiomyopathy. Preoperative evaluation of cardiac function, often with echocardiography, is essential to assess myocardial function. Patients with preexisting cardiac dysfunction may require careful intraoperative fluid management, the use of cardioprotective agents, and the avoidance of excessive myocardial depression from anesthetics. Taxanes, while less directly cardiotoxic, have been associated with arrhythmias and autonomic instability, necessitating vigilant intraoperative hemodynamic monitoring [37].

Taxane-based chemotherapy is associated with peripheral neuropathy, which may complicate the use of regional anesthesia. Patients experiencing chemotherapy-induced neuropathy may be at higher risk of nerve injury or prolonged sensory deficits following peripheral nerve blocks. However, regional anesthesia remains a valuable option, as it is associated with decreased surgical stress, reduced opioid requirements, and shorter hospital stays [38]. Careful preoperative neurologic assessment and dose modifications in local anesthetics may be necessary when employing these techniques. Patients should be counseled on the risks of nerve injury when considering a regional anesthetic technique.

Mastectomy is an umbrella term that encompasses a wide array of surgeries that remove the entire breast tissue on one side of the body. Mastectomy can include just the removal of breast tissue, nipple or skin sparing mastectomy, or modified radical mastectomy. A modified radical mastectomy is the most invasive and aggressive of the above options, combining breast tissue removal with axillary lymph node dissection. In most cases, radical mastectomies require general anesthesia. Partial mastectomies with or without sentinel node biopsies may be done under monitored anesthesia care with local anesthesia on the field.

If a patient's tumor burden has decreased following chemotherapy administration, a lumpectomy may be considered instead of a full mastectomy. In a lumpectomy, a small incision is made in the skin overlying the tumor, and the tumor and its margin are excised. This can be done under general anesthesia. As regional techniques evolve, more are being completed under regional. Now, it is common to utilize a pectoral nerve block, also known as a PECS block. A PECS I block targets the pectoral nerves, which are a branch from the brachial plexus cords. Specifically, it targets the lateral and medial pectoral nerves, which innervate the pectoralis major and can be helpful in tumor resection in the upper anterior chest wall. A PECS II block is a more comprehensive regional technique and can be used for more invasive operations. It targets the anterior and lateral divisions of the thoracic intercostal nerves T2-6, the long thoracic nerve, and the thoracodorsal nerve.

A developing alternative for the PECS I and II block is a serratus anterior plane block. This affects the lateral cutaneous branch of the intercostal nerves T2-9, thoracodorsal nerve, and the long thoracic nerve, which provide anesthesia to the anterior and lateral walls of the chest. The serratus anterior plane block can lend itself well as the sole anesthetic technique for less invasive breast operations such as lumpectomy, as well as for control of postoperative pain. These regions are an important tool to consider and utilize in appropriate patients.

An essential part of a patient's anesthetic plan is evaluation of their risk for postoperative nausea and vomiting (PONV). Patients who have previously received chemotherapy may be at a higher risk for PONV than a similar patient who has not been treated with chemotherapy [39]. Therefore, empiric treatment of PONV for patients who have undergone neoadjuvant chemotherapy should be considered as part of their anesthetic plan. Dexamethasone is an effective treatment for PONV in patients undergoing radical mastectomy who have received neoadjuvant chemotherapy [40].

Colorectal Cancers

Patients with colorectal cancer often require surgery following neoadjuvant chemotherapy. Colorectal cancer encompasses a large array of tumor types and locations, with adenocarcinoma being the most frequent cell type.

Most colon cancers are treated first with endoscopic or surgical removal of the tumor. Further investigation of this tissue sample is completed to determine the grade and type of tumor to further guide treatment. For stage III colonic adenocarcinoma, the standard recommended adjuvant therapy is an oxaliplatin-containing regimen such as FOLFOX (leucovorin, Fluorouracil (5-FU), and Oxaliplatin), XELOX (Oxaliplatin and Capecitabine), or FLOX (fluorouracil and oxaliplatin). Capecitabine or 5-FU/LV monotherapy is used if the patient has preexisting neuropathy.

There is developing research on the utility of neoadjuvant chemotherapy in colorectal cancer, specifically the Fluoropyrimidine Oxaliplatin and Targeted Receptor Preoperative Therapy (FOxTROT) trial. This new research has shown that a 6-week course of neoadjuvant oxaliplatin-fluoropyrimidine chemotherapy treatment can lead to histopathologic down-staging, fewer incomplete resections, and better 2-year disease control [41]. As oncologic medicine integrates this practice, more colorectal cancer patients will present for surgical treatment following neoadjuvant therapy.

Oxaliplatin may contribute to autonomic neuropathy, which can affect hemodynamic stability and increase the risk of intraoperative hypotension. It also has nephrotoxic effects, which can compromise renal function and alter drug clearance. Preoperative assessment of renal function is crucial for adjusting medication dosages, particularly for nephrotoxic agents such as NSAIDs and certain antibiotics. Both effects demand optimization of fluid status and vigilance in managing hemodynamic fluctuations during surgery.

Fluoropyrimidine-based regimens are associated with endothelial dysfunction and increased thromboembolic risk. In particular, 5-fluorouracil (5-FU) and capecitabine have been linked to coronary vasospasm, myocardial ischemia, and cardiomyopathies, necessitating careful cardiovascular monitoring, especially in patients with preexisting cardiac disease. Fluoropyrimidines are also associated with hepatotoxicity, including steatosis and sinusoidal injury, which may impair hepatic metabolism of anesthetic agents. Preoperative liver function tests can help guide drug selection and dosing, particularly for hepatically metabolized agents like volatile anesthetics and opioids.

Surgical removal of the diseased colon involves locating the primary tumor, excision of the tumor with 5cm margins, and lymphadenectomy. A minimum of 12 lymph nodes must be sampled to ensure accurate staging of the disease [42]. Because of the invasive nature of these procedures, bowel surgery is performed with general anesthesia. A patient's post-operative course can be augmented with regional techniques for ongoing pain control. This may be complicated by exposure to fluoropyrimidines and oxaliplatin, as well as their associated neurotoxicity. The presence of existing neuropathy of any source (ischemic, toxin, metabolic, *etc.*) may place patients at higher risk for secondary neurologic injury with the administration of regional anesthesia. This is known as the "double crush phenomenon," first noted by Upton and McComas in 1973. With the adoption of neoadjuvant chemotherapy in more colorectal cancer patients, the use of regional anesthesia techniques must be carefully weighed.

Neurosurgery

Neurosurgical oncology can be complicated by the need for invasive procedures to procure tissue diagnosis. Therefore, neoadjuvant chemotherapy is not a hallmark of treatment for most cases. In adults, glioblastoma multiforme is the most common primary brain tumor, and the mainstay of its treatment is surgical resection. This diagnosis is primarily based on CT/MRI imaging findings.

Depending on the tumor location and feasibility, a surgeon may opt for gross total resection or supramaximal resection. Gross total resection refers to the surgical removal of all visible tumor tissue, whereas supramaximal resection involves the removal of all visible tumor as well as surrounding brain tissue seen on imaging. Gross total resection has been shown to increase 1- and 2-year survival rates compared to supramaximal resection. Following resection, radiation treatment is completed to eradicate remaining microscopic disease. Because surgical outcomes are heavily weighted on the ability to resect the tumor burden, there is continuing research about the utility of neoadjuvant chemotherapy to shrink tumor size in hopes of enabling adequate surgical resection. There have also been developments in noninvasive diagnostics, such as serum or CSF analysis, that can identify circulating tumor cells and circulating tumor DNA. The ability to diagnose glioblastoma without direct biopsy, as well as the opportunity to shrink tumor size prior to surgical intervention, can provide a more straightforward operation with less damage to surrounding healthy tissue. In a review conducted by Nabian *et al.*, which examined the growing body of research on neoadjuvant chemotherapy for glioblastoma multiforme, the most frequently used regimen was temozolomide plus bevacizumab [43].

One of the primary drugs in this regimen, temozolomide, is an alkylating agent with hematologic and neurologic side effects. As expected with other alkylating agents, marked immunosuppression is a prevalent concern [44]. Resultant neutropenia and even aplastic anemia can increase a patient's risk of infection. During a stressful event, such as a brain tumor resection, the risk is even higher. Steroids, which are frequently used to decrease brain edema perioperatively, also play a role in patients' susceptibility to infection. The neurological side effects of temozolomide include seizures, cerebral hemorrhage, and cerebral edema.

The other primary drug being investigated for its use in the treatment of primary brain malignancies is bevacizumab. This drug is used to decrease tumor vasculature by directly affecting vascular endothelial growth factor, thereby reducing the tumors' ability to spread and grow. Because of these anti-angiogenic effects, bevacizumab has been associated with alterations in vascular integrity and can predispose patients to intracranial hemorrhage. Its actual effect on the rate of intracranial hemorrhage continues to be investigated, with some studies finding a dose-dependent risk of intracranial hemorrhage [45], and others finding no significant relationship [46].

In the setting of general anesthesia, the risk of seizure is low due to the generalized slowing of neuronal activity. However, not all neurosurgical procedures are conducted under general anesthesia, particularly those requiring intraoperative brain mapping to preserve critical motor and language functions. Awake craniotomies, for instance, are often performed to facilitate real-time cortical and subcortical mapping, allowing surgeons to identify and avoid essential functional areas while resecting pathologic tissue. The use of direct cortical stimulation for brain mapping has been associated with an increased risk of seizure activity, likely due to the focal excitation of neuronal circuits. Additionally, pharmacologic agents used in the perioperative period can further modulate seizure risk. Notably, dexmedetomidine, a sedative commonly utilized in awake craniotomies for its anxiolytic and analgesic properties while preserving respiratory drive, has been implicated in lowering the seizure threshold [47]. This suggests that careful titration is essential to minimize the likelihood of seizure occurrence during functional neurosurgery.

Thoracic Surgery

Thoracic surgery is frequently indicated for the treatment of patients with lung cancer. This is planned as a primary method of treatment followed by adjuvant chemotherapy or following neoadjuvant treatments to facilitate downstaging. Surgical care may consist of a lymph node biopsy, wedge resection, lobe resection, or pneumonectomy.

There are several approaches that can be taken for intrathoracic procedures. These operations may be thoracoscopic, robotic, video-assisted, or with open thoracotomy techniques. Utilizing minimally invasive robotic or video-assisted approaches can result in decreased pain, decreased hospital length of stay, and reduced overall cost. Despite the advancements in minimally invasive procedures, there are still cases where a thoracotomy may be a better surgical approach. Considerations include tumor location, small chest volume, dense adhesions, or the surgeon's clinical judgement.

Regardless of the surgical technique planned, one-lung ventilation with the patient in the lateral decubitus position is utilized for optimizing access to the surgical field. The one-lung ventilation technique can be accomplished *via* a dual-lumen endotracheal tube or with a bronchial blocker. There are inherent concerns associated with one-lung ventilation, including increased tidal volumes and elevated ventilatory pressures. At baseline, patients requiring thoracic surgery, such as those with lung cancer and frequently a significant tobacco history, may already have compromised pulmonary compliance and diffusion capacity, which may result in increased ventilatory pressures and hypoxia. In patients who have previously been treated with bleomycin, carmustine, or cyclophosphamide, side effects such as pulmonary fibrosis may develop years later. The preoperative evaluation of these patients should include pulmonary function testing to accurately quantify the risk to the patient. A forced expiratory volume (FEV1)less than 60% of predicted has been found to be the strongest predictor of postoperative complications, including death, and can be used as a benchmark for predicting a patient's ability to tolerate one-lung ventilation [48].

There has been investigative use of the chemoimmunotherapy drug nivolumab in the treatment of lung cancer. As this neoadjuvant therapy is being studied, investigators are seeing its effects during operative intervention. One of the biggest concerns is its potential to cause dense adhesions and fibrosis, particularly at the lung fissures or in the vicinity of hilar and mediastinal nodal stations [49]. These changes can complicate surgical access and increase the difficulty of intubation and ventilation. The fibrosis and adhesions that nivolumab may cause can distort normal anatomy, making tracheal or bronchial manipulation more challenging. Additionally, the drug's immune-modulating effects can heighten the risk of inflammatory airway responses, such as bronchospasm. Preoperative imaging should be carefully reviewed to assess the extent of fibrotic changes, and the anesthetic plan may need to be adjusted based on the patient's specific anatomical alterations. Furthermore, nivolumab-induced fibrosis may also reduce pulmonary compliance and contribute to compromised lung function.

Another new and developing immunotherapy is tumor-infiltrating lymphocyte (TIL) therapy. Currently, TIL has been approved for the treatment of metastatic melanoma, but it holds promise for treating lung cancer. TIL therapy involves harvesting a patient's own immune cells, specifically lymphocytes, which can recognize and attack cancer cells. These lymphocytes are isolated from the tumor tissue, expanded in the lab to increase their number and strength, and then reinfused into the patient's body to help fight the malignancy. The FDA's recent approval of TIL therapy for metastatic melanoma offers a hopeful glimpse into how this innovative treatment can provide a more personalized and targeted approach to cancer care. Researchers are optimistic that ongoing studies will refine this method for broader applications, such as lung cancer, which could significantly improve treatment outcomes for patients with this difficult-to-treat disease. Patients undergoing TIL therapy often experience immune-related side effects, including fever and inflammatory reactions. Refer to Chapter 4 for additional details on immunotherapy.

In the context of lung cancer, where treatments typically involve a combination of surgery, chemotherapy, and radiation, the introduction of TIL therapy adds a novel layer of complexity. As the role of TIL therapy expands in lung cancer treatment, the collaboration between oncologists, surgeons, and anesthesiologists will be essential in optimizing patient care and enhancing the overall effectiveness of cancer treatments.

CONCLUSION

The intersection of chemotherapy and anesthesia presents a complex and evolving challenge in modern oncologic care. As cancer treatments have become more sophisticated, so too has our understanding of how chemotherapeutic agents can interact with anesthetic planning and influence perioperative outcomes. Chemotherapy can lead to a wide array of organ-specific toxicities—cardiac, pulmonary, hepatic, renal, and neurological—that may increase perioperative risk and require tailored anesthetic strategies. Agents like doxorubicin, cisplatin, and vincristine have well-documented side effect profiles that must be considered when evaluating a patient for surgery.

Anesthesiologists play a crucial role in the multidisciplinary care of oncology patients, particularly by anticipating complications, optimizing organ function preoperatively, and choosing anesthetic techniques that minimize additive toxicity. A detailed understanding of the pharmacodynamics of both chemotherapy and anesthetic agents is crucial, particularly in managing patients who are immunosuppressed or thrombocytopenic. Furthermore, the timing of surgery in relation to chemotherapy cycles remains a critical consideration to reduce postoperative morbidity.

Ultimately, improving outcomes for cancer patients undergoing surgery requires close collaboration between oncologists, anesthesiologists, and surgical teams. Through comprehensive preoperative assessment and vigilant intraoperative and postoperative care, clinicians can mitigate risks and support better recovery trajectories for this vulnerable patient population.

REFERENCES

[1] Watson J, Ninh MK, Ashford S, *et al.* Anesthesia Medications and Interaction with Chemotherapeutic Agents. Oncol Ther 2021; 9(1): 121-38. [http://dx.doi.org/10.1007/s40487-021-00149-1] [PMID: 33861416]

[2] Wecker L, Taylor DA, Theobald RJ, Eds. Brody's human pharmacology: molecular to clinical. 6th

ed., Philadelphia, PA: Elsevier, Inc 2019.

[3] Brenner GM, Stevens CW. Pharmacology. 5th ed., Philadelphia, PA: Elsevier 2018.

[4] American association for cancer research, editor. Holland-Frei cancer medicine 8: an approved publication of the American association for cancer research. 8th ed. Shelton, Conn: People's medical publ; 2010.

[5] Zucca E, Conconi A, Martinelli G, *et al.* Final Results of the IELSG-19 Randomized Trial of Mucosa-Associated Lymphoid Tissue Lymphoma: Improved Event-Free and Progression-Free Survival With Rituximab Plus Chlorambucil Versus Either Chlorambucil or Rituximab Monotherapy. J Clin Oncol 2017; 35(17): 1905-12.
[http://dx.doi.org/10.1200/JCO.2016.70.6994] [PMID: 28355112]

[6] Mateos MV, Dimopoulos MA, Cavo M, *et al.* Daratumumab plus Bortezomib, Melphalan, and Prednisone for Untreated Myeloma. N Engl J Med 2018; 378(6): 518-28.
[http://dx.doi.org/10.1056/NEJMoa1714678] [PMID: 29231133]

[7] Xiao ZZ, Wang ZF, Lan T, *et al.* Carmustine as a Supplementary Therapeutic Option for Glioblastoma: A Systematic Review and Meta-Analysis. Front Neurol 2020; 11: 1036.
[http://dx.doi.org/10.3389/fneur.2020.01036] [PMID: 33041980]

[8] van den Bent MJ, Brandes AA, Taphoorn MJB, *et al.* Adjuvant procarbazine, lomustine, and vincristine chemotherapy in newly diagnosed anaplastic oligodendroglioma: long-term follow-up of EORTC brain tumor group study 26951. J Clin Oncol 2013; 31(3): 344-50.
[http://dx.doi.org/10.1200/JCO.2012.43.2229] [PMID: 23071237]

[9] Moertel CG, Lefkopoulo M, Lipsitz S, Hahn RG, Klaassen D. Streptozocin-doxorubicin, streptozocin-fluorouracil or chlorozotocin in the treatment of advanced islet-cell carcinoma. N Engl J Med 1992; 326(8): 519-23.
[http://dx.doi.org/10.1056/NEJM199202203260804] [PMID: 1310159]

[10] Griffiths G, Hall R, Sylvester R, Raghavan D, Parmar MK. International phase III trial assessing neoadjuvant cisplatin, methotrexate, and vinblastine chemotherapy for muscle-invasive bladder cancer: long-term results of the BA06 30894 trial. J Clin Oncol 2011; 29(16): 2171-7.
[http://dx.doi.org/10.1200/JCO.2010.32.3139] [PMID: 21502557]

[11] Rollins KD, Lindley C. Pemetrexed: A multitargeted antifolate. Clin Ther 2005; 27(9): 1343-82.
[http://dx.doi.org/10.1016/j.clinthera.2005.09.010] [PMID: 16291410]

[12] Levine MN, Pritchard KI, Bramwell VHC, Shepherd LE, Tu D, Paul N. Randomized trial comparing cyclophosphamide, epirubicin, and fluorouracil with cyclophosphamide, methotrexate, and fluorouracil in premenopausal women with node-positive breast cancer: update of National Cancer Institute of Canada Clinical Trials Group Trial MA5. J Clin Oncol 2005; 23(22): 5166-70.
[http://dx.doi.org/10.1200/JCO.2005.09.423] [PMID: 16051958]

[13] Le Rhun E, Wallet J, Mailliez A, *et al.* Intrathecal liposomal cytarabine plus systemic therapy versus systemic chemotherapy alone for newly diagnosed leptomeningeal metastasis from breast cancer. Neuro-oncol 2020; 22(4): 524-38.
[http://dx.doi.org/10.1093/neuonc/noz201] [PMID: 31637444]

[14] Gehan EA, Freireich EJ. The 6-MP versus placebo clinical trial in acute leukemia. Clin Trials 2011; 8(3): 288-97.
[http://dx.doi.org/10.1177/1740774511407358] [PMID: 21730077]

[15] Arthur C, Jeffrey A, Yip E, *et al.* Prolonged administration of low-dose cytarabine and thioguanine in elderly patients with acute myeloid leukaemia (AML) achieves high complete remission rates and prolonged survival. Leuk Lymphoma 2020; 61(4): 831-9.
[http://dx.doi.org/10.1080/10428194.2019.1697876] [PMID: 31809629]

[16] Rossi JF, Van Hoof A, De Boeck K, *et al.* Efficacy and safety of oral fludarabine phosphate in previously untreated patients with chronic lymphocytic leukemia. J Clin Oncol 2004; 22(7): 1260-7.

[http://dx.doi.org/10.1200/JCO.2004.05.012] [PMID: 15051774]

[17] Yu KD, Ye FG, He M, *et al.* Effect of Adjuvant Paclitaxel and Carboplatin on Survival in Women With Triple-Negative Breast Cancer. JAMA Oncol 2020; 6(9): 1390-6. [http://dx.doi.org/10.1001/jamaoncol.2020.2965] [PMID: 32789480]

[18] Grill J, Brard C, Picton S, *et al.* PDCT-05. FINAL RESULTS OF THE VINILO OPEN-LABEL PHASE II RANDOMIZED TRIAL FOR PEDIATRIC LOW-GRADE GLIOMAS (pLGG) COMPARING THE COMBINATION VINBLASTINE-NILOTINIB WITH VINBLASTINE ALONE. Neuro-oncol 2019; 21 (Suppl. 6): vi184-4. [http://dx.doi.org/10.1093/neuonc/noz175.769]

[19] Lee DH, Kim SW, Suh C, *et al.* Belotecan, new camptothecin analogue, is active in patients with small-cell lung cancer: results of a multicenter early phase II study. Ann Oncol 2008; 19(1): 123-7. [http://dx.doi.org/10.1093/annonc/mdm437] [PMID: 17823384]

[20] Cowan JD, Neidhart J, Mcclure S, *et al.* Randomized trial of doxorubicin, bisantrene, and mitoxantrone in advanced breast cancer: a Southwest Oncology Group study. J Natl Cancer Inst 1991; 83(15): 1077-84. [http://dx.doi.org/10.1093/jnci/83.15.1077] [PMID: 1875415]

[21] Bajetta E, Valagussa P, Bonadonna G, *et al.* Combined modality treatment for stage I–II non-hodgkin's lymphomas: CVP versus BACOP chemotherapy. Int J Radiat Oncol Biol Phys 1988; 15(1): 3-12. [http://dx.doi.org/10.1016/0360-3016(88)90340-9] [PMID: 2455701]

[22] Osborne RJ, Filiaci V, Schink JC, *et al.* Phase III trial of weekly methotrexate or pulsed dactinomycin for low-risk gestational trophoblastic neoplasia: a gynecologic oncology group study. J Clin Oncol 2011; 29(7): 825-31. [http://dx.doi.org/10.1200/JCO.2010.30.4386] [PMID: 21263100]

[23] Fisher B, Costantino J, Redmond C, *et al.* A randomized clinical trial evaluating tamoxifen in the treatment of patients with node-negative breast cancer who have estrogen-receptor-positive tumors. N Engl J Med 1989; 320(8): 479-84. [http://dx.doi.org/10.1056/NEJM198902233200802] [PMID: 2644532]

[24] Vergote I, Robertson J F R. Fulvestrant is an effective and well-tolerated endocrine therapy for postmenopausal women with advanced breast cancer: results from clinical trials. Br J Cancer 2004; 90(S1) (Suppl. 1): S11-4. [http://dx.doi.org/10.1038/sj.bjc.6601631] [PMID: 15094759]

[25] Shipley WU, Seiferheld W, Lukka HR, *et al.* Radiation with or without Antiandrogen Therapy in Recurrent Prostate Cancer. N Engl J Med 2017; 376(5): 417-28. [http://dx.doi.org/10.1056/NEJMoa1607529] [PMID: 28146658]

[26] Crawford ED, Eisenberger MA, McLeod DG, *et al.* A controlled trial of leuprolide with and without flutamide in prostatic carcinoma. N Engl J Med 1989; 321(7): 419-24. [http://dx.doi.org/10.1056/NEJM198908173210702] [PMID: 2503724]

[27] Goodman RS, Johnson DB, Balko JM. Corticosteroids and Cancer Immunotherapy. Clin Cancer Res 2023; 29(14): 2580-7. [http://dx.doi.org/10.1158/1078-0432.CCR-22-3181] [PMID: 36648402]

[28] Li L, Duan W, Zhang L, *et al.* The efficacy and safety of gemcitabine, cisplatin, prednisone, thalidomide versus CHOP in patients with newly diagnosed peripheral T□cell lymphoma with analysis of biomarkers. Br J Haematol 2017; 178(5): 772-80. [http://dx.doi.org/10.1111/bjh.14763] [PMID: 28597542]

[29] Labar B, Suciu S, Willemze R, *et al.* Dexamethasone compared to prednisolone for adults with acute lymphoblastic leukemia or lymphoblastic lymphoma: final results of the ALL-4 randomized, phase III trial of the EORTC Leukemia Group. Haematologica 2010; 95(9): 1489-95. [http://dx.doi.org/10.3324/haematol.2009.018580] [PMID: 20378563]

[30] de Castro G Jr, Kudaba I, Wu YL, *et al.* Five-Year Outcomes With Pembrolizumab Versus Chemotherapy as First-Line Therapy in Patients With Non–Small-Cell Lung Cancer and Programmed Death Ligand-1 Tumor Proportion Score ≥ 1% in the KEYNOTE-042 Study. J Clin Oncol 2023; 41(11): 1986-91.
[http://dx.doi.org/10.1200/JCO.21.02885] [PMID: 36306479]

[31] Kirkwood JM, Del Vecchio M, Weber J, *et al.* Adjuvant nivolumab in resected stage IIB/C melanoma: primary results from the randomized, phase 3 CheckMate 76K trial. Nat Med 2023; 29(11): 2835-43.
[http://dx.doi.org/10.1038/s41591-023-02583-2] [PMID: 37845511]

[32] Yennurajalingam S, Bruera E. Do Patients Benefit from a Trial of Corticosteroids at the End of Life? Curr Treat Options Oncol 2022; 23(6): 796-805.
[http://dx.doi.org/10.1007/s11864-022-00977-x] [PMID: 35362799]

[33] Vardy J, Chiew KS, Galica J, Pond GR, Tannock IF. Side effects associated with the use of dexamethasone for prophylaxis of delayed emesis after moderately emetogenic chemotherapy. Br J Cancer 2006; 94(7): 1011-5.
[http://dx.doi.org/10.1038/sj.bjc.6603048] [PMID: 16552437]

[34] Bhagat A, Kleinerman ES. Anthracycline-Induced Cardiotoxicity: Causes, Mechanisms, and Prevention. In: Kleinerman ES, Gorlick R, Eds. Current Advances in Osteosarcoma (Internet). Cham: Springer International Publishing 2020; pp. 181-92. Available from: http://link.springer.com/10.1007/978-3-030-43032-0_15
[http://dx.doi.org/10.1007/978-3-030-43032-0_15]

[35] Smit-Fun V, Buhre WF. The patient with chronic heart failure undergoing surgery. Curr Opin Anaesthesiol 2016; 29(3): 391-6.
[http://dx.doi.org/10.1097/ACO.0000000000000335] [PMID: 26978592]

[36] Nettlefold C, Chakraborty P, Al Shaheen A, *et al.* A Primer on the Evolving Subspecialty of Onco-Electrophysiology. Can J Cardiol 2025; 41(2): 181-94.
[http://dx.doi.org/10.1016/j.cjca.2024.11.005] [PMID: 39521053]

[37] Huettemann E, Sakka SG. Anaesthesia and anti-cancer chemotherapeutic drugs. Curr Opin Anaesthesiol 2005; 18(3): 307-14.
[http://dx.doi.org/10.1097/01.aco.0000169240.14056.19] [PMID: 16534356]

[38] Vanni G, Costanzo G, Pellicciaro M, *et al.* Awake Breast Surgery: A Systematic Review. In Vivo 2023; 37(4): 1412-22.
[http://dx.doi.org/10.21873/invivo.13225] [PMID: 37369489]

[39] Abut Y, Bolat K, Yanık N, *et al.* Previous chemotherapy can cause PONV. Adv Clin Exp Med 2023; 32(1): 113-6.
[http://dx.doi.org/10.17219/acem/157242] [PMID: 36603139]

[40] Li ZH, Liu D, He ZJ, Fan ZY. [Influence of dexamethasone on the incidence of postoperative nausea and vomiting in breast cancer patients with neoadjuvant chemotherapy]. Beijing Da Xue Xue Bao 2015; 47(4): 685-9.
[PMID: 26284410]

[41] Morton D, Seymour M, Magill L, *et al.* Preoperative Chemotherapy for Operable Colon Cancer: Mature Results of an International Randomized Controlled Trial. J Clin Oncol 2023; 41(8): 1541-52.
[http://dx.doi.org/10.1200/JCO.22.00046] [PMID: 36657089]

[42] Benson AB, Venook AP, Al-Hawary MM, *et al.* Colon Cancer, Version 2.2021, NCCN Clinical Practice Guidelines in Oncology. J Natl Compr Canc Netw 2021; 19(3): 329-59.
[http://dx.doi.org/10.6004/jnccn.2021.0012] [PMID: 33724754]

[43] Nabian N, Ghalehtaki R, Zeinalizadeh M, Balaña C, Jablonska PA. State of the neoadjuvant therapy for glioblastoma multiforme—Where do we stand? Neurooncol Adv 2024; 6(1): vdae028.
[http://dx.doi.org/10.1093/noajnl/vdae028] [PMID: 38560349]

[44] Zhou Q, Rokita SE. A general strategy for target-promoted alkylation in biological systems. Proc Natl Acad Sci USA 2003; 100(26): 15452-7.
[http://dx.doi.org/10.1073/pnas.2533112100] [PMID: 14673113]

[45] Lim S, Clarke NH, Maloney SL, *et al.* Bevacizumab exerts dose-dependent risk for intracranial hemorrhage in patients with malignant gliomas. J Neurooncol 2025; 172(1): 273-80.
[http://dx.doi.org/10.1007/s11060-024-04916-8] [PMID: 39747716]

[46] Yang L, Chen CJ, Guo XL, *et al.* Bevacizumab and risk of intracranial hemorrhage in patients with brain metastases: a meta-analysis. J Neurooncol 2018; 137(1): 49-56.
[http://dx.doi.org/10.1007/s11060-017-2693-4] [PMID: 29170906]

[47] Paquin-Lanthier G, Subramaniam S, Leong KW, *et al.* Risk Factors and Characteristics of Intraoperative Seizures During Awake Craniotomy: A Retrospective Cohort Study of 562 Consecutive Patients With a Space-occupying Brain Lesion. J Neurosurg Anesthesiol 2023; 35(2): 194-200.
[http://dx.doi.org/10.1097/ANA.0000000000000798] [PMID: 34411059]

[48] Keagy BA, Lores ME, Starek PJK, Murray GF, Lucas CL, Wilcox BR. Elective pulmonary lobectomy: factors associated with morbidity and operative mortality. Ann Thorac Surg 1985; 40(4): 349-52.
[http://dx.doi.org/10.1016/S0003-4975(10)60065-3] [PMID: 4051616]

[49] Ugalde Figueroa P, Lacroix V, Van Schil PE. Neoadjuvant Chemoimmunotherapy Complicates Subsequent Surgical Resection and Adjuvant Immunotherapy Is Preferable From the Surgical Standpoint. J Thorac Oncol 2024; 19(6): 858-61.
[http://dx.doi.org/10.1016/j.jtho.2024.02.009] [PMID: 38849165]

CHAPTER 4

Immunotherapy - Anesthetic Considerations

Dylan Windle-Puente[1], **Osheen Abramian**[2] and **Grace Abramian**[3,*]

[1] *Mount Sinai Hospital, New York, USA*

[2] *Jefferson Einstein Montgomery Hospital, Thomas Jefferson University, Philadelphia, USA*

[3] *Department of Anesthesiology, Cooper Medical School of Rowan University, Cooper University Health Care, Camden, NJ, USA*

Abstract: This chapter provides an overview of cancer immunotherapy, tracing its evolution from historical observations to cutting-edge therapies like immune checkpoint inhibitors, CAR T-cell therapy, and bispecific T-cell engagers. We explain how these treatments harness or modify the immune system to target cancer, detailing their mechanisms, clinical applications, and associated toxicities across multiple organ systems. Key agents include CTLA-4 and PD-1/PD-L1 inhibitors, high-dose IL-2, interferons, and therapeutic vaccines like Sipuleucel-T. As these drugs can potentially impact every organ system, thoughtful anesthetic planning for the care of cancer patients is critical for minimizing complications. We emphasize the importance of assessing immune-related adverse events (irAEs) such as pneumonitis, myocarditis, neurotoxicity, and endocrinopathies through preoperative planning and throughout the perioperative period. We advocate for close coordination with oncology and surgical teams to optimize perioperative care. Emerging therapies and future directions—including novel checkpoint inhibitors, CAR-NK cells, and oncolytic viruses—are also discussed, highlighting the field's rapid growth and evolving clinical impact.

Keywords: Anesthetic risk stratification, Bispecific T-cell engagers, BiTEs, Chimeric Antigen Receptor Cells, CAR T-Cells, Immunosuppression, Myasthenia Gravis-like syndrome, Neuropathy, Oncologic anesthesia, Regional anesthesia, Tumor immunology, Vaccines.

INTRODUCTION

History

Cancer immunotherapy is rapidly advancing and has evolved greatly throughout the ages, with anecdotal reports of tumors disappearing after an infection in anci-

* **Corresponding author Grace Abramian:** Department of Anesthesiology, Cooper Medical School of Rowan University, Cooper University Health Care, Camden, NJ, USA; E-mail: abramian-grace@cooperhealth.edu

Bharathi Gourkanti, Irwin Gratz, William Marion, Rajiv Lingaraju & Grace Abramian (Eds.)

ent Egypt [1]. Busch and Fehleisen were German physicians who noticed the regression of tumors in cancer patients that were unintentionally infected with erysipelas [2]. In 1868, Busch purposefully infected a cancer patient with erysipelas and noted the subsequent shrinkage of the tumor. William Coley, a surgeon in New York, is often cited as the first to attempt immunotherapy. He injected heat-inactivated bacteria called Coley's toxins into patients who were not surgical candidates, noting significant tumor regression [2].

In 1957, the Cancer Immunosurveillance Hypothesis was proposed by Burnet and Thomas, suggesting that the immune system patrols for cancer cells [3]. This eventually formed the basis for tumor immunology and helped explain spontaneous tumor regressions, which guided later research. Shortly after this, the use of Bacillus Calmette-Guerin (BCG), a weakened form of the bacteria that causes tuberculosis, for bladder cancer demonstrated that the resultant immune stimulation could fight tumors [3]. There were several early cytokine therapies, such as interferon-alpha and interleukin-2 (IL-2) that were explored in the 1970s-1980s as cancer treatments. This was an important step that showed evidence of ramping up T-cells to induce remission of cancer. IL-2 is a T-cell growth factor that was FDA-approved for the treatment of metastatic melanoma and renal cell carcinoma in the 1990s [4].

In 1992, Tasuku Honjo identified PD-1 (programmed cell death-1), a protein that acts as a brake on the immune system by regulating T-cell activity [5]. This helped give rise to immune checkpoint inhibitors, which block the interactions between PD-1 and its ligands, allowing the immune system to fight cancer. In 1996, James Allison also contributed to this cause by discovering that CTLA-4 acts similarly as an immune brake, preventing T cells from attacking cancer cells. He developed antibodies to block CTLA-4, allowing T cells to attack tumors. In 2011, Ipilimumab, an immune checkpoint inhibitor, was FDA-approved for the treatment of metastatic melanoma [3]. Combination therapy using anti-CTLA-4 and anti-PD-1 antibodies is often used to improve remission rates. In 2017, the first chimeric antigen receptor (CAR) T-cell therapies were approved for refractory lymphoma [6]. This involves genetically engineering a patient's T cells to express a CAR that recognizes a specific cancer antigen, allowing T cells to target cancer cells.

Current Practice Overview

Immunotherapy has become a mainstay in cancer treatment for a variety of malignancies. Immune checkpoint inhibitors (ICIs) are monoclonal antibodies that block inhibitory receptors like CTLA-4, PD-1, or ligand PD-L1. These are approved for numerous cancers (melanomas, lung cancer, renal cancer, lymphoma, *etc*). Adoptive cellular therapies, such as CAR T-cell therapy, involve personalized genetic engineering of a patient's T cells to attack tumor cells. T-cell receptor (TCR)- engineered T cells, on the other hand, are engineered to express a modified TCR that recognizes antigens presented on tumor cells by major histocompatibility complex (MHC) molecules. Cytokine therapies, such as high-dose IL-2 and interferon, are older forms of immunotherapy that boost the immune response non-specifically. Cancer vaccines involve exposure to tumor antigens to activate a humoral immune response to tumor-specific antigens [7]. Lastly, bispecific T-cell engagers (BiTEs) are substances that form a bridge by binding T cells with a target antigen on cancer cells, allowing the T cell to destroy the tumor cell [8].

NATIVE ANTITUMOR IMMUNITY

These are the therapies that enhance the body's existing immune response against tumors. "Native" antitumor immunity refers to the immune system's capacity to recognize and destroy cancer cells. Since tumors can evade or suppress this response, the following therapies help overcome this by boosting intrinsic immune functions or removing inhibitory mechanisms.

Immune Checkpoint Inhibitors (ICIs)

ICIs are monoclonal antibodies that block inhibitory receptors or ligands on T-cells and other immune cells, preventing the ability of tumors to evade immune attack.

- ***Mechanism of Action***: CTLA-4 on T-cells downregulates the immune response by competing with CD28 for binding B7 ligands on antigen-presenting cells. Tumor cells can increase CTLA-4 activity to help prevent T-cell activation. Anti-CTLA-5 antibodies block this inhibition, leading to increased T-cell activation in lymph nodes. PD-1 on T-cells is a "brake" on activated T-cells in peripheral tissues. When PD-1 binds ligand PD-L1 on tumor or immune cells, the T-cell becomes inactive. Anti-PD-1 and anti-PD-L1 antibodies prevent this from happening, allowing T cells to attack tumor cells (Fig. **1**). This enhanced immune activity helps control tumors but also causes autoimmune side effects because of the increased immune activity that has the potential to attack normal organs. Combinations of these different drugs can improve remission at the cost of higher toxicity.
- ***Common Agents and Clinical Use***: Some examples of anti-CTLA-4 monoclonal antibodies are Ipilimumab and Tremelimumab, though the latter has no clinical indication. Anti-PD-1 monoclonal antibodies include Pembrolizumab and Nivolumab. Lastly, anti-PD-L1 monoclonal antibodies include

Atezolizumab, Avelumab, and Durvalumab. ICIs have become the standard of care in many cancers, including numerous locally advanced, metastatic, and unresectable cancers [8].

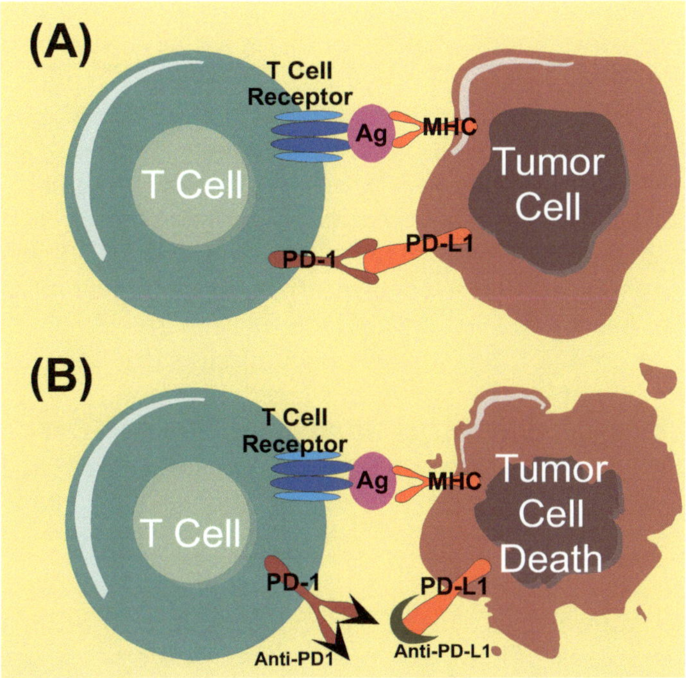

Fig. (1). Mechanism of PD-1 and PD-L1 in the activation of T Cell immunity. PD-1, programmed cell death-1; PD-L1, programmed death ligand 1. Ag, Antigen, MHC, major histocompatibility complex.

Cytokines

Cytokine therapy involves administering proteins that stimulate the immune system nonspecifically. These therapies are now less common as standalone treatments, though they may be encountered as they are sometimes used in combination trials.

- ***High-Dose IL-2 Therapy***: IL-2 is a T-cell growth factor that was FDA-approved for the treatment of metastatic melanoma and renal cell carcinoma in the 1990s. High doses of IL-2, a T-cell growth factor, can increase the ability of cytotoxic T-cells and NK cells to attack cancer cells. NK cells achieve this *via* direct cytotoxicity, cytokine secretion, induction of apoptosis, and their contribution to antibody-dependent cell-mediated cytotoxicity [9]. Of note, IL-2 also increases regulatory T-cells and has a short half-life, meaning it requires intensive administration protocols [9]. Since IL-2 can activate endothelial cells and increase permeability of the endothelium, it can lead to vascular leak syndrome, which is associated with fluids shifting out of the bloodstream. This can manifest as fluid retention, peripheral edema, hypotension, pulmonary edema, multi-organ dysfunction, and arrhythmias. Because of this potential to cause life-threatening side effects, IL-2 treatment is usually given in an ICU setting, though its use is limited today as newer therapies have surpassed it in efficacy and safety. A recent history of IL-2 therapy is important to note, as patients may have residual organ damage. Of note, IL-15 is being studied as an alternative to IL-2 since it can stimulate T-cells and NK cells with less T-reg activation.

- ***Interferons***: Interferon-alpha was approved for the treatment of melanoma, AIDS-related Kaposi's sarcoma, and hairy cell leukemia, but it is not used commonly, as there are newer, more effective therapies. Interferon-alpha can boost immune responses and has anti-proliferative effects on tumors much like IL-2, but it also has significant side effects such as flu-like symptoms, fatigue, depression, liver toxicity, and thyroid dysfunction [9]. Interferon-gamma has been tested but did not show efficacy in cancer remission.
- ***Granulocyte-Macrophage Colony-Stimulating Factor (GM-CSF)***: GM-CSF can recruit dendritic cells and macrophages. It is sometimes used as an immune stimulant in combination with other therapies, such as with a cancer vaccine [9].

Vaccines

Cancer vaccines stimulate a patient's immune system to recognize and attack tumor-specific antigens. There are prophylactic vaccines, such as the HPV vaccine, to prevent cervical cancer. There are also therapeutic vaccines that treat existing cancer. Therapeutic vaccines are the focus of this section, as they are considered a form of immunotherapy administered to cancer patients. Generally, they have fewer systemic side effects compared to ICIs or CAR-T therapies.

- ***Sipuleucel-T (Provenge)***: This was the first FDA-approved therapeutic cancer vaccine, which was used for metastatic castration-resistant prostate cancer [9]. It is an autologous cellular vaccine, meaning the patient's antigen-presenting cells (dendritic cells) are exposed to a prostate tumor antigen fused with an immune stimulant, then reinfused to induce an immune response against cancer cells. This modest improvement in survival rates is observed in prostate cancer. Significant adverse effects include acute infusion reactions and thromboembolic events, though they are rare [9].
- ***Other Vaccines***: Success has been limited with cancer vaccine trials. Related to vaccine therapy Talimogene laherparepvec (T-VEC) is the only FDA-approved oncolytic virus for the treatment of unresectable melanoma [9]. It is an engineered herpesvirus that infects tumor cells and releases tumor antigens along with GM-CSF to induce a robust immune response.

TUMOR-REACTIVE IMMUNE CELLS

These are therapies in which immune cells are engineered or directed to attack tumor cells. Unlike checkpoint inhibitors or cytokines, these therapies involve preparing immune effector cells that specifically target the tumor.

Chimeric Antigen Receptor (CAR) T-cells

This therapy is a form of adoptive cell transfer immunotherapy.

- ***Mechanism of Action*:** T-lymphocyte (both CD4+ and CD8+) are collected from a patient and genetically engineered to express an artificial chimeric antigen receptor (CAR) that recognizes a specific tumor antigen [9]. It is then expanded and reinfused into the patient. Once the CAR binds a specific tumor antigen, it triggers the T-cell to destroy the cancer cell. This bypasses the need for traditional antigen presentation, making this process MHC-independent.
- ***Current Uses*:** There are currently five FDA-approved CAR-T therapies for hematologic malignancies: lo tisagenlecleucel, lisocabtagene maraleucel, brexacubtagene autoleucel, and idecabtagene vicluecel. Idecabtagene vicleucel targets B-cell maturation antigen for multiple myeloma, while the other therapies target the CD19 antigen found on B-cell lineage malignancies [9]. These have found favorable results in refractory cancers, with some patients achieving long-term remission.
- ***Cytokine Release Syndrome*:** The most common toxicity (75-90% of patients) is cytokine release syndrome (CRS), which can occur due to the massive release of cytokines (IFN-gamma, IL-6 from macrophages, *etc*.) from activated CAR T-cells [10]. Common symptoms resemble sepsis and can include fevers, hypotension (due to vasodilation), hypoxia, and multi-organ failure within days of infusion (median onset is 2 days). If severe, patients can require supplemental oxygen and vasopressors for blood pressure support. Tocilizumab, an IL-6 blocker, can reverse these adverse effects while maintaining CAR T-cells' cancer-fighting ability. This is first-line therapy for grade 2+ CRS; corticosteroids are added if CRS is not responsive to tocilizumab [11]. If a patient shows signs of CRS and needs emergency surgery, the patient should be managed much like a patient with septic shock– with invasive monitoring and aggressive hemodynamic support. Otherwise, surgeries should be delayed for as much recovery time as possible.
- ***Immune Effector Cell-Associated Neurotoxicity Syndrome (ICANS)*:** ICANS is a neurotoxic syndrome associated with encephalopathy, confusion, seizures, and, in severe cases, cerebral edema, brain herniation, and death. It often follows CRS by a few days. Of note, CAR T can also lead to prolonged B-cell aplasia (since it may target CD19, killing normal B cells) and cytopenias. Due to all of

these risks, elective surgery is generally avoided in the immediate period of CAR T infusion.

T-Cell Receptor (TCR) Engineered T-cells

TCR-engineered T-cells are another form of adoptive cell therapy. However, instead of an artificial CAR, the T cell is given a new traditional T-cell receptor that targets a specific tumor antigen presented by MHC molecules.

- ***Mechanism of Action***: T-cells *via* their TCR recognize peptides bound to HLA (MHC) on cell surfaces. TCR genes that recognize a tumor-specific peptide are identified, and the T-cells are then genetically modified to express those TCRs. These TCR-engineered T-cells can then recognize tumor cells presenting that specific antigen on their HLA and kill them.
- ***Clinical Status***: TCR-engineered T-cells are mostly experimental. There is no current FDA-approved therapy using TCR-engineered T-cells.
- ***Toxicities***: Similar to CAR T, though off-target effects is a rare toxicity where there is cross-reactivity.

Bispecific T-cell Engagers (BiTEs)

- ***Mechanism***: BiTEs can bind a tumor antigen and a T-cell (usually CD3) at the same time. This physically brings T-cells into contact with tumor cells, activating T cells to kill the tumor cells. BiTEs effectively create a bridge connecting T-cells to cancer cells.
- ***Current Uses***: Blinatumomab was the first approved BiTE for relapsed B-ALL in 2014 [9]. Amivantanab was later approved for NSCLC in 2021.
- ***Toxicities***: Like CAR T-cells, BiTEs can cause cytokine release syndrome and neurotoxicity. BiTEs can be managed with the interruption of the infusion and supportive care, while CAR T-cell effects persist.

TOXICITY BY SYSTEM

Immunotherapy toxicities often occur due to an overactive immune response that damages normal tissues. This is different from what is seen with chemotherapy, which includes neutropenia and nausea.

Pulmonary

- ***Immune-Mediated Pneumonitis***: Checkpoint inhibitors can cause pneumonitis [9]. Presentation can range from asymptomatic to severe diffuse pneumonitis with respiratory failure. However, it is important to note that patients with even mild pneumonitis are at increased risk of postoperative pulmonary complications, including respiratory failure with the need for prolonged ventilatory support. Symptoms can include cough, shortness of breath, and wheezing.

- ***Diagnosis/Management*:** Chest x-ray and CT scan of the chest. The most common findings are ground-glass opacities with multifocal consolidations. High-dose corticosteroids are the first-line treatment [12]. If refractory to steroids, additional immunosuppressants such as infliximab can be used.
- ***Other Pulmonary Issues*:** CRS due to CAR T-cell therapy can lead to pulmonary edema, capillary leak, and ARDS. CRS patients often require supplemental oxygen or even intubation. IL-2 can cause a capillary leak syndrome that has the potential to lead to respiratory failure.
- ***Perioperative Considerations*:** In patients with current or past pneumonitis, pulmonary function tests should be completed. Preoperative evaluations should include discussions about new or worsening respiratory symptoms like dyspnea or cough. Elective surgeries should be delayed if there is active inflammation or worsening respiratory status. Patients should be advised regarding the risk of postoperative pulmonary complications and the potential need for postoperative respiratory support. Intraoperatively, lung-protective ventilation strategies should be utilized. Avoid excess fluids due to the risk of pulmonary edema.

Cardiovascular

- ***Myocarditis*:** Immune checkpoint inhibitors (ICIs) can also cause autoimmune myocarditis. While it is uncommon, autoimmune myocarditis has a high mortality rate. Patients present with symptoms related to heart failure, chest pain, life threatening arrhythmias due to conduction abnormalities, or sudden cardiac death. It often occurs within weeks of beginning ICI. Current recommendations are to check baseline EKG and consider troponin monitoring for patients on ICIs. BNP, echocardiogram, and chest x-ray can also be considered. Other testing to be guided by cardiology include stress testing, cardiac catheterization, and cardiac MRI [12].
- ***Other ICI Cardiac Issues*:** Pericarditis and vasculitis are rare but possible [10]. Vasculitis could present like giant cell arteritis with risk of aortic inflammation. ICI-induced vasculitis can present as fevers, elevated inflammatory markers, jaw claudication (if the temporal artery is affected), *etc*. If the patient had an episode of vasculitis, they may require long-term steroids.
- ***CAR T-cell Related CV Issues*:** If severe CRS develops, these patients can develop hypotensive shock requiring vasopressors [11]. Tachyarrhythmias are common in CRS due to high fever and elevated circulating catecholamines. Patients can also develop cardiomyopathy, though this is usually reversible.
- ***Management*:** Immune myocarditis is usually treated with high-dose corticosteroids, and often with additional immunosuppressants like infliximab or

tocilizumab if refractory [11]. If identified preoperatively, surgery should be delayed if possible until myocarditis is resolved or well-controlled. If proceeding with surgery, a cardiology consult, echocardiogram, EKG, and troponins should be ordered. Intraoperatively, consider placing an arterial line for continuous blood pressure monitoring and have vasoactive medications prepared. Avoid or use caution with medications that are cardiodepressive. Ensure defibrillator pads are available if there is a history of serious dysrhythmias or heart block. Postoperatively, patients should be monitored with telemetry and/or ICU admission.

Central Nervous System

- ***Checkpoint Inhibitors***: Immune-related adverse events (irAEs) are less common, with an incidence of around 5%. However, the incidence of severe (grade 3 or higher) neurologic irAEs is 1.5% [12]. Neurologic, along with cardiac irAEs, have a higher fatality rate than other irAEs. Typical management includes steroids and discontinuation of immunotherapy.
    1. ***Encephalitis***: Patients can present with confusion, seizures, or focal deficits. Work-up may include a neurologic consultation, an MRI of the brain with and without contrast, a lumbar puncture with CSF analysis, an EEG, and serum studies (CBC, metabolic panel, inflammatory markers, and ANCA) [12]. Treatment often requires immunosuppressive treatment while holding the ICI.
    2. ***Aseptic Meningitis***: Patients present with headache, photophobia, and neck stiffness. Work-up includes MRI brain with and without contrast and lumbar puncture with CSF analysis [12]. It is usually treatable with steroids.
    3. ***Demyelinating Syndrome***: ICI-associated Guillain-Barré Syndrome and transverse myelitis have been reported. These can cause weakness or paralysis. The work-up includes a neurologic consultation, an MRI of the spine with and without contrast, and a lumbar puncture with CSF analysis [12]. It is important to note the potential for autonomic instability, sensitivity to neuromuscular blockade, and possible need for postoperative ventilatory support.
    4. ***Myasthenia Gravis-Like Syndrome***: ICIs can induce myasthenia gravis, presenting with symptoms such as ptosis, muscle weakness, and respiratory failure in severe cases [12]. Work-up can include AChR and antistriated muscle antibodies (if negative, consider MuSK and LPR4 antibodies) and pulmonary function tests. Again, it is important to note the altered sensitivity to neuromuscular blockers in this case, and the potential need for postoperative ventilation.

5. ***Peripheral Neuropathies***: Patients present with pain, weakness, or a change in sensorium. They present an increased risk for perioperative positioning injury and should be carefully positioned and padded.

- ***CAR T-Cell Neurotoxicity***: Immune effector Cell-Associated Neurotoxicity Syndrome (ICANS) is seen predominantly with CAR T therapies and sometimes BiTEs. The mechanism is not fully understood, but it may involve endothelial dysfunction and blood-brain barrier leak, along with increased cytokine release, leading to inflammation in the CNS. It usually occurs within a week after infusion and can overlap with or follow CRS. Symptoms usually begin with encephalopathy, where patients become confused, obtunded, and develop expressive aphasia [11]. Eventually, symptoms can progress to seizures, weakness, elevated intracranial pressure, cerebral edema, and coma or death. Severe presentations often require ICU-level care, with intubation, seizure control, and measures to reduce intracranial pressure.
  1. ***Management***: Unlike in CRS, IL-6 blockers like tocilizumab can not treat neurotoxicity because they do not cross the blood-brain barrier [11]. Treatment for grade 2+ ICANS is high-dose corticosteroids and antiseizure prophylaxis. If severe, measures to reduce ICP, like head elevation and hypertonic saline, are indicated. Most ICANS are reversible with supportive treatment.
  2. ***Anesthetic Considerations***: Intraoperatively, standard measures for reducing intracranial pressure include hyperventilation, an elevated head of the bed if the procedure allows, continuation of ICP monitoring if used, and consideration of TIVA. Antiepileptics should be readily available. If a patient has a history of ICANS, consider avoidance of drugs that lower the seizure threshold.
- • ***Anesthetic implications summary***: A focused neurologic examination should be performed preoperatively in patients taking these forms of immunotherapy. If the patient has MG, GBS, or neuropathy, plan any necessary administration of neuromuscular blockade accordingly. If they have active encephalitis or neurotoxicity, delay elective surgeries if possible. Consider short-acting agents to limit postoperative sedation, which will enable prompt assessment of mental status.

Renal

• ***Checkpoint Inhibitor-Related Nephritis***: While uncommon, autoimmune activation due to ICIs can cause acute renal injury, usually secondary to acute interstitial nephritis. Median time to onset is 14 weeks from administration. Patients present with symptoms such as urinary frequency, fluid retention with edema, weight gain, nausea or vomiting, high blood pressure, or a change in mental status [12]. Urinalysis shows inflammatory cells or mild proteinuria. Of note, the checkpoint blockade can precipitate acute rejection in kidney transplant patients.

1. ***Management***: Management with corticosteroids while holding the ICI is standard. Most patients recover kidney function if treated promptly.

- ***CAR T and Others***: CAR T therapy does not directly cause nephritis, but during severe CRS, there can be a reduction in renal perfusion with resultant injury. It can also cause TLS in leukemia. IL-2 can cause acute renal injury *via* capillary leak and hypotension.
- ***Anesthetic Implications Summary***: Preoperatively, review a basic metabolic panel for creatinine trend and electrolytes in all patients on immunotherapy. If creatinine is newly elevated, consultation with a nephrologist may be indicated for early optimization and treatment. Intraoperatively, avoid nephrotoxic agents and ensure adequate hydration. Dose-adjust medications that are renally excreted in the setting of AKI or elevated creatinine. Lastly, be sure to monitor urine output closely for procedures longer than two hours or involving significant anticipated fluid shifts.

Gastrointestinal

- ***Colitis***: GI toxicities are common complications of ICIs. Immune-mediated colitis is one of the most common serious irAEs associated with CTLA-4 inhibitors. Onset usually occurs within 5-10 weeks of initiation of ICI therapy [12]. Patients can present with diarrhea, abdominal pain, bleeding, or acute perforation. Immune-mediated colitis pathologically resembles inflammatory bowel disease with T-cell infiltration of colonic mucosa. Grade 3+ colitis (7+ stools per day over baseline or with bleeding) requires corticosteroids and ICI discontinuation. Infliximab (anti-TNF) or vedolizumab (gut-specific anti-integrin) can also be used in patients with inadequate response to steroids [12]. Anticipate electrolyte derangements in the setting of diarrhea. If colitis is active or worsening, unrelated elective surgery should be delayed if possible.
- ***Hepatitis***: Immune-related hepatitis is more likely to occur with the combination of ICIs. Although rare, severe cases can present with jaundice and acute hepatic failure. Preoperatively, liver enzymes should be checked. If AST/ALT are elevated significantly and suspected to be related to immunotherapy, elective surgery should be postponed. If surgery must proceed, dose-adjust drugs with significant hepatic metabolism. Of note, severe hepatitis can cause coagulopathy and low albumin, impacting drug binding and bleeding risk. Lastly, CAR T does not typically cause autoimmune hepatitis; however, during CRS, liver enzymes

can become quite elevated. Typically, this resolves with treatment of CRS. IL-2 can also elevate LFTs secondary to hypoperfusion in the setting of capillary leak.

- ***Pancreatitis***: Less common, but ICI-induced pancreatitis can occur. Anticipate delayed gastric emptying, electrolyte disturbances, sepsis, and potential pulmonary involvement if severe.
- ***Upper GI***: ICIs also rarely cause esophagitis or gastritis, but checkpoint therapy can commonly worsen reflux or cause ulcerations secondary to inflammation or steroid use.
- ***Anesthetic Considerations Summary***: For any GI irAE, nutrition and hydration status should be optimized preoperatively, as chronic diarrhea or hepatitis can contribute to acute dehydration, malnutrition, and low serum albumin. Ensure to anticipate coagulopathies in the setting of severe liver dysfunction. If the patient is on long-term steroid therapy, a stress dosing regimen should be discussed with the patient's oncologic or endocrine team.

Endocrine

- ***Overview***: Endocrine gland injury is a common side effect of treatment with checkpoint inhibitors. Median time to onset of endocrine toxicities is 14.5 weeks [12]. Unlike other irAEs, many endocrine derangements in the setting of checkpoint inhibitor therapy result in permanent hormone deficiencies since the inflammatory injury can destroy glandular tissue. Patients may require chronic hormone replacement therapy and stress dose steroid considerations.
- ***Hypophysitis***: Hypophysitis can occur with CTLA-4 inhibitors, most commonly with ipilimumab, with an incidence of about 10% [12]. The inflammation of the pituitary gland leads to secondary adrenal insufficiency with low ACTH, and often concomitant hypothyroidism and hypogonadism. Patients can present with vague systemic symptoms of headaches, fatigue, and nausea. Treatment includes high-dose steroids and then long-term hormone replacement as indicated. It is important to note their long-term steroid dependency as they are ACTH-deficient.
- ***Thyroid Dysfunction***: PD-1 inhibitors can commonly cause thyroiditis. There is typically a transient hyperthyroid phase (as active inflammation causes hormone release), followed by hypothyroidism as the gland is destroyed. Many patients require exogenous thyroid hormone in the long term. Checkpoint-induced hypothyroidism is one of the most common irAEs.
- ***Adrenalitis***: Primary adrenal insufficiency is less common, but it is known to occur. Patients may have mineralocorticoid loss. Patients typically present with fatigue, low blood pressure, and electrolyte imbalance. Treatment is analogous to the management of Addison's disease.

- ***Type 1 Diabetes Mellitus*:** Anti-PD-1 agents can cause destruction of pancreatic islet cells, leading to insulin-dependent diabetes [12]. Though this is relatively rare, awareness is important as patients can present in diabetic ketoacidosis. These patients will require insulin management perioperatively.
- ***Others*:** Checkpoint therapy can rarely cause hypoparathyroidism or SIADH indirectly. Immunotherapy can also affect the gonadal axis, leading to low testosterone/estrogen.
- ***CAR T-Cell Therapy Considerations*:** CAR T-cell therapy generally does not directly cause endocrine autoimmunity. However, CRS can cause endocrine gland derangement indirectly, through hypoperfusion, systemic inflammation, and/or the stress of acute critical illness. Long-term steroids given for CRS/ICANS can also cause Cushingoid features and adrenal suppression.
- ***Anesthetic Considerations Summary*:** Symptoms of endocrine dysfunction in the perioperative period should be investigated, and the patient should be optimized as appropriate. Thyroid and adrenal derangements are common after immune therapy, and care should be taken to ensure that patients are euthyroid. Medical management should include a plan for perioperative steroid administration with stress dose as appropriate. Diabetic patients, whether their insulin deficiency is immunotherapy mediated or otherwise, should be managed as is standard of care with insulin sliding scale or infusion, and glucose levels should be closely monitored perioperatively. Adrenal insufficiency should be considered in the differential diagnosis when perioperative hemodynamic instability occurs, and patients should be treated with IV steroids if there is a high suspicion.

Dermatological

- ***Overview*:** Dermatologic conditions due to checkpoint inhibitors are among the most commonly observed side effects [10]. They frequently occur with CTLA-4 inhibitors, though they can present in the setting of anti-PD-1 and PD-L1 therapies. The majority of these conditions are mild, and they typically include rash, pruritus, or vitiligo. The median time to onset of skin conditions is 4 weeks [12].
- ***Severe Cutaneous Adverse Reactions (SCAR)*:** SCAR includes Stevens-Johnson syndrome, toxic epidermal necrolysis (TEN), and acute generalized exanthematous pustulosis. Bullous pemphigoid, an autoimmune blistering disease, can also be triggered by ICIs. Symptoms of SCAR may include fever, widespread rash, skin pain, skin sloughing, facial or upper-extremity edema, pustules, blisters, or erosions [12]. These conditions require dermatology evaluation and high-dose steroids or immune globulin treatment.

- ***Anesthetic Considerations Summary***: For mild rashes, it is important to differentiate between immunotherapy-mediated reactions and symptoms of drug allergy or early anaphylaxis. Use caution with drugs that can release histamine, and consider premedication with an antihistamine. A history of healed SJS can cause difficulty with airway management secondary to scarring and distortion of normal anatomy after mucosal involvement, and can make IV access challenging as well. Note that patients may be prescribed chronic steroids or other immunosuppressants for a skin irAE.
- *CAR T-Cell Therapy Considerations*: Patients can present with a transient rash during CRS (usually a blotchy, erythematous rash with a fever). Otherwise, chronic dermatologic changes are uncommon with CAR T-cell therapy.

Musculoskeletal

- ***Overview***: ICIs commonly cause rheumatologic complications such as an inflammatory arthritis that resembles rheumatoid arthritis. The median time to onset is 38 weeks [12], and this tends to be non-severe. Rheumatologic involvement can occur with either form of ICI treatment, though this is generally more frequent with PD-1 and PD-L1 antagonists. Many musculoskeletal irAEs are managed with NSAIDs or low-dose steroids while continuing immunotherapy if the tumor response is adequate. More severe cases may require interruption of ICI therapy and treatment with methotrexate or biologic agents.
- ***Inflammatory Arthritis***: Inflammatory arthritis can present as joint pain, stiffness, or swelling in the small joints of the hands, wrists, or larger joints. It occasionally requires rheumatologic treatment (NSAIDs, steroids, or even TNF inhibitors if severe). Arthralgia without obvious inflammation and myalgias are also common with ICI therapy.
- ***Myositis***: An autoimmune attack on muscles is rare but would present as proximal muscle weakness, elevated CK enzyme, and myalgias. In severe cases, checkpoint-induced myositis can cause myocarditis and even myasthenia gravis, which could impair respiration or sensitivity to neuromuscular blocking agents.
- ***Polymyalgia Rheumatica-Like Syndrome***: Older patients on ICIs have reported shoulder and hip girdle aching and stiffness, most prominent in the morning, similar to polymyalgia rheumatica. This is usually responsive to low-dose steroids.
- ***CAR T-Cell Considerations***: CRS can cause myalgias, though usually no long-term musculoskeletal issues are caused by CAR T-cell therapy.
- ***Anesthetic Implications Summary***: Active arthritis can call for emphasis on patient positioning. Additionally, joint pain can limit mobility postoperatively, so pain control regimen should be planned accordingly. Care should be taken to avoid hyperextension or extreme mandibular subluxation during airway

management. Myositis or muscle weakness can complicate neuromuscular blockade, so neuromuscular agents should be used cautiously, and return of full function should be monitored closely.

Hematologic

- ***Overview***: Hematologic irAEs from ICIs are less common. The median time to onset is 5.7 weeks [12]. Immune thrombocytopenic purpura, in which platelet destruction leads to low platelet can occur. Patients present with petechiae and bruising and are treated with steroids or IVIG. Hemophagocytic Lymphohistiocytosis (HLH)/macrophage activation syndrome (MAS) is an inflammatory reaction where immune cells consume blood cells and cause cytopenias. Patients present with fever, cytopenias, elevated ferritin, and organ failure. Patients can also get autoimmune hemolytic anemia and aplastic anemia. Of note, mild neutropenia or thrombocytopenia can occur.

CAR-T-Cell Therapy Considerations

1. Patients tend to have prolonged cytopenias after therapy, as lymphodepleting chemotherapy is given before CAR T in addition to the CAR T effect on marrow and cytokines [11]. Neutropenia and thrombocytopenia put the patient at risk for infection and bleeding, respectively. Blood counts are frequently monitored, and patients are given growth factors such as G-CSF or transfusions as needed.
2. For CD19 CAR T, B-cell aplasia occurs, leading to low immunoglobulin levels for months to years [11]. Patients often receive IVIG therapy periodically, which should be maintained perioperatively, in consultation with the oncology team. Additional perioperative antibiotics or extended regimens can be considered.
3. Severe CRS can consume clotting factors, causing a DIC-like state. Liver dysfunction during CRS can also contribute. A coagulation profile should be monitored in a patient recovering from CRS.
4. HLH/MAS can also rarely occur, overlapping with CRS. HLH can cause long-term organ damage if severe.

- ***Anesthetic Considerations Summary***: Obtain a CBC preoperatively in patients with current or previous immunotherapy. Changes to standard antibiotic prophylaxis may be required in neutropenic patients. If neutrophil counts are less than 1000/microliter, consider delaying surgery if possible for treatment with G-CSF. If the patient is thrombocytopenic, platelets should be ready for transfusion in anticipation of major surgery if <50k or if there is active bleeding. If severely anemic, optimize with transfusion. If the patient has ITP or AIHA on therapy, consider avoiding drugs that further impair platelets. If the patient has a history of HLH, ensure all organ function has been re-evaluated since they were likely critically ill. Of note, if the patient is receiving IVIG, perioperative volume overload is a potential consequence depending on cardiorenal status and other fluids administered.

Other Systems

- ***Ocular***: Uveitis, iritis, and episcleritis can uncommonly occur due to ICI therapy [12]. Uveitis typically presents with eye pain, redness, and visual changes. It is uncommon, but it can put a patient's vision at risk if severe.
- ***Ototoxicity***: Very rarely, autoimmune labyrinthitis can occur, leading to hearing loss and balance issues.
- ***Preexisting Autoimmune Disease***: If a patient has an autoimmune condition such as lupus, immunotherapy can worsen the preexisting disease process.

PREOPERATIVE CONSIDERATIONS FOR PATIENTS ON IMMUNOTHERAPY

Organ System Review and Screening: In order to ensure optimized medical condition and planning preoperatively, it is important to obtain a thorough review of systems. Screen for any immunotherapy-related organ toxicities as described in section 4. Inquire about present and past toxicities, system by system. Perform a focused physical exam assessing organ systems at risk. Additional specialists should be involved, and additional testing and optimization performed based on history and physical examination findings (Table **1**).

- ***Cardiac***: A baseline EKG and consider a troponin and BNP level. An echocardiogram and/ or consultation with a cardiologist is warranted if a patient has a history of myocarditis or symptoms suggestive of new or worsening cardiac dysfunction.
- ***Pulmonary***: Consider a chest x-ray or a CT scan if the patient has a history of pneumonitis and evolving or worsening symptoms. PFTs should be performed if there is a history of severe pneumonitis, oxygen dependency, or respiratory failure. The patient's primary pulmonologist should be involved in perioperative optimization and planning prior to major surgery.
- ***Endocrine***: Thyroid function should be monitored routinely, and changes in symptoms investigated further prior to elective surgery. Ensure glucose is controlled as with any other diabetic patient. Morning cortisol can be considered if adrenal function is in doubt. Ensure patients are on an appropriate steroid dose and plan stress coverage if there is suspicion or risk for adrenal insufficiency.

- ***Renal/Liver*****:** electrolytes, liver function, and nutritional status should be assessed.
- ***Hematologic*****:** If a patient has had CAR T therapy or a known cytopenia, check a CBC.
- ***Neurologic*****:** If there is a history of neurotoxicity, review prior neuroimaging and consider involving a neurology specialist for documenting a baseline cognitive, motor, and/or sensory status.

Medication Overview

• ***Immunotherapy drugs*****:** It is important to know which immunotherapy drug regimen the patient has been receiving and when the last dose was given.

1. ***Checkpoint inhibitors*****:** Often given every 2-4-6 weeks. Elective surgeries are scheduled thoughtfully in order to differentiate surgical complications from irAEs.
2. ***CAR T Therapy*****:** It is important to note that if the patient received a dose within the last two months, they are still susceptible to late CRS or neurotoxicities.

• ***Corticosteroids*****:** Many patients who have a history of severe irAEs may be maintained on a prolonged steroid taper. This can cause adrenal suppression (possible need for stress-dose steroid), increased infection risk (possible need for antibiotic prophylaxis), poor wound healing (risk for dehiscence), hypertension, and hyperglycemia.

• ***Other Immunosuppressants*****:** As discussed previously, patients may be taking several other medications to treat any irAEs they might have, including but not limited to infliximab, IVIG, tocilizumab, *etc.* Any changes to the medication regimen in the perioperative period should be planned in conjunction with the patient's oncology team.

• ***Concurrent Medications for Cancer*****:** Some patients get immunotherapy combined with other chemotherapeutic agents. See Chapter 5 for additional details. In general, most cancer and supportive meds should be continued as per the patient's oncologic care plan.

Oncologist Coordination

- ***Timing of Surgery Relative to Immunotherapy*****:** For elective cases, it is important to coordinate with the oncologist for an optimal window (finding a window that manages toxicity but does not postpone definitive cancer management). The patient should have time to recover from any high-grade toxicities before surgery, and oncologists may want the patient to completely taper off immunosuppressants treating irAEs before the stress of surgery. If the patient is in the middle of an immunotherapy cycle, consider scheduling surgery when the drug is at a lower activity level. Discuss with oncology if any changes should be made to chemotherapeutic timing to allow for postoperative recovery. If immunotherapy is continued into the perioperative period, more vigilance is needed for irAEs post-operatively. If the surgery is urgent or emergent and the patient has had recent immunotherapy, it is important to note the potential consequences. If a patient has recently received CAR T-cells (within 1-2 months) and has a surgical emergency, they are at high risk for CRS and ICANS during the perioperative course. The oncologist should be immediately available to consult regarding perioperative management.

Table 1. Preoperative considerations for patients on immunotherapy.

Category	Details
Organ System Screening	Thorough review of systems to screen for immunotherapy-related organ toxicities. Focused physical exam. Involve specialists and consider special testing.
Cardiac	Baseline EKG, consider troponin and BNP levels. Echocardiogram or cardiologist consultation if history of myocarditis or otherwise indicated.
Pulmonary	Review of recent imaging for the history of pneumonitis. Pulmonologist consultation for severe pneumonitis, oxygen dependence, or acute respiratory failure.
Endocrine	Assess organ-specific symptoms and monitor thyroid function. Ensure glucose control. Consider morning cortisol if adrenal function is uncertain. Plan stress-dose steroids for adrenal insufficiency risk.
Renal/Liver	Assess electrolytes, liver function, and nutritional status.
Hematologic	Check CBC for patients with CAR-T therapy or known cytopenia.
Neurologic	Review neuroimaging if prior neurotoxicity. Consider a neurology consult to document baseline neurologic function.
Immunotherapy Drugs	Review regimen and last administration. If possible, time surgery to differentiate irAEs from surgical complications.
CAR-T Therapy	Patients within 2 months of administration are at risk for late CRS and neurotoxicity.
Corticosteroids	May require stress-dose steroids. Risks include infection, poor wound healing, hypertension, and hyperglycemia.
Other Immunosuppressants	Patients may be on infliximab, IVIG, tocilizumab, *etc*. Coordinate perioperative changes with oncology.
Oncologist Coordination	Coordinate surgery timing with the oncologist. Schedule during lower drug activity. Postpone surgery if high-grade toxicities. Emergency surgery after recent CAR T-cell therapy carries high CRS/ICANS risk.

INTRAOPERATIVE MANAGEMENT

- ***Ventilatory Strategies*:** If the patient has a history of pneumonitis or lung injury, consider using ARDS-protocol-style ventilation (low tidal volumes, adequate PEEP, and limit plateau pressures) to mitigate risk of barotrauma or exacerbation of inflammatory processes. If the patient suffers neuromuscular complications like MG, plan for possible postoperative ventilation.
- ***Hemodynamic Management*:** If the patient has a history of myocarditis or reduced ejection fraction, maintain adequate perfusion pressure and avoid significant drops in blood pressure to ensure organ perfusion. Consider invasive hemodynamic monitoring if the patient has a significant cardiac history such as myocarditis. For patients with adrenal insufficiency, have IV steroids and vasopressor infusion available. For patients with capillary leak issues such as recent CRS, be judicious with IV fluid administration to avoid fluid overload.

Anesthetic Drug Considerations

- ***Drug Interactions with Immunotherapy*:** For the most part, immunotherapy drugs do not have direct interactions with anesthetic agents. However, it is important to consider the impact of immunotherapy-induced organ damage on drug metabolism and uptake if liver, renal, or endocrine systems are involved.
- ***Anesthetic Technique*:** Volatile anesthetics and opioids can suppress immune function, while propofol intravenous anesthesia and regional anesthesia might preserve immune function [13]. Consider using multimodal analgesia to minimize opioids, and if feasible, consider total intravenous anesthesia (TIVA) with propofol instead of inhalational agents (such as sevoflurane) [14]. However, further research is needed on whether TIVA would improve oncological outcomes significantly compared to inhalational agents. There is no current recommendation supported by evidence.
- ***Neuromuscular Blockers*:** If the patient had previous neuromuscular pathology such as myositis or myasthenia gravis, consider short-acting or easily titratable muscle relaxants and ensure to monitor with a peripheral nerve stimulator. Consider using sugammadex for reversal if there are signs of prolonged neuromuscular blockade. Consider avoiding muscle relaxants entirely, utilizing regional techniques whenever possible. Succinylcholine should be avoided in patients with prior Guillain-Barré as it can cause hyperkalemia and cardiac arrhythmias.
- ***Analgesics*:** NSAIDs should be avoided if the patient has active colitis or gastritis. Acetaminophen is generally safe, but should be used with caution in immune hepatitis patients (Table 2).

Table 2. Intraoperative considerations for patients on immunotherapy.

Category	Details
Ventilator Management	**Mitigate risk of barotrauma** • Lower airway pressures • Use of PEEP for oxygenation • Minimize atelectasis **Avoid hyperoxia** • Minimize FiO2 Glucocorticoids for reactive airways
Hemodynamics	Avoid large fluctuations in blood pressure Invasive monitoring if reduced ejection fraction or history of myocarditis Glucocorticoids and vasopressors for possible adrenal insufficiency
	Consider TIVA over volatile gases Multimodal analgesics Short acting neuromuscular blockers if history of neuromuscular disease Utilization of sugammadex Prioritize neuraxial anesthesia over general if feasible If history of Guillain-Barre syndrome avoid succinylcholine and use volatile anesthetics with caution Minimize NSAID usage if history of colitis or severe gastritis

POSTOPERATIVE CARE AND MONITORING

- ***Monitoring for irAEs*:** Be mindful of potential irAEs postoperatively, which can occur unexpectedly, as many irAEs have a delayed onset. Keep immunotherapy-related toxicity as part of the differential diagnosis, and involve the patient's oncology team immediately if unusual complications arise.
- ***Resuming Immunotherapy*:** Typically, immunotherapy is resumed (if previously held) postoperatively once the patient has recovered from surgery, as planned in collaboration with the oncology team.
- ***ICU Needs*:** If the patient has a history of severe cardiac, pulmonary, or neurological preoperative toxicities, consider planned ICU admission postoperatively.
- ***Infection Precautions*:** Since this patient population is at higher risk for infection, ensure to follow standard infection protocols and use appropriate antibiotic prophylaxis as indicated.
- ***Wound Healing*:** As previously discussed, if the patient is on chronic steroids, monitor surgical wounds closely for dehiscence or infection. Coordinate with surgery and oncology on steroid management during the perioperative period.

EMERGING THERAPIES AND FUTURE DIRECTIONS

New Checkpoint Inhibitors

- ***LAG-3 Inhibitors*:** Relatlimab was recently FDA-approved in combination with nivolumab for melanoma [15]. LAG-3 is another T-cell "brake," blocking it significantly enhances T-cell activity with a modest increase in toxicity. Anesthetic considerations will likely remain similar, but unique side effects may arise. TIGIT and TIM-3 inhibitors are currently in trial.
- ***Costimulatory Agonists*:** CD40 agonists, 4-1BB agonists, OX40 agonists are drugs that activate stimulatory receptors on T-cells and are currently in trials [16]. These can have a high risk of severe cytokine release.

Cellular Therapies

- ***CAR-T for Solid Tumors*:** There is ongoing research for CAR-T therapy to be used for solid tumors [17]. However, they have had many hurdles due to toxicity (such as organ damage if the target antigen is in normal tissues).
- ***CAR-NK Cells*:** Engineering natural killer cells with CAR could cause less CRS/ICANS since they produce different cytokines [18].
- ***Tumor Infiltrating Lymphocytes (TIL) Therapy*:** TIL therapy involves surgically harvesting a patient's own lymphocytes from the tumor, expanding them, and reinfusing after chemo (often with IL-2 support) [19]. Adverse events are due to the surgery, high-dose IL-2, and immunosuppression from chemotherapy.

Bispecific and Multispecific Antibodies:

- Bispecific full antibodies like Teclistamab target BCMA on myeloma and CD3 and T cells and were recently approved for multiple myeloma [20]. CRS and ICANS are associated with toxicities.
- Trispecific antibodies (such as a T cell with two different tumor antigens) are in development [21].

Oncolytic Viruses and Vaccines

- ***Oncolytic Viruses*:** T-VEC for melanoma is already in use, and others are in trials. Generally, their side effects are flu-like symptoms and injection-site inflammation. Theoretically, they can cause infection symptoms such as herpetic lesions.
- ***Cancer Vaccines*:** Many personalized vaccine approaches are in trials. They tend to have minimal side effects and are unlikely to complicate anesthesia.

- ***Managing Toxicity***: Therapies to manage adverse effects are being studied, such as IL-1 for refractory CRS [22]. In the future, management of immunotherapy complications may become more effective.

CONCLUSION

Cancer immunotherapy represents a transformative frontier in oncology, with therapies such as immune checkpoint inhibitors, CAR T-cell therapy, and bispecific T-cell engagers redefining the therapeutic landscape. As these agents become increasingly integrated into clinical practice, they present new challenges and considerations for perioperative and anesthetic care. We have outlined the mechanisms, clinical applications, and toxicities associated with key immunotherapeutic modalities, emphasizing the necessity of multidisciplinary collaboration to anticipate and manage immune-related adverse events. As the field continues to evolve with the development of next-generation therapies, anesthesiologists and perioperative clinicians must remain informed and adaptable, ensuring safe and effective care for this complex and growing patient population.

The key challenge lies not in drug interactions per se, but in recognizing and managing immune-related adverse events (irAEs) that can compromise multiple organ systems. Preoperative evaluation must be thorough and systems-based, incorporating appropriate lab work, imaging, specialist consultation, and risk stratification tailored to the patient's immunotherapy history. Particular attention should be paid to prior myocarditis, pneumonitis, endocrinopathies (*e.g.*, adrenal insufficiency, thyroiditis), and neurologic events, all of which can profoundly alter anesthetic risk.

Intraoperative ventilation strategies should reflect any underlying pulmonary inflammation, while hemodynamic goals should account for cardiac dysfunction or steroid dependence. Multimodal, opioid-sparing analgesia and the judicious use of total intravenous anesthesia (TIVA) may offer theoretical immunologic advantages. Neuromuscular blockade must be cautiously managed in patients with prior myositis, myasthenia gravis, or other immune-mediated neuromuscular complications.

Coordination with oncology is essential for determining appropriate surgical timing relative to immunotherapy cycles and for managing perioperative immunosuppressive regimens. For patients recently treated with CAR T-cell therapy, heightened vigilance for delayed cytokine release syndrome (CRS) or neurotoxicity (ICANS) is warranted, even weeks after infusion.

As immunotherapy continues to evolve rapidly—with novel agents like CAR-NK cells, new checkpoint inhibitors, and oncolytic viruses entering clinical practice—anesthesiologists must stay informed and agile. This chapter equips anesthesiologists with the clinical tools and interdisciplinary perspective necessary to navigate this evolving landscape and provide safe, individualized perioperative care to patients receiving cancer immunotherapy.

REFERENCES

[1] Rouse BT. Tumor immunology: a historical perspective. Nat Rev Cancer 2005; 5(4): 277-87.

[2] Nauts HC, Swift WE, Coley BL. The treatment of malignant tumors by bacterial toxins as developed by the late William B. Coley, M.D., reviewed in the light of modern research. Cancer Res 1946; 6(4): 205-16.
[PMID: 21018724]

[3] Dunn GP, Old LJ, Schreiber RD. The immunobiology of cancer immunoediting and immunotherapy. Immunity 2004; 21(2): 137-48.
[http://dx.doi.org/10.1016/j.immuni.2004.07.017] [PMID: 15308095]

[4] Rosenberg SA, Lotze MT, Muul LM, *et al.* Observations on the systemic administration of autologous lymphokine-activated killer cells and recombinant interleukin-2 to patients with metastatic cancer. N Engl J Med 1985; 313(23): 1485-92.
[http://dx.doi.org/10.1056/NEJM198512053132327] [PMID: 3903508]

[5] Ishida Y, Agata Y, Shibahara K, Honjo T. Induced expression of PD-1, a novel member of the immunoglobulin gene superfamily, upon programmed cell death. EMBO J 1992; 11(11): 3887-95.
[http://dx.doi.org/10.1002/j.1460-2075.1992.tb05481.x] [PMID: 1396582]

[6] National Cancer Institute. FDA Approves CAR T-Cell Therapy for Certain Lymphomas. 2017. Available from: https://www.cancer.gov/news-events/cancer-currents-blog/2017/yescarta-fda-lymphoma

[7] Melero I, Gaudernack G, Gerritsen W, *et al.* Therapeutic vaccines for cancer: an overview of clinical trials. Nat Rev Clin Oncol 2014; 11(9): 509-24.
[http://dx.doi.org/10.1038/nrclinonc.2014.111] [PMID: 25001465]

[8] National Cancer Institute. Bispecific T-cell engager. Available from: https://www.cancer.gov/publications/dictionaries/cancer-terms/def/bispecific-t-cell-engager

[9] Willsmore ZN, Coupland H, Mahbubani KT, Thomas SJ, Larkin J, Lee RWJ. Immunotherapy-associated toxicities: implications for perioperative management. Br J Anaesth 2022; 128(3): 456-72.
[PMID: 35803756]

[10] Brudno JN, Kochenderfer JN. Toxicities of chimeric antigen receptor T cells: recognition and management. Blood 2016; 127(26): 3321-30.
[http://dx.doi.org/10.1182/blood-2016-04-703751] [PMID: 27207799]

[11] Neelapu SS, Tummala S, Kebriaei P, *et al.* Chimeric antigen receptor T-cell therapy — assessment and management of toxicities. Nat Rev Clin Oncol 2018; 15(1): 47-62.
[http://dx.doi.org/10.1038/nrclinonc.2017.148] [PMID: 28925994]

[12] Martins F, Sofiya L, Sykiotis GP, *et al.* Adverse effects of immune-checkpoint inhibitors: epidemiology, management and surveillance. Nat Rev Clin Oncol 2019; 16(9): 563-80.
[http://dx.doi.org/10.1038/s41571-019-0218-0] [PMID: 31092901]

[13] Snyder GL, Greenberg S. Effect of anaesthetic technique and other perioperative factors on cancer recurrence. Br J Anaesth 2010; 105(2): 106-15.
[http://dx.doi.org/10.1093/bja/aeq164] [PMID: 20627881]

[14] Makito K, Matsui H, Fushimi K, Yasunaga H. Volatile versus intravenous anesthesia for cancer surgery: a retrospective cohort study. Anesthesiology 2020; 132(3): 508-20.

[15] Tawbi HA, Schadendorf D, Lipson EJ, *et al.* Relatlimab and nivolumab versus nivolumab in untreated advanced melanoma. N Engl J Med 2022; 386(1): 24-34. [http://dx.doi.org/10.1056/NEJMoa2109970] [PMID: 34986285]

[16] Beatty GL, Gladney WL. Immune escape mechanisms as a guide for cancer immunotherapy. Clin Cancer Res 2015; 21(4): 687-92. [http://dx.doi.org/10.1158/1078-0432.CCR-14-1860] [PMID: 25501578]

[17] Newick K, O'Brien S, Moon E, Albelda SM. CAR T cell therapy for solid tumors. Annu Rev Med 2017; 68(1): 139-52. [http://dx.doi.org/10.1146/annurev-med-062315-120245] [PMID: 27860544]

[18] Rezvani K. Engineering natural killer cells for cancer immunotherapy. Mol Ther 2020; 28(1): 1-3. [PMID: 31864908]

[19] Sarnaik A, Hamid O, Khushalani NI, *et al.* Lifileucel, a tumor-infiltrating lymphocyte therapy, in metastatic melanoma. J Clin Oncol 2023; 41(6): 1130-40. [PMID: 33979178]

[20] Moreau P, Garfall AL, van de Donk NWCJ, *et al.* Teclistamab in relapsed or refractory multiple myeloma. N Engl J Med 2022; 387(6): 495-505. [http://dx.doi.org/10.1056/NEJMoa2203478] [PMID: 35661166]

[21] Labrijn AF, Janmaat ML, Reichert JM, Parren PWHI. Bispecific antibodies: a mechanistic review of the pipeline. Nat Rev Drug Discov 2019; 18(8): 585-608. [http://dx.doi.org/10.1038/s41573-019-0028-1] [PMID: 31175342]

[22] Grupp SA, Maude SL, Shaw PA, *et al.* Durable remissions in children with relapsed/refractory acute lymphoblastic leukemia treated with T cells engineered with a CD19-specific chimeric antigen receptor. Blood 2016; 127(26): 3321-30. [PMID: 27207799]

CHAPTER 5

Radiation Therapy - Anesthetic Considerations

Marcus Ryan Dal Nogare[1,*] and **Eric You**[1]

[1] *Department of Anesthesiology, Cooper Medical School of Rowan University, Cooper University Health Care, Camden, NJ, USA*

Abstract: This chapter will provide an in-depth review of radiation therapy and its implications on anesthetic management. It will begin with a brief overview of cancer and the history of radiation therapy's progression into an essential tool in cancer treatment. Next, the mechanism behind radiation therapy's effectiveness in targeting cancer cells will be explored. Lastly, a systems-based approach to radiation therapy and its impact on anesthetic planning will be discussed.

Keywords: Direct DNA damage, Indirect DNA damage, Ionization, Linear accelerators, Linear energy transfer, Mitotic catastrophe, Radiation therapy, Radiotherapy, Radiation oncology, Radiobiology.

INTRODUCTION

Over the past few decades, cancer treatment modalities have advanced exponentially, driven by large global cancer research and development initiatives. Despite significant advancements in early detection, diagnostic tools, and targeted multimodal therapies, cancer continues to impose a significant burden on healthcare systems worldwide. The International Agency for Research on Cancer (IARC) estimates that there were 20 million new cancer cases with 9.7 million deaths in 2022. By the year 2050, IARC predicts over 35 million new cancer cases yearly, representing a 77% increase from the 20 million cases of 2022 [1]. Given the significant burden of cancer globally, researchers and clinicians must continue to develop and implement these lifesaving advancements in cancer therapies to improve outcomes.

Modern cancer treatment is often tailored specifically to the individual patient based on factors such as comorbidities, age, tumor type, tumor genetics, stage, and location within the body. Although each patient's treatment plan is unique, the overarching principle of therapy remains the same: targeted eradication of

* **Corresponding author Marcus Ryan Dal Nogare:** Department of Anesthesiology, Cooper Medical School of Rowan University, Cooper University Health Care, Camden, NJ, USA; E-mail: dalnogare-marcus@cooperhealth.edu

Bharathi Gourkanti, Irwin Gratz, William Marion, Rajiv Lingaraju & Grace Abramian (Eds.)

cancer cells while causing the least amount of damage to surrounding healthy tissues. Currently, cancer treatments can target malignant cells through a variety of modalities. These include radiation therapy, chemotherapy, immunotherapy, and hormonal therapy. Radiation therapy, also called radiotherapy, is one of the oldest and most extensively utilized cancer treatment options available. Its success is evidenced by its use in up to 50% of all cancer treatment plans [2]. The implementation of radiation therapy is utilized in a diverse number of cancer types, including breast, lung, prostate, head and neck, cervix, and brain, among others. Radiation therapy can serve as the primary treatment, in combination with systemic therapy and/or surgery, or in a palliative role to relieve symptoms such as pain and obstructions caused by large tumors. Over the years, its effectiveness and widespread use have led to the establishment of radiation oncology, a medical subspecialty dedicated entirely to the application of radiation therapy.

History of Radiation Therapy

The origins of radiation therapy date back to the revolutionary work of German physicist Wilhelm Roentgen (Fig. **1**). In 1895, while experimenting with cathode ray tubes in his laboratory, Dr. Roentgen discovered a new form of electromagnetic radiation. This radiation could penetrate solid materials such as limbs, leaving behind an image on photographic plates [3]. This discovery, later named X-rays, formed the foundation for modern radiology and early radiation therapy. Shortly after Roentgen's work, the work of a Nobel prize-winning physicist couple, Marie and Pierre Curie on radiation-producing uranium salts led to the discovery of the radioactive element radium [3]. The high levels of radiation emitted from radium were used in the treatment of various cutaneous cancers, yielding promising results. These two discoveries accelerated the application of radiation in the treatment of numerous medical conditions.

Likely the most important advancement in the field of radiation therapy was the clinical application of linear accelerators (linac). Decades prior to this, high-energy particle accelerators were theorized and eventually developed by physicists. As these devices became more efficient, they were adopted by early pioneers of radiation oncology for their use in cancer treatment. In 1953, the first clinical linac was installed at the Hammersmith Hospital in London, England [4]. The success of clinical linacs is due to their ability to deliver high-energy radiation beams in a more precise manner to maximize tumor damage while limiting damage to healthy tissues. Around the time linear accelerators were making their way into hospitals, scientists and clinicians began to deepen their understanding of the interaction between radiation and living cells. This is known as the study of radiobiology. The decades following these milestone events have produced numerous advancements in the field of radiation oncology.

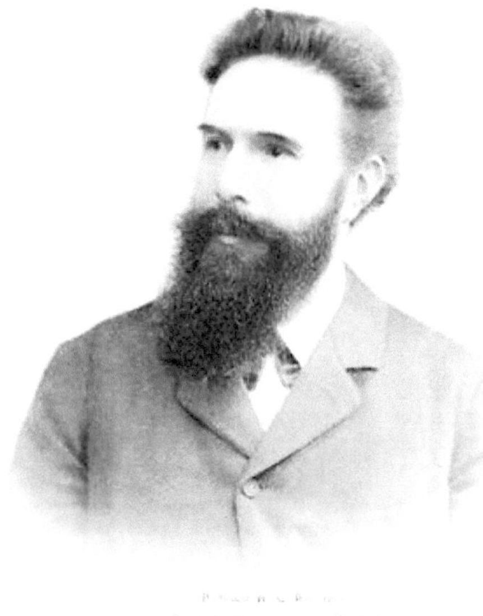

Fig. (1). Portrait of Wilhelm Roentgen, late 19th century(Commercial license purchased for image through istockphoto.com).

Mechanisms of Radiation Therapy

Effective DNA repair mechanisms are an important safety net in healthy cells to preserve their genome from the estimated 100 thousand spontaneous or induced DNA lesions that occur daily [5]. The study of radiobiology has shown that cancerous cells are more susceptible to lethal DNA damage from radiation compared to their healthy counterparts. This is a result of unique characteristics found in a majority of cancer cells that aid in their ability to proliferate.

Sensitivity to DNA damage changes with the cell cycle phases; G2 and M phases are the most sensitive, while S phase is the most resistant due to active DNA synthesis and increased activity of DNA repair mechanisms (Fig. **2**) [6]. Due to the rapid proliferation of most cancer cells, they can be found in these sensitive phases more often, making them susceptible targets for radiation-induced DNA damage. When DNA damage occurs, cancer cells typically have a reduced ability to repair it compared to healthy cells [7]. This is largely due to mutations in genome segments responsible for DNA repair that cancer cells take advantage of to progress into a more aggressive state. An example of this is the well-studied BRCA1 or BRCA2 genes, which are crucial for repairing double-strand DNA breaks and are commonly found in breast and ovarian cancers, leading to increased genetic instability [8].

Cell cycle checkpoints play an important role in the regulation of cellular reproduction, making sure that each phase is correctly executed before moving forward. This system of checks helps reduce potential genomic instability. Cancer cells often possess mutations in important checkpoint proteins [9]. Radiation therapy can utilize these failed safety mechanisms in the cell cycle to induce DNA damage that will go unrepaired and lead to apoptosis or mitotic catastrophe in cancerous cells. Common checkpoint mutations in cancer cells usually involve the G1/S checkpoint, which ensures the cell is ready for S phase DNA replication and surveys for DNA damage before replication can begin. The G2/M checkpoint confirms that DNA replication was completed successfully without significant DNA damage before mitosis can begin. Lastly, the spindle assembly checkpoint verifies that all chromosomes are properly aligned and attached to the spindle before cell division occurs (Fig. **2**) [9].

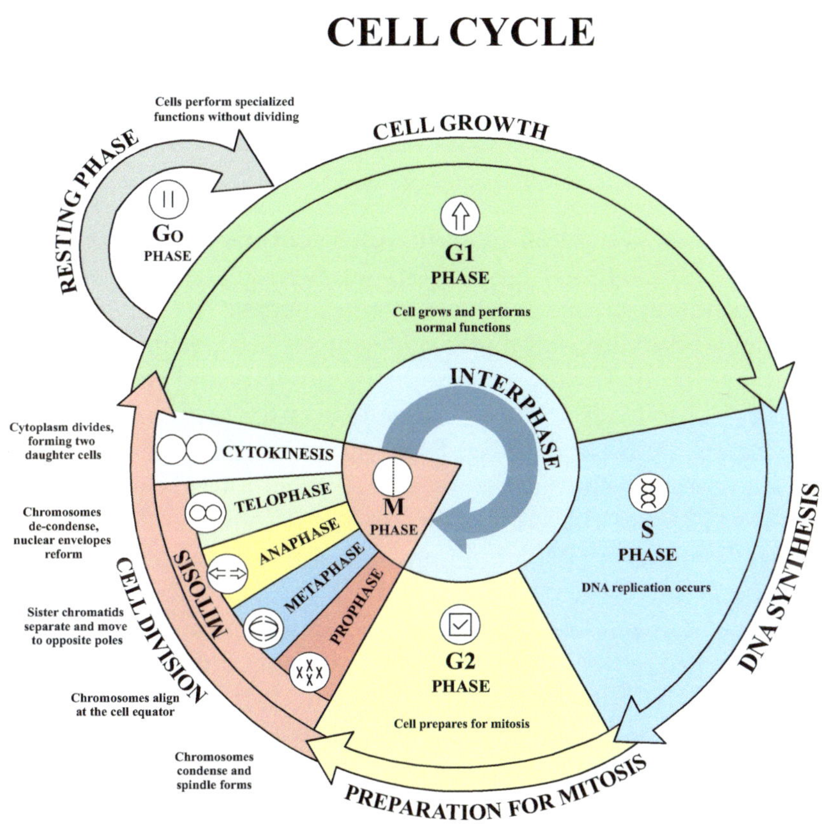

Fig. (2). Stages of the cell cycle. (Image will need to be acquired through the publisher's Shutterstock account, Image ID 2483833465).

On a molecular level, radiation therapy in the form of high-energy waves or particles, such as photons (gamma rays and X-rays), or particles (electrons and protons) is directed at inducing DNA damage through direct or indirect mechanisms. The energy generated from radiation therapy is transferred to cells through ionization, where electrons located in DNA atoms are displaced, leading to the creation of volatile charged particles capable of severe molecular damage [10].

The mechanism of direct DNA damage occurs when ionizing radiation interacts directly with the DNA molecule (Fig. **3**). The energy is transferred to atoms within cellular DNA, resulting in ionization, excitation, and subsequent destabilization of the molecule [10]. This destabilization eventually manifests as DNA damage in the form of single-strand breaks (SSBs), double-strand breaks (DSBs), and base modifications. Of the various direct DNA damage mechanisms, DSBs are the most effective at stopping the proliferation of cancer cell lines due to the highly cytotoxic nature of these lesions and their potential to cause disastrous genomic instability if left unrepaired [11]. Direct DNA damage is often the result of high linear energy transfer (LET) radiation subtypes, such as heavy ions like carbon. High LET radiation characteristically delivers higher amounts of energy over shorter distances and is more likely to strike DNA molecules within the nucleus directly.

Indirect DNA damage is created from the interaction between ionizing radiation and cellular water molecules (Fig. **3**). This interaction results in the radiolysis of water and the production of reactive oxygen species (ROS) such as hydroxyl radicals, hydrogen peroxide, and superoxide anions [10]. Highly volatile ROS can exert their damage by diffusing into the cell's nucleus and reacting directly with DNA molecules. This leads to DNA damage similar to that found in high LET therapies, including DSBs and SSBs. ROS-mediated DNA damage is commonly associated with therapies that utilize low LET radiation subtypes such as X-rays and gamma rays [12]. For these therapy types, it is important to note that relative biological effectiveness (RBE), which is a measure of biological damage per unit of radiation absorbed, is directly affected by the cancerous cell's antioxidant capacity and local oxygen concentrations. Solid malignancies often generate an environment of hypoxia due to rapid growth, inadequate angiogenesis, and high metabolic demand. The hypoxic environment will decrease the RBE of numerous radiation therapies that rely heavily on indirect DNA damage through the generation of ROS, leading to a resistance to treatment [13, 14].

Both direct and indirect DNA damage activate the cell's DNA damage response (DDR) pathways. DDR is essential for the coordination of DNA repair, cell cycle arrest, and potential apoptosis. Common DNA repair pathways include base excision repair (BER), nucleotide excision repair (NER), mismatch repair (MMR), homologous recombination (HR), and non-homologous end joining

(NHEJ) [15]. Ionizing radiation seeks to induce DNA damage that overwhelms the DDR DNA repair capabilities, if still functional and not mutated, leading to mitotic catastrophe or apoptosis.

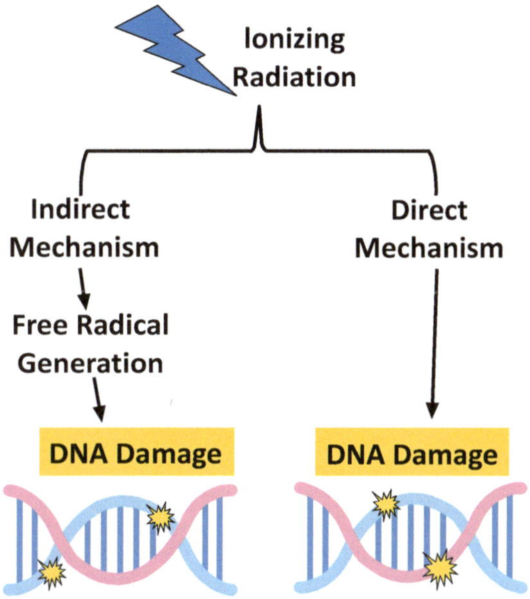

Fig. (3). Mechanisms of DNA damage from radiation therapy.

Radiation Therapy Types

Radiation therapy can be classified into two main categories: external beam radiation therapy (EBRT) and internal radiation therapy. EBRT delivers high-energy radiation from a radiation source located outside of the body [12]. This method is known for its accurate delivery of radiation, made possible by sophisticated radiation equipment and advanced mapping techniques. The EBRT method has wider applications compared to internal radiation therapy and is therefore utilized more often in cancer treatment plans. Internal radiation therapy involves placing radioactive material inside the body to deliver continuous radiation to cancerous tissues. This can be accomplished by inserting radioactive implants directly into or near the tumor, or by administering radioactive substances orally or intravenously, allowing them to circulate systemically and eventually reach the targeted cancerous tissues [12]. Both methods aim to deliver ionizing radiation to cancerous tissue in an attempt to cause DNA damage significant enough to limit further growth and spread while still preserving healthy tissue. Examples of specific therapies include:

External Radiation

- Three-Dimensional Conformal Radiation Therapy (3D-CRT) – 3D images of tumors are created using CT or MRI scans to aid in the mapping and aiming of radiation beams [16].
- Intensity Modulated Radiation Therapy (IMRT) - This is an advanced form of 3D-CRT that allows modulation of radiation beam intensity within each field. This helps in delivering a more calculated dose while limiting healthy tissue exposure, especially when tumors are close to vulnerable organs [16].
- Volumetric Modulated Arc Therapy (VMAT) – A form of IMRT that uses a single 360-degree arc motion around the patient during radiation delivery. This arc motion is unique when compared to the fixed-angle radiation beam found in standard IMRT [16].
- Proton Beam Therapy – Proton therapy is a form of particle therapy that utilizes protons rather than the more traditional X-rays. By utilizing unique characteristics of particle radiation, this technique allows for better dose distribution in deep-seated tumors and limits damage to surrounding tissues [16]. Other forms of particle therapy include boron neutron capture therapy (BNCT) and carbon ion radiotherapy (CIRT).
- Stereotactic Radiation Therapy – This is a highly precise external beam therapy used in the treatment of smaller and well-demarcated tumors. It delivers higher doses of radiation, which allow therapy completion in one to five sessions on average [16]. There are two main subtypes, including stereotactic radiosurgery (SRS) used for brain tumors and stereotactic body radiation therapy (SBRT) used in body cancers of the lung, prostate, spine, and pancreas.
- Electron Beam Therapy – Although technically a form of particle therapy, electron beam therapy is often treated as a separate modality. This form of radiation therapy utilizes electrons, which have limited tissue penetration, making it useful for cancers involving the skin and superficial tissues [17].
- Total Body Irradiation (TBI) – Total body radiation is a less precise therapy that exposes almost the entire body to radiation. This large field therapy is usually combined with chemotherapy in patients with hematologic cancers in preparation for a stem cell transplant by destroying cancerous cells and suppressing the immune system to prevent rejection [18].

Internal Radiation Therapy

Brachytherapy – This simple method of delivering radiation is accomplished through the placement of radioactive implants such as seeds or capsules within or adjacent to cancerous tissues [19]. These radioactive materials allow for the continuous emission of low-dose radiation to the target tissues. Brachytherapy can be used temporarily or left in place for life and is commonly utilized in prostate and cervical cancers.

Systemic Radiation Therapy (SRT) – Systemic radiation therapy is a treatment modality where radioactive substances are given to patients *via* oral or intravenous routes. These radioactive substances eventually accumulate in their target tissues, leading to the destruction of cancerous cells. The most common application of SRT is radioactive iodine (I-131) in the treatment of certain thyroid cancers.

SYSTEMIC RADIATION EFFECTS AND ANESTHESIA CONSIDERATIONS

Central Nervous System Radiation Complications and Anesthesia Considerations

Radiation therapy is widely used to treat a range of malignant and benign conditions of the brain, skull base, and adjacent structures such as the pituitary gland. CNS radiation is dependent on the size and location of the tumor. For example, small tumors such as vestibular schwannomas and meningiomas can be treated with a single session. Larger tumors, such as gliomas, require multiple therapies over the span of three to six weeks [20]. Side effects from CNS radiation can be categorized as early and late clinical manifestations. Early complications typically occur within six months after completing radiation therapy. Acute radiation encephalopathy appears within two weeks of therapy (although some cases can occur hours after initial therapy). Early-delayed encephalopathy occurs between two weeks and six months after starting therapy. Common symptoms include fatigue, lethargy, memory/attention deficits, nausea, and anorexia. The hypothesized pathophysiology is transient demyelination caused by blood-brain barrier disruption or oligodendroglial injury [21].

For anesthesia considerations, the disruption of the blood-brain barrier can increase the risk of seizures during and after administering anesthesia. Providers will need to closely monitor for seizure-like activities and use anticonvulsants as needed. Another consideration, especially in the pediatric population, is that prolonged exposure to anesthesia can contribute to neurocognitive decline. Additionally, a thorough preoperative neurocognitive exam should be performed to assess patients' baseline cognitive function and status.

Radiation can also damage intracranial or extracranial vasculature, leading to ischemic or hemorrhagic strokes. Abnormal anastomosis can occur, resulting in diseases such as moyamoya disease or vascular AV malformations. The carotid arteries can become stenotic after cervical radiotherapy [20]. These radiation-induced vasculopathies are typically an accelerated form of atherosclerosis, and complications tend to occur many years after treatment (7 years for intracranial arteries, 20 years for extracranial arteries). The vasculopathy typically occurs in unusual locations, such as the distal internal carotid arteries [22]. The baroreceptor response can also be altered, leading to drastic hemodynamic shifts intraoperatively.

Patients who have a remote history of CNS radiation, especially in the cervical region, should be evaluated for possible carotid vasculopathy. Hemodynamics should be monitored closely with invasive monitoring for patients who are at high risk for developing cerebral hypoperfusion, especially patients who also have malfunctioning baroreceptor reflexes. Intraoperative hypertension should also be avoided due to potential intracranial AV malformations that can lead to hemorrhagic stroke conversion. Carotid endarterectomy might be considered appropriate for the patient prior to undergoing additional surgeries.

Head and Neck Radiation Complications and Anesthesia Considerations

Radiation therapy in the head and neck region is typically targeted at the oral, pharyngeal, and laryngeal regions of the human body. Squamous cell carcinoma (SCC) accounts for approximately 90% of cases. Radiation therapy improves clinicaland functional outcomes of up to 75% of cancer patients as a primary or adjuvant therapy [23]. In addition to squamous cell carcinoma, head and neck radiation can be utilized for a variety of thyroid carcinomas [24].

Radiation therapy causes dose-dependent tissue damage as described before, leading to inflammation and eventual apoptosis of the tissues. This damage can also lead to fibrosis in the head and neck region. Acute toxicity can result in mucositis, dermatitis, dysphagia, odynophagia, and hoarseness. Chronic toxicity can result in, but is not limited to, xerostomia, dental caries, malnutrition, trismus, thyroid dysfunction, radiation fibrosis syndrome, vocal cord restriction, and subglottic narrowing [23]. Anatomical changes in the pharyngeal and laryngeal can result in significant airway challenges. Physiological changes can occur in the thyroid that impact perioperative care. Intensity modulated radiation therapy (IMRT) became a common technique for SCC due to its ability to target the primary tumor burden and lymph node regions while decreasing dosage to healthy adjacent tissues [23]. However, despite the advancements of localized targeting therapy, radiation-induced toxicity remains a challenge for anesthesiologists during the perioperative period [24].

Radiation-induced hypothyroidism can often be undetected due to its subclinical course, but it can progress to clinical hypothyroidism. Clinical hypothyroidism manifests with slow mentation, possible pleural and pericardial effusion, decreased gastrointestinal motility, weight gain, congestive heart failure, and delayed wound healing [25].

Pre-operative assessment of thyroid function is critical before elective surgeries for patients with head and neck radiation. Non-specific symptoms such as lethargy and fatigue can be attributed to cancer treatment side effects that delay the diagnosis of thyroid disease. If hypothyroidism is suspected, patients should be optimized with thyroid hormone supplements prior to surgery. During emergent cases where hypothyroidism is not corrected, the major concern is cardiovascular instability and collapse. Intraoperative pressor support may be needed for patients with uncorrected hypothyroidism.

Another major concern for anesthesiologists in patients post-head and neck radiation is securing the airway. Temporomandibular joint fibrosis and non-compliant neck tissues significantly increase the difficulty of masked ventilation. Trismus and neck fibrosis can make direct laryngoscopy, and thus intubation, difficult [26]. Subtle voice changes, dysphagia, and new onset of stridor may be signs of airway compromise [27]. Patients with a history of head and neck radiation are at high risk for difficult ventilation and difficult intubation situations upon induction, which will require a surgical airway to be established. Anesthesiologists must be familiar with the difficult airway algorithm when encountering patients with head and neck radiation (Fig. **4**). Advanced techniques such as awake fiberoptic intubation should be utilized to secure the airway before induction in known or suspected difficult airways.

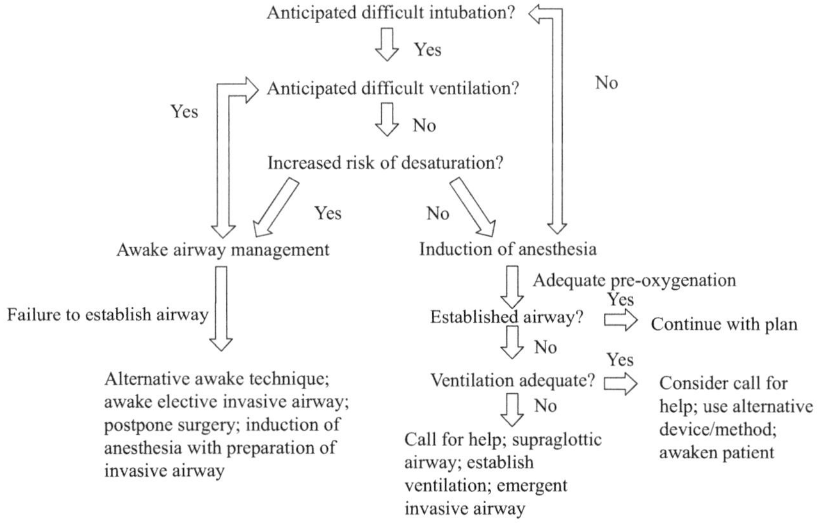

Fig. (4). Difficult airway algorithm for difficult intubation and/or ventilation

Thoracic Radiation Complications and Anesthesia Considerations

Patient populations receiving thoracic radiation typically involve the following malignancies: lung, breast, esophageal, and mediastinal lymphoma [28]. The risk of developing radiation-induced lung disease depends on numerous factors, such as the total dose administered (greater than 20 Gy), concurrent chemotherapy, smoking history, tumor location, and tumor size.

Radiation disrupts the alveolar barrier function *via* destruction of epithelial and endothelial cells within the lungs. This induces an inflammatory response, leading to increased vascular permeability and cytokine release, which results in pulmonary edema and alveolar dysfunction [29]. This acute manifestation results in radiation pneumonitis. Once macrophages accumulate and activate the inflammatory cascade, they contribute to the development of hypoxia and the production of reactive oxygen/nitrogen species. Further proinflammatory, profibrogenic, and proangiogenic cytokines produce a non-healing tissue response that leads to chronic radiation injury of radiation fibrosis [30]

Acute radiation pneumonitis typically occurs in 4-12 weeks, but can manifest within 1 week if radiation dosage is high or if concurrent chemotherapy is given [28]. Non-specific symptoms such as cough, dyspnea, low-grade fevers, and pleuritic chest pain are often associated. In severe cases of hypoxia, subsequent right-sided heart failure can occur. Treatment involves systemic oral or IV steroid therapy depending on the severity of the disease [31]. Radiation fibrosis, which typically develops over months to years, is proportional to the area of radiation. Patients may develop restrictive lung disease presenting with cough, shortness of breath, a reduction in oxygen diffusion capacity, and a decrease in respiratory volumes. Pulmonary function testing and potentially chest imaging are essential pre-operatively to evaluate lung compliance and gas exchange/diffusion properties.

Due to the restrictive nature of the disease, many anesthesia considerations are applied in the perioperative period. Masked ventilation could be challenging, and patients can desaturate quickly due to reduced residual functional capacity. Intraoperatively, patients have a higher risk of respiratory complications due to decreased compliance. Lung protective ventilation should be utilized to minimize barotrauma. Factors that can precipitate pulmonary hypertension should be avoided, such as hypercarbia, hypoxia, acidosis, and/or pain [32].

Thoracic radiation, especially in the mediastinum region, can also lead to radiation-induced heart disease by the cytotoxic effects of radiation [33]. The process begins with a disruption of the coronary arterial endothelial barriers. Local inflammation with platelet aggregation results in microvascular injury, tissue ischemia, and oxidative stress in the cardiomyocytes. These damaged cells are removed and replaced, which contributes to myocardial scar formation. Radiation-induced heart disease can be seen in all structures in the heart, such as the coronary arteries, myocardium, cardiac valves, conduction system, and pericardium.

A comprehensive preoperative cardiac risk stratification should be performed appropriately prior to elective surgeries (Fig. **5**). Coronary artery disease was reported in approximately 85% of patients 5 to 10 years after radiation therapy. Valvular heart disease was reported in 2 to 6% of patients 10 years after radiation [34]. Myocardial scar formation can also lead to ventricular systolic and diastolic dysfunction [33]. An echocardiogram and 12-lead ECG should ideally be performed for a full cardiac evaluation. Nuclear stress tests and possible cardiac catheterization should be performed for those with suspected ischemic diseases. Coronary-CT scans can also be utilized to monitor accelerated calcification and atherosclerosis. Intraoperative hemodynamic shifts should be closely monitored with invasive blood pressure measurement methods. If hemodynamics require vasopressor support, the drug of choice should be carefully selected based on any presenting valvular or cardiac pathologies (ie, phenylephrine to maintain afterload for aortic stenosis; norepinephrine to maintain heart rate and forward flow for aortic regurgitation). Hemoglobin should be maintained above 8 for adequate oxygenation of the myocardium, especially if patients are afflicted with ischemic heart disease.

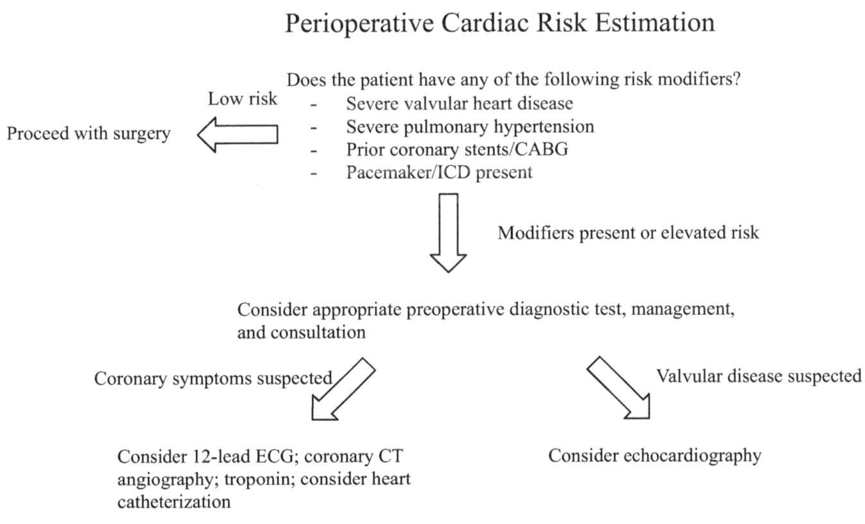

Fig. (5). Cardiac risk stratification and evaluation for patients with a history of thoracic radiation

Gastrointestinal Radiation Complications and Anesthetic Considerations

Radiation to the abdomen and pelvic region can be used for rectal, ovarian, cervical, and prostate cancer. The epithelial cells within the bowels are highly susceptible to damage from radiation therapy. Acute gastrointestinal toxicity typically occurs 2-3 weeks after therapy, starting with nonspecific symptoms such as anorexia, nausea, vomiting, and diarrhea [35]. Chronic toxicity manifests in chronic diarrhea, malabsorption, proliferative mucosal telangiectasias, strictures, bowel adhesions, and/or ulceration. Chronic diarrhea and malabsorption can lead to electrolyte abnormalities that should be evaluated appropriately. Ulceration and mucosal telangiectasias can contribute to GI bleeds and anemia that requires transfusion therapy. Patients who experience excessive nausea and vomiting or have signs and symptoms of bowel obstructions may require rapid sequence induction techniques for intubation to minimize aspiration risk upon induction of anesthesia.

Although radiation traditionally has not been used for liver lesions, modern radiation therapy, such as stereotactic body therapy or yttrium 90 transarterial radioembolization, has proven an effective therapeutic option for liver malignancies [36, 37]. Despite the advancement of treatments, radiation-induced liver disease can still be observed in external radiation or radioembolization therapies. For radiation-induced liver disease, patients often experience symptomatic ascites, inflammation-induced liver enzyme elevations, and coagulopathies from liver dysfunction [38]. Hepatic injury may occur within a few weeks, months, or years of radiation therapy. It is hypothesized that veno-occlusive damage occurs secondary to the destruction of central vein lumina, leading to congestion damage. Liver function tests and coagulation studies should be performed before surgical cases, especially if fibrotic changes are suspected in the liver. Fresh frozen plasma and other coagulation products may be necessary to correct any coagulation abnormalities prior to surgery. Given the proximal location of the liver to the lungs, patients with a history of liver radiation who develop new onset of respiratory symptoms should be suspected of having possible radiation-induced lung injuries. In addition, numerous anesthetic drugs are metabolized in the liver by oxidation, reduction, hydrolysis, and conjugation mechanisms. Careful dosing of anesthetics, paralytics, and narcotics should be considered before administering drugs.

Musculoskeletal Radiation Complications and Anesthetic Considerations

Primary musculoskeletal system tumors are not usually associated with radiation therapy. However, the musculoskeletal and peripheral nerve systems can have collateral consequences from the radiation therapy to other parts of the body.

Similar to other organ systems, radiation induces tissue thickening, loss of elasticity, and parenchymal atrophy along with impaired function. Muscle weakness and atrophy can be seen in patients who have had exposure to chronic radiation therapy [39]. In addition to the weakness or atrophy, the fibrosis in the soft tissues can lead to a limited range of motion, stiffening, and asymmetric peripheral neuropathies, including the brachial plexus [40].

A detailed musculoskeletal strength exam should be performed preoperatively to establish a baseline level of function. This can also be used in the post-operative evaluation of any new-onset weakness. The patient's positioning before surgery can be challenging due to the limited range of motion and contractures. Extra care and planning should be taken when positioning and padding patients to limit any injuries to the skeletal system. Quantitative neuromuscular monitors should be applied to areas with minimal pathology to accurately quantify muscle paralysis intraoperatively so the correct reversal dose can be given. Although neuropathies are not an absolute contraindication to regional anesthesia, peripheral and neuraxial blocks should be carefully considered in these patients due to the risk of worsening symptoms. A baseline functional exam should be performed before administering any form of regional anesthesia.

CONCLUSION

Radiation therapy is one of the most extensively utilized cancer treatment options available due to its broad application and ability to cause lethal DNA damage to cancerous cells. Its success is evidenced by its use in up to 50% of all cancer treatment plans. Advances in modern radiation technology have allowed precise targeting of cancerous tissues, limiting exposure and damage to healthy adjacent structures. Despite this, significant anatomical and physiological changes to healthy tissues can still occur. Additional workup might be necessary prior to surgery for patients with a history of radiation therapy. Anesthesiologists must take special precautions in this patient population, as these changes can significantly impact the anesthesia management.

REFERENCES

[1] World Health Organization. Global cancer burden growing, amidst mounting need for services [Internet]. Geneva: World Health Organization; 2024 Feb 1 [cited 2025 Apr 30]. Available from: https://www.who.int/news/item/01-02-2024-global-cancer-burden-growing--amidst-mou-ting-need-for-services

[2] Baskar R, Lee KA, Yeo R, Yeoh KW. Cancer and radiation therapy: current advances and future directions. Int J Med Sci 2012; 9(3): 193-9. [http://dx.doi.org/10.7150/ijms.3635] [PMID: 22408567]

[3] Rose C, Lichter AS. History of radiation oncology in the United States. The ASCO Post. 2022 Jun 25 [cited 2025 Feb 1]. Available from: https://ascopost.com/issues/june-25-2022/history-of-radia-ion-oncology-in-the-united-states/

[4] Thwaites DI, Tuohy JB. Back to the future: the history and development of the clinical linear accelerator. Phys Med Biol 2006; 51(13): R343-62.
[http://dx.doi.org/10.1088/0031-9155/51/13/R20] [PMID: 16790912]

[5] Smith J, Doe A. The role of DNA repair in cancer therapy. Front Genet 2015; 6: 157.

[6] Pawlik TM, Keyomarsi K. Role of cell cycle in mediating sensitivity to radiotherapy. Int J Radiat Oncol Biol Phys 2004; 59(4): 928-42.
[http://dx.doi.org/10.1016/j.ijrobp.2004.03.005] [PMID: 15234026]

[7] Hubenak JR, Zhang Q, Branch CD, Kronowitz SJ. Mechanisms of injury to normal tissue after radiotherapy: a review. Plast Reconstr Surg 2014; 133(1): 49e-56e.
[http://dx.doi.org/10.1097/01.prs.0000440818.23647.0b] [PMID: 24374687]

[8] Gorodetska I, Kozeretska I, Dubrovska A. BRCA genes: the role in genome stability, cancer stemness and therapy resistance. J Cancer 2019; 10(9): 2109-27.
[http://dx.doi.org/10.7150/jca.30410] [PMID: 31205572]

[9] Molinari M. Cell cycle checkpoints and their inactivation in human cancer. Cell Prolif 2000; 33(5): 261-74.
[http://dx.doi.org/10.1046/j.1365-2184.2000.00191.x] [PMID: 11063129]

[10] Grant WB. The physics of radiation therapy. Johns Hopkins APL Tech Dig 1983; 4(1): 1-14.

[11] Morgan MA, Lawrence TS. Molecular pathways: overcoming radiation resistance by targeting DNA damage response pathways. Clin Cancer Res 2015; 21(13): 2898-904.
[http://dx.doi.org/10.1158/1078-0432.CCR-13-3229] [PMID: 26133775]

[12] National Cancer Institute. Radiation therapy for cancer [Internet]. Bethesda (MD): National Cancer Institute; 2020 [cited 2025 Feb 1]. Available from: https://www.cancer.gov/about-cancer/treatment/types/radiation-therapy

[13] Beckers C, Pruschy M, Vetrugno I. Tumor hypoxia and radiotherapy: A major driver of resistance even for novel radiotherapy modalities. Semin Cancer Biol 2024; 98: 19-30.
[http://dx.doi.org/10.1016/j.semcancer.2023.11.006] [PMID: 38040401]

[14] Wang H, Jiang H, Van De Gucht M, De Ridder M. Hypoxic radioresistance: can ROS be the key to overcome it? Cancers (Basel) 2019; 11(1): 112.
[http://dx.doi.org/10.3390/cancers11010112] [PMID: 30669417]

[15] Chatterjee N, Walker GC. Mechanisms of DNA damage, repair, and mutagenesis. Environ Mol Mutagen 2017; 58(5): 235-63.
[http://dx.doi.org/10.1002/em.22087] [PMID: 28485537]

[16] Koka K, Verma A, Dwarakanath BS, Papineni RVL. Technological advancements in external beam radiation therapy (EBRT): an indispensable tool for cancer treatment. Cancer Manag Res 2022; 14: 1421-9.
[http://dx.doi.org/10.2147/CMAR.S351744] [PMID: 35431581]

[17] Renard S, Parent L, de Marzi L, Tsoutsou P, Kirova Y. Electron radiation therapy: Back to the future? Cancer Radiother 2024; 28(6-7): 553-9.
[http://dx.doi.org/10.1016/j.canrad.2024.07.013] [PMID: 39389842]

[18] Quast U. Whole body radiotherapy: A TBI-guideline. J Med Phys 2006; 31(1): 5-12.
[http://dx.doi.org/10.4103/0971-6203.25664] [PMID: 21206634]

[19] National Cancer Institute. Brachytherapy to treat cancer [Internet]. Bethesda (MD): U.S. Department of Health and Human Services; [cited 2025 Feb 1]. Available from:https://www.cancer.gov/about-cancer/treatment/types/radiation-therapy/brachytherapy

[20] Kosmin M, Rees J. Radiation and the nervous system. Pract Neurol 2022; 22(6): 450-60.
[http://dx.doi.org/10.1136/pn-2022-003343] [PMID: 35995554]

[21] Young DF, Posner JB, Chu F, Nisce L. Rapid-course radiation therapy of cerebral metastases: Results and complications. Cancer 1974; 34(4): 1069-76.
[http://dx.doi.org/10.1002/1097-0142(197410)34:4<1069::AID-CNCR2820340416>3.0.CO;2-4] [PMID: 4418812]

[22] Smith ER, Scott RM. Moyamoya: epidemiology, presentation, and diagnosis. Neurosurgery Clinics 2010; 21(3): 543-51.
[PMID: 20561502]

[23] Alfouzan AF. Radiation therapy in head and neck cancer. Saudi Med J 2021; 42(3): 247-54.
[http://dx.doi.org/10.15537/smj.2021.42.3.20210660] [PMID: 33632902]

[24] Khan Joad SA, Jain D. Head and neck radiotherapy - A risk factor for anaesthesia? Indian J Anaesth 2020; 64(6): 488-94.
[http://dx.doi.org/10.4103/ija.IJA_864_19] [PMID: 32792713]

[25] Diaz R, *et al.* Hypothyroidism as a consequence of intensity-modulated radiotherapy with concurrent taxane-based chemotherapy for locally advanced head-and-neck cancer. International Journal of Radiation Oncology* Biology* Physics. 2010 Jun 1;77(2):468-76.
[http://dx.doi.org/10.1016/j.ijrobp.2009.05.018]

[26] Balakrishnan M, Kuriakose R, Koshy RC. Radiation induced changes in the airway—anaesthetic implications. Southern African Journal of Anaesthesia and Analgesia 2004; 10(2): 19-21.
[http://dx.doi.org/10.1080/22201173.2004.10872356]

[27] Muthukumar A, Dong W, Zheng G. Effects of head and neck radiotherapy on airway management outcomes. JCA Advances 2024; 1(3-4): 100039.
[http://dx.doi.org/10.1016/j.jcadva.2024.100039]

[28] Gaillard F, Campos A, Murphy A, *et al.* Radiation-induced lung disease. Reference article, Radiopaedia.org (Accessed on 28 Nov 2024).
[http://dx.doi.org/10.53347/rID-9273]

[29] Kainthola A, Haritwal T, Tiwari M, *et al.* Immunological aspect of radiation-induced pneumonitis, current treatment strategies, and future prospects. Front Immunol 2017; 8: 506.
[http://dx.doi.org/10.3389/fimmu.2017.00506] [PMID: 28512460]

[30] Tsoutsou PG, Koukourakis MI. Radiation pneumonitis and fibrosis: mechanisms underlying its pathogenesis and implications for future research. International Journal of Radiation Oncology* Biology* Physics. 2006 Dec 1;66(5):1281-93.
[http://dx.doi.org/10.1016/j.ijrobp.2006.08.058]

[31] Jain V, Berman A. Radiation pneumonitis: old problem, new tricks. Cancers (Basel) 2018; 10(7): 222.
[http://dx.doi.org/10.3390/cancers10070222] [PMID: 29970850]

[32] Restrictive Lung Disease Considerations | considerations [Internet]. considerations. 2016 [cited 2025 Apr 29]. Available from: https://www.anesthesiaconsiderations.com/restrictive-lung-disea-e-considerations

[33] Banfill K, Giuliani M, Aznar M, *et al.* Cardiac toxicity of thoracic radiotherapy: existing evidence and future directions. J Thorac Oncol 2021; 16(2): 216-27.
[http://dx.doi.org/10.1016/j.jtho.2020.11.002] [PMID: 33278607]

[34] Chang HM, Okwuosa TM, Scarabelli T, *et al.* Cardiovascular Complications of Cancer Therapy. J Am Coll Cardiol 2017; 70(20): 2552-65.
[http://dx.doi.org/10.1016/j.jacc.2017.09.1095] [PMID: 29145955]

[35] O'Brien PC. Radiation injury of the rectum. Radiother Oncol 2001; 60(1): 1-14.
[http://dx.doi.org/10.1016/S0167-8140(01)00378-4] [PMID: 11410298]

[36] Vernuccio F, Godfrey D, Meyer M, *et al.* Local tumor control and patient outcome using stereotactic body radiation therapy for hepatocellular carcinoma: iRECIST as a potential substitute for traditional

criteria. AJR Am J Roentgenol 2019; 213(6): 1232-9.
[http://dx.doi.org/10.2214/AJR.18.20842] [PMID: 31613663]

[37] Yuan H, Liu F, Li X, Guan Y, Wang M. Transcatheter arterial chemoembolization combined with simultaneous DynaCT-guided radiofrequency ablation in the treatment of solitary large hepatocellular carcinoma. Radiol Med (Torino) 2019; 124(1): 1-7.
[http://dx.doi.org/10.1007/s11547-018-0932-1] [PMID: 30132184]

[38] Sangro B, Gil-Alzugaray B, Rodriguez J, *et al.* Liver disease induced by radioembolization of liver tumors: description and possible risk factors. Cancer 2008; 112(7): 1538-46.

[39] Stubblefield MD. Radiation fibrosis syndrome: neuromuscular and musculoskeletal complications in cancer survivors. PM R 2011; 3(11): 1041-54.
[http://dx.doi.org/10.1016/j.pmrj.2011.08.535] [PMID: 22108231]

[40] Fijardo M, Kwan JYY, Bissey PA, Citrin DE, Yip KW, Liu FF. The clinical manifestations and molecular pathogenesis of radiation fibrosis. EBioMedicine 2024; 103: 105089.
[http://dx.doi.org/10.1016/j.ebiom.2024.105089] [PMID: 38579363]

CHAPTER 6

Effects of Anesthesia on Cancer

Siddhi Desai[1,*], **Michael Mahrous**[1] and **Bharathi Gourkanti**[1]

[1] *Department of Anesthesiology, Cooper Medical School of Rowan University, Cooper University Health Care, Camden, NJ, USA*

Abstract: The aim of this chapter is to explore the effects of perioperative anesthetic choices on cancer biology and recurrence. By looking at current research, this chapter compares how different anesthetic agents can affect immune function, inflammatory processes, and tumor progression. This chapter compares the effects of intravenous and volatile anesthetics, as well as the effects of commonly used analgesics. The goal of this chapter is to equip clinicians with basic knowledge on these effects to guide the creation of tailored anesthetic strategies in this relatively large patient population. This chapter also emphasizes the need for further research on these effects due to the relative lack of randomized controlled trials.

Keywords: Opioids, Anesthesia, Blood product transfusion, Cancer progression, Ketamine, Propofol, Volatile anesthetics, Wound healing.

INTRODUCTION

The perioperative period is a crucial period for patients undergoing surgery for cancer treatment. Surgery causes systemic inflammation, immunosuppression, and metabolic changes in the body- all of which create an environment susceptible to tumor growth. In addition to surgical stress, anesthetics and analgesics can also influence immune system response, tumor cell angiogenesis, and proliferation, which can potentially lead to tumor recurrence and metastasis. This chapter reviews current evidence on the immunological and oncologic effects of various anesthetics, including volatile and intravenous agents, regional anesthesia, opioids, and adjunctive medications. By exploring the mechanisms through which these agents affect tumor biology—such as changes in immune cell activity, cytokine production, angiogenesis, and gene expression—anesthesiologist can better tailor their plan to optimize perioperative cancer care.

* **Corresponding author Siddhi Desai:** Department of Anesthesiology, Cooper Medical School of Rowan University, Cooper University Health Care, Camden, NJ, USA; E-mail: desai-siddhi@cooperhealth.edu

Bharathi Gourkanti, Irwin Gratz, William Marion, Rajiv Lingaraju & Grace Abramian (Eds.)

Volatile Anesthetics and Cancer Progression

Research on the link between volatile anesthetics and cancer development is still in progress. Recent research, however, has revealed that *via* several biological mechanisms, volatile anesthetics may affect cancer outcomes. Volatile anesthetics can compromise the immune system and encourage tumor growth, therefore increasing the chance of metastases and worsening the long-term cancer prognosis [1].

Proinflammatory Effects and Immunomodulatory Actions

Volatile anesthetics such as isoflurane and sevoflurane impact the immune system by changing the balance between T-helper 1 (Th1) and T-helper 2 (Th2) cells. While Th1 cells more actively contribute to anti-inflammatory actions, Th2 cells help to induce inflammation. Research on volatile anesthetics has revealed a stronger drive toward a Th2-dominant immune response [2]. For instance, research by Ji *et al.* revealed that during surgery, the Th1/Th2 ratio was much reduced by sevoflurane [3]. In a similar context, Saha *et al.* found that isoflurane lowered CD4+ T-helper cell numbers, most likely in response to elevation of anti-inflammatory cytokines, creating a Th2-dominant immunological response that might promote tumor growth and spread [4]. Volatile anesthetics have also been shown to reduce another key lymphocyte of the innate immune system, natural killer (NK) cells. NK cells play a crucial role in tumor surveillance and control of infections. This suppression is partly mediated through the inhibition of adhesion molecules such as leukocyte function-associated antigen-1 (LFA-1). LFA-1 is crucial for natural killer (NK) cell activation and their ability to kill target cells. It facilitates the formation of the immunological synapse and promotes adhesion between NK cells and their targets [5]. Though they do not change the degranulation process, volatile anesthetics reduce NK cell activity by interfering with their capacity to form efficient conjugations and polarizations with target cells [5]. Reduced NK cell activity during the perioperative phase could help to explain higher susceptibility to tumor spread and infections.

Using volatile anesthetics lowers the quantity and activity of circulating natural killer (NK) cells both during and after surgery, therefore perhaps causing immunosuppression [6].

Impact of Cellular Apoptosis and Tumor Proliferation

Volatile anesthetics have been shown to induce apoptosis in major components of the immune system, such as T cells and B cells, *via* a mitochondria-dependent caspase-mediated pathway [7]. The mitochondria-dependent caspase pathway is a critical apoptotic process in which mitochondria cause cell death by releasing proteins into the cytoplasm, which activates caspases [7]. These effector caspases subsequently execute cell death by cleaving a range of proteins, resulting in DNA breakage and cell shrinkage [7, 8].

Across several cell types and tissues, volatile anesthetics have been demonstrated to potentially upregulate hypoxia-inducible factors (HIFs), particularly HIF-1α. HIFs a transcription factor that enables cells to tolerate low oxygen levels (hypoxia), specifically fast-expanding tumors that exceed their blood supply [9]. In a study by *Qi Fang Li*, Hep3b cells, a human hepatocellular carcinoma (HCC) cell line, were exposed to volatile anesthetics [9]. In their study, when Hep3B cells were exposed to isoflurane, it stimulated a time- and concentration-dependent increase in HIF-1α protein levels [9]. This upregulation of HIF-1α enhances the expression of several downstream target genes, including heme oxygenase 1, inducible nitric oxide synthase, and vascular endothelial growth factor (VEGF) [9]. Furthermore, the elevation of VEGF helps new blood vessels to develop. These new capillaries stimulate additional development and provide routes for tumor cells to enter the bloodstream (metastasis).

Volatile anesthetics have also been shown to enhance the transcription of pro-metastatic factors such as MMP-2 and MMP-9. MMP2 and MMP9 are matrix metalloproteinases, a type of enzyme that is essential for tissue remodeling and breakdown [10]. Both take part in a number of physiological and pathological processes, such as angiogenesis, cancer metastasis, and wound healing. It has been observed that sevoflurane and isoflurane increase MMP-2 and MMP-9 expression [10 - 12]. On the other hand, conflicting results also imply that volatile anesthetics like desflurane and sevoflurane can inhibit tumor cell invasion and lower MMP-9 secretion in specific situations, like colorectal cancer cells [13]. Depending on the cancer type and anesthetic used, these two studies demonstrate the intricate and context-dependent effects of volatile anesthetics on the transcription of pro-metastatic factors, which may either encourage or inhibit tumor progression.

The ability of volatile anesthetics to upregulate the expression of PD-L1 on tumor-associated macrophages supports the immunosuppressive properties of volatile anesthetics. PD-L1 stands for Programmed Death-Ligand 1, a protein that helps regulate immune responses [14]. It is a type of immune checkpoint molecule that helps control how strong the immune system's attack on cancer cells. Essentially, PD-L1 acts as a brake on the immune system [14]. This modification of the tumor microenvironment fosters an immunosuppressive milieu, which may promote the survival of tumor cells and facilitate metastasis in the post-surgical period.

In addition, volatile anesthetics and angiogenesis, as well as cell migration, also have a complex and context-dependent relationship whereby the anesthetic agent and the cellular environment affect the effects. It has been demonstrated that different mechanisms influence angiogenesis and cell migration in volatile anesthetics, including isoflurane and sevoflurane. By means of the HIF-signaling pathway, which comprises upregulation of VEGF-A and enhancement of cell migration, isoflurane has been reported to enhance renal cancer growth and malignant potential [15]. Likewise, sevoflurane has been shown to enhance migration, invasion, and colony-forming capacity of human glioblastoma cells, presumably by means of higher expression of the cell surface protein CD44 [16]. On the other hand, research indicates that some volatile anesthetics could have inhibitory effects on angiogenesis and cell migration. Unlike sevoflurane, which did not affect migration in the same study, xenon, another volatile anesthetic, has been shown to lower cell migration and the release of pro-angiogenic factors in breast adenocarcinoma cells [17]. Volatile anesthetics have generally complex effects on angiogenesis and cell migration; responses depend much on the anesthetic used and the cellular context.

After analyzing the several studies listed above, definitive conclusions cannot be formed, even if experimental and clinical data suggest that volatile anesthetics may accelerate cancer development. Further study is needed to guide evidence-based anesthetic approaches in oncologic surgery.

Propofol

Anti-inflammatory and Immunomodulatory Properties

Propofol, a widely utilized intravenous anesthetic, has considerable anti-inflammatory and immunomodulating action.

Propofol has been proven to stimulate a Th1 response, therefore changing the T-helper 1 (Th1)/T-helper 2 (Th2) balance, unlike several volatile anesthetics. Propofol anesthesia, according to Ji *et al.*, stimulates T-helper cell development toward the Th1 phenotype, hence raising the Th1/Th2 ratio during surgical operations [3]. Under general anesthesia, a Th1 reaction facilitates the expansion and preservation of the cell-mediated immune response. Moreover, unlike isoflurane, which was linked to a notable decline in the Th1/Th2 ratio, Inada *et al.* discovered that propofol anesthesia has no influence on this ratio following surgery [18]. These results, especially considering volatile anesthetics, imply that propofol might have an immunological benefit in either preserving or boosting Th1-mediated responses.

Suppression of Prostaglandin and Inflammatory Cytokine Production

Propofol has been reported to exert anti-tumor effects through several molecular mechanisms. Specifically, it downregulates the expression of pro-inflammatory cytokines, including interleukin-6 (IL-6) and interleukin-8 (IL-8), as well as cyclooxygenase-2 (COX-2), and prostaglandin E2 (PGE2) [19]. Propofol inhibits COX-2, an inducible enzyme involved in the synthesis of prostaglandins, which leads to decreased production of prostaglandin E2 (PGE2) as evidenced in studies utilizing murine peritoneal macrophages and human monocytic cells [18 - 20]. Given the immunosuppressive role of PGE2 in the tumor microenvironment, its downregulation by propofol may enhance antitumor immune responses [20]. Notably, the diminished expression of PGE2 has been associated with increased levels of interferon-gamma (IFN-γ) produced by natural killer (NK) cells, thereby augmenting their cytotoxic activity and enhancing the immune-mediated tumor surveillance activity [20]. Additionally, inhibition of COX-2 leads to decreased levels of VEGF, which is critical for endothelial cell proliferation and neovascularization within the tumor microenvironment. By inhibition of VEGF, propofol works to reduce tumor angiogenesis, proliferation, and metastasis, ultimately suppressing tumor development and metastatic potential [19].

Stimulation of NK Cell Proliferation and Suppression of Cytotoxic T Lymphocyte Activity

Propofol has been shown to have both inhibitory and stimulatory effects on NK cell function. Vulcano *et al*., found that exposure to propofol significantly reduced the fraction of CD56^dimCD16^bright natural killer (NK) cells, which are the most cytotoxic phenotype of NK cells [5]. This data shows propofol's possible immunosuppressive mechanism, which is similar to the effects of volatile anesthetics on NK cell function. '

Clinical studies, notably in perioperative situations involving cancer patients, have shown that propofol administration enhances NK cell function and tumor cytotoxicity. Propofol has been shown in colon cancer patients to boost natural killer (NK) cell activity and tumoricidal efficacy [5]. Propofol specifically boosted the expression of NK cell activation receptors and cytotoxic effector molecules, while also increasing NK cell proliferation [5]. These data suggest that propofol promotes NK cell function throughout the perioperative phase, potentially boosting immune surveillance and outcomes in cancer surgeries.

Propofol inhibits T cell function through multiple routes. First, it inhibits T cell glycolytic metabolism, which is required for T cell activation and function [21]. By limiting T cell activation, T cells differentiate into effectors, which leads to a decrease in cytokine production, reducing the anti-tumor effectiveness of CD8+ T cells [21]. Propofol has also been demonstrated to prevent the binding of lymphocyte function-associated antigen-1 (LFA-1) to intercellular adhesion molecule-1 (ICAM-1), which is essential for T cell proliferation and interleukin-2 production [22]. This inhibition works by a competitive mechanism, which directly reduces T cell proliferation and IL-2 production [22]. These immunosuppressive effects may impair both antitumor immunity and the host's ability to respond effectively to viral threats.

Modulation of Genetic Signaling Pathways and Inhibition of Histone Acetylation

Propofol primarily regulates cancer cell gene expression by inhibiting histone acetylation, specifically *via* the sirtuin deacetylase SIRT2. Propofol inhibits SIRT2, which regulates the cell cycle, apoptosis, and stress responses by deacetylating histones and other substrates [23]. Propofol may alter the acetylation landscape within cancer cells by inhibiting SIRT2, which could contribute to its anti-cancer properties, such as decreased cell proliferation, migration, and invasion [23].

In conclusion, propofol has largely anti-tumor effects, although some pro-tumor effects have been observed, emphasizing the need for more clinical research.

Ketamine

Ketamine, an anesthetic and analgesic medicine, has been demonstrated to directly affect cancer cells by inhibiting growth, activating death, and, in some instances, augmenting ferroptosis [24]. According to a growing number of *in vitro* and *in vivo* studies, ketamine appears to be able to inhibit the proliferation and migration of many cancer cell types, including neuroglioma, lung, colorectal, breast, and liver cancer cells, by blocking the N-methyl-D-aspartate (NMDA) receptor and subsequent downstream signaling [25 - 27].

Ketamine-induced mortality in glioma cells was observed as a result of NMDA receptor inhibition [28]. Apoptosis has also been observed in lung cancer due to elevated CD69 expression levels [28]. Furthermore, in preclinical models of breast and liver cancer, ketamine has been shown to induce ferroptosis, a type of controlled cell death characterized by iron-dependent lipid peroxidation [29].

However, not all of the studies support a protective effect. Long-term ketamine usage may promote tumor growth in some circumstances, such as breast cancer, where it has been proven to increase metastases [30]. It works by activating oncogenic signaling pathways in the tumor microenvironment [30]. These findings highlight the context-dependent nature of ketamine's effects on cancer, which vary depending on tumor type, dosage, and exposure time. Although its role in oncology is being studied, no clinical guidelines from major oncologic or anesthesiology organizations recommend ketamine as an anti-cancer treatment at this time. Although its postoperative use for anesthesia and analgesia in cancer patients is not restricted based on known evidence, the long-term oncologic effects of ketamine exposure remain unknown and necessitate more prospective investigation [31].

To summarize, ketamine has both anti- and pro-tumor actions. Its influence varies depending on the situation, highlighting the importance of ongoing clinical research before recommending treatments.

Thiopental

Though less commonly used, thiopental has been shown to have significant immunosuppressive effects, particularly in the perioperative setting. Thiopental has been shown in experimental studies to decrease leukocyte cytotoxic activity against tumor cells *in vitro*, thereby impairing tumor immune surveillance and response [32]. Furthermore, in mice models, thiopental has been related to a higher incidence of lung metastases, showing that its immunosuppressive effects may contribute to metastatic progression [33].

Thiopental inhibits the activation of NF-κB, a transcription factor that regulates proinflammatory gene expression [34]. Inhibition of this pathway reduces cytokine production, particularly TNF-α, in human glioma cells [34]. Furthermore, thiopental has been shown to promote lymphocyte mortality, which may explain perioperative lymphopenia and increased susceptibility to infection [35]

These findings indicate that thiopental can lower immunity, limit inflammatory reactions, and improve metastatic potential, hence influencing clinical outcomes in cancer patients.

Dexmedetomidine

Dexmedetomidine, a commonly used anesthetic and selective α2-adrenergic receptor agonist, has been linked to increased immune response against cancer cells. Preclinical studies on mice models of colorectal cancer found increased $CD4^+$ and $CD8^+$ T-cell function and activity, leading to decreased tumor growth [36]. In lung cancer models, dexmedetomidine increased NK cell function, which slowed tumor growth [37].

Clinical trials, particularly in women undergoing uterine cancer surgery, have demonstrated its immunomodulating capabilities. Dexmedetomidine administration has been linked to reduced opioid use, increased postoperative interferon-gamma (IFN-γ), and improved early postoperative recovery [38].

Several studies, however, have raised concerns regarding dexmedetomidine's potential pro-metastatic effects. Dexmedetomidine increased metastatic burden in mice models of breast, lung, and colon cancer *via* α2 adrenergic signaling pathways, potentially altering tumor cell adhesion, migration, and evasion in the tumor microenvironment [39].

Dexmedetomidine can cause metastatic illness in some cancers but can also induce anti-tumor immunity in others. More research is needed to determine its impact on perioperative strategies for oncological surgery.

Opioids

Increased Mu Opioid Receptor and the Effects on Tumor Growth

Although opioids are commonly used to relieve perioperative pain, their role in cancer growth has piqued researchers' interest. Opioids trigger the sympathetic nervous system. High amounts of catecholamine and cortisol suppress cytotoxic T lymphocytes (CTLs) and natural killer (NK) cells, decreasing innate immunity [40]. This neuroendocrine-immune relationship is critical for immunological surveillance, particularly under physically demanding conditions and during the perioperative phase.

Cancer cells have been found to have greater levels of the mu-opioid receptor (MOR), which may explain tumor cell proliferation, migration, invasion, and epithelial-mesenchymal transitions [41]. MOR overexpression has been associated with increased tumor growth and metastasis in non-small cell lung cancer (NSCLC) [42]. MOR activation has been shown in both *in vitro* and *in vivo* models of head and neck squamous cell carcinoma (HNSCC) to promote tumor formation and metastatic potential [43]. In hepatocellular carcinoma (HCC), increased MOR expression and activity are associated with aggressive tumor features, metastasis, and a poor prognosis [[44]. The findings demonstrate the importance of MOR in the genesis and spread of malignancies across a wide range of cancer types.

Immunosuppressive Effects

MOR expression in combination with Toll-like receptor 4 (TLR4) has also been shown to have immunomodulatory effects on NK cells [45]. Morphine, methadone, and buprenorphine have been shown to reduce NK cells' cytotoxic activity, limiting their ability to recognize and destroy cancer cells [45]. Fentanyl and tramadol have minimal to no suppressive effects, implying that the degree of immunosuppression is determined by the opioid's receptor binding location [46].

Furthermore, activation of the MOR inhibits the manufacture of pro-inflammatory cytokines such as tumor necrosis factor (TNF) and interleukin-6 (IL-6), which is particularly evident with morphine [47].

Opioids have an effect on chemokine production in addition to lowering cytokines. Morphine has been shown to reduce chemokine release, particularly interleukin-8 (IL-8), which contributes to opioid immunosuppressive effects [48].

Impact on Wound Healing and Tumor Growth

Regular morphine usage has been associated with decreased immune cell recruitment to the wound site, delaying tissue regeneration and increasing susceptibility to infection [49]. Reducing physical and immunological barriers allows the immunosuppressive impact to indirectly promote metastatic processes.

Opioids have also been shown to have an effect on extracellular matrix remodeling and cell migration. Lowering matrix metalloproteinase-9 (MMP-9) activity and increasing tissue inhibitors of metalloproteinases (TIMPs) reduce endothelial and breast cancer cell chemotactic capacity [50]. These changes may limit invasion in some cases; however, the kind of tumor and the microenvironment will alter the overall impact on metastases [50, 51].

Opioids are also angiogenesis mediators, which are important for tumor formation and wound healing. Opioids in breast cancer cells increase HIF-1α and COX-2 expression, leading to increased angiogenesis and metastasis [52].

These findings highlight the importance of judicious opioid use in cancer patients, as they balance effective analgesia with the potential implications of tumor formation and insufficient wound healing.

Regional Anesthesia and Local Anesthetics

Local anesthetics, such as lidocaine, bupivacaine, and ropivacaine, have been demonstrated in studies to induce cancer cell death by increasing both internal (mitochondria-related cytochrome c release) and external (death receptor-related) pathways [53].

Aside from death receptor-mediated pathways, local anesthetics can cause a stress reaction in the cell, directing it to death [54]. Furthermore, local anesthetics increase the activation of genes that promote cell death [55].

Inhibition of Tumor Cell Growth and Migration

Local anesthetics are known for their ability to prevent tumor cell proliferation, migration, and invasion. Amide-type local anesthetics, such as lidocaine and ropivacaine, have been found to reduce cancer cell motility and invasiveness by influencing metastasis-related signaling pathways [56]. Furthermore, local anesthetics suppress matrix metalloproteinase (MMP) secretion, which leads to extracellular matrix breakdown and a reduction in metastatic potential [57]. Finally, they can alter the tumor microenvironment by blocking chemokine-mediated cell movement, which reduces tumor migration and invasion [56].

Immune Function Enhancement

Local anesthetics, like volatile and intravenous anesthetics, affect both innate and adaptive immune responses by affecting NK and T-helper ($CD4^+$) cells [58]. *In vitro* studies have shown that lidocaine can boost NK cell cytotoxicity by upregulating activating surface receptors and increasing lytic granule release [59]. In contrast, NK cell cytotoxicity may be suppressed at higher concentrations or when using more lipophilic local anesthetics such as bupivacaine and ropivacaine [60].

Lidocaine has been shown to increase the number of $CD4^+$ T cells in peripheral blood, as well as the $CD4^+/CD8^+$ ratio and the frequency of $CD29^+$ (helper-inducer) T cells, hence increasing adaptive immunity [61]. Lidocaine has been shown to reduce T cell proliferation and cytokine production by blocking IL-2 and TNF-α [58].

Preservation of Th1/Th2 Ratio and IFN-gamma Levels

Local anesthetics can preserve the Th1/Th2 ratio and IFN-γ levels, especially during surgical stress and inflammation, promoting a stronger immune response [62].

Reduction of Pro-inflammatory Cytokines like IL-10, IL-8, and TNF-alpha

Local anesthetics have been shown to reduce pro-inflammatory cytokines such as TNF-α and IL-8 [62]. In addition to blocking pro-inflammatory mediators, lidocaine has been shown in animal models to increase anti-inflammatory cytokine levels in plasma and lung tissue [63]. The shift to an anti-inflammatory cytokine profile, particularly in the context of tissue injury or infection, indicates a rebalancing of the immune response. Suppressing pro-inflammatory signaling pathways, such as NF-κB, increases anti-inflammatory effects [64].

Local anesthetics reduce inflammation by increasing anti-inflammatory mediators such as IL-10 and decreasing cytokine production (*e.g.*, TNF-α, IL-8).

The Role of NSAIDs and COX Inhibitors

Inhibition of Cyclooxygenase (COX-2) and Prostaglandins (PGE)

COX-2, which is frequently overexpressed in many cancers, is critical for carcinogenesis because it promotes cell proliferation, angiogenesis, invasion, metastases, and resistance to death [65]. The principal output of COX-2 activity, prostaglandin E2 (PGE2), largely mediates these effects [66]. Pharmacological suppression of COX-2, using either nonsteroidal anti-inflammatory drugs (NSAIDs) or COX-2 inhibitors, suppresses PGE2 synthesis and thereby downregulates these carcinogenic pathways [67]. This results in decreased tumor cell proliferation and angiogenesis, decreased metastatic capacity, increased death signaling, and improved susceptibility to chemotherapy and radiotherapy.

Reduction in Prostaglandin Synthesis, Limiting Inflammation, and Possibly Tumor Growth

Additionally, changing the tumor microenvironment by reducing inflammatory cytokines and modifying immune cell recruitment, as well as by blocking COX-2 and so lowering PGE2 levels, would all help to produce antitumor effects [[68]. Furthermore, implicated in the modulation of tumor angiogenesis and lymphangiogenesis is prostaglandin signaling *via* certain receptors [[68]. Tumor development and metastases depend on these mechanisms, which emphasizes the need for prostaglandin generation in the malignant cells [69].

Effects of Perioperative Blood and Crystalloid Transfusion on CancerRecurrence

Blood Transfusion Effect

Perioperative blood transfusion, particularly allogeneic red blood cell transfusion, has been repeatedly related to a higher risk of cancer recurrence and a worse survival rate across numerous solid tumor types [70]. Patients undergoing curative-intent surgery for malignancies such as colorectal and lung cancer provide very strong evidence [71]. Significantly, the association appears to be dose-dependent; larger transfusion volumes are associated with a higher likelihood of recurrence and poorer long-term results [70]. Despite these consistent findings, the quality of the evidence remains limited because patients who receive transfusions typically have more advanced disease, experience more intraoperative blood loss, or have significant comorbidities—all of which independently increase the risk of cancer recurrence [70].

Translocation-related immunomodulation (TRIM) has been proposed as a biological explanation for the association between transfusion and cancer recurrence [72]. TRIM may involve cytokine profile alterations, suppression of cell-mediated immunity, and increased regulatory T cell activity [73]. Though a causal link between transfusion and oncologic outcomes has not been established, the clinical significance of these immunologic changes is debated [73]. Furthermore, while recent results demonstrate that reducing leukocytes in transfused blood products does not eliminate the relationship with poor oncologic outcomes, the initial assumptions predicted that it would lessen potential immunosuppressive effects [74].

Current best practice recommends limiting perioperative transfusions until more conclusive data is available [70].

Crystalloid Transfusion Effect

There is no established association between crystalloid administration and cancer recurrence. All available data and concerns regarding recurrence risk pertain to blood transfusions, not to crystalloid administration, therefore suggesting that crystalloid administration does not impact the progression of cancer. More data and research are needed to better understand if a correlation exists.

Albumin and Its Dual Effects on Cancer Progression

Albumin shows different, context-dependent effects on cancer progression that change depending on tumor type and microenvironment. Albumin suppresses tumor growth and invasion in hepatocellular carcinoma (HCC), hence preventing development [75]. Clear cell renal cell carcinoma has also been linked to similar tumor-suppressive effects, presumably mediated by production of endoplasmic reticulum stress and resulting tumor cellular death [76].

On the other hand, albumin could help tumors grow, as shown in B-cell chronic lymphocytic leukemia [77]. Albumin triggers AKT signaling, therefore shielding cells from radiation and chemotherapy-induced death [77].

In conclusion, albumin can suppress or promote cancer cell growth depending on tumor type and cellular context.

CONCLUSION

During the perioperative phase, anesthetics and analgesics have complex impacts on the immune system, inflammation, and tumor biology. Volatile anesthetics, opioids, and drugs like thiopental have been linked to immunosuppressive effects that may promote tumors to grow and spread. On the other hand, intravenous drugs like propofol, local anesthetics, and some adjuncts like NSAIDs have been shown to exhibit anti-tumor properties. However, these effects are highly context-dependent, varying across cancer types and patient-specific factors.

Understanding the relationship between anesthetics, immune surveillance, and cancer progression is critical for creating perioperative therapies that reduce oncological risk. While precise clinical guidelines are still being developed, available research suggests that anesthetic procedures have the potential to alter long-term cancer outcomes. Future research, particularly prospective, randomized clinical trials, is needed to validate these findings and inform evidence-based anesthetic procedures for oncologic patients.

REFERENCES

[1] Yang W, Cai J, Zabkiewicz C, Zhang H, Ruge F, Jiang WG. The Effects of Anesthetics on Recurrence and Metastasis of Cancer, and Clinical Implications. World J Oncol 2017; 8(3): 63-70. [http://dx.doi.org/10.14740/wjon1031e] [PMID: 29147437]

[2] Schreiber S, Hammers CM, Kaasch AJ, Schraven B, Dudeck A, Kahlfuss S. Metabolic Interdependency of Th2 Cell-Mediated Type 2 Immunity and the Tumor Microenvironment. Front Immunol 2021; 12: 632581. [http://dx.doi.org/10.3389/fimmu.2021.632581] [PMID: 34135885]

[3] JI, Fu-hai; WANG, Yu-lan; YANG, Jian-ping. Effects of propofol anesthesia and sevoflurane anesthesia on the differentiation of human T-helper cells during surgery. Chinese Medical Journal 124(4): p 525-529, February 2011. [http://dx.doi.org/10.3760/cma.j.issn.0366-6999.2011.04.008]

[4] Saha P, Das D, Behera SK, *et al.* Management of T cell responses by anesthetic drugs-propofol & isoflurane in perioperative breast cancer patients: A prospective hospital-based study. Indian J Med Res 2024; 160(5): 489-500. [http://dx.doi.org/10.25259/ijmr_2382_23] [PMID: 39737515]

[5] Vulcano TJ, Abdulahad WH, van Meurs M, Jongman RM, Struys MMRF, Bosch DJ. The impact of different anesthetics on the distribution and cytotoxic function of nk cell subpopulations: An *in vitro* study. Int J Mol Sci 2024; 25(20): 11045. [http://dx.doi.org/10.3390/ijms252011045] [PMID: 39456827]

[6] Liu S, Wang B, Li S, *et al.* Immune cell populations decrease during craniotomy under general anesthesia. Anesth Analg 2011; 113(3): 572-7. [http://dx.doi.org/10.1213/ANE.0b013e3182278237] [PMID: 21813628]

[7] Loop T, Dovi-Akue D, Frick M, *et al.* Volatile anesthetics induce caspase-dependent, mitochondria-mediated apoptosis in human T lymphocytes *in vitro.* Anesthesiology 2005; 102(6): 1147-57. [http://dx.doi.org/10.1097/00000542-200506000-00014] [PMID: 15915027]

[8] Matsuoka H, Kurosawa S, Horinouchi T, Kato M, Hashimoto Y. Inhalation anesthetics induce apoptosis in normal peripheral lymphocytes *in vitro.* Anesthesiology 2001; 95(6): 1467-72.

[http://dx.doi.org/10.1097/00000542-200112000-00028] [PMID: 11748407]

[9] Li QF, Wang XR, Yang YW, Su DS. Up-regulation of hypoxia inducible factor 1α by isoflurane in Hep3B cells. Anesthesiology 2006; 105(6): 1211-9. [http://dx.doi.org/10.1097/00000542-200612000-00021] [PMID: 17122584]

[10] Song Z, Wang J, Su Q, Luan M, Chen X, Xu X. The role of MMP-2 and MMP-9 in the metastasis and development of hypopharyngeal carcinoma. Rev Bras Otorrinolaringol (Engl Ed) 2021; 87(5): 521-8. [Internet]. [PMID: 31882379]

[11] Chen Y, Ouyang W, Lv H, Chen W. Exploring the mechanisms by which common inhalational anesthetics influence malignant tumor metastasis: A data mining study based on comparative toxicogenomic databases. Ecotoxicol Environ Saf 2025; 289: 117660-0. [http://dx.doi.org/10.1016/j.ecoenv.2024.117660] [PMID: 39765114]

[12] Iwasaki M, Zhao H, Jaffer T, *et al.* Volatile anaesthetics enhance the metastasis related cellular signalling including CXCR2 of ovarian cancer cells. Oncotarget 2016; 7(18): 26042-56. [http://dx.doi.org/10.18632/oncotarget.8304] [PMID: 27028996]

[13] Müller-Edenborn B, Roth-Z'graggen B, Bartnicka K, *et al.* Volatile anesthetics reduce invasion of colorectal cancer cells through down-regulation of matrix metalloproteinase-9. Anesthesiology 2012; 117(2): 293-301. [http://dx.doi.org/10.1097/ALN.0b013e3182605df1] [PMID: 22739763]

[14] Zhang H, Liu L, Liu J, *et al.* Roles of tumor-associated macrophages in anti-PD-1/PD-L1 immunotherapy for solid cancers. Mol Cancer 2023; 22(1): 58. [http://dx.doi.org/10.1186/s12943-023-01725-x] [PMID: 36941614]

[15] Benzonana LL, Perry NJS, Watts HR, *et al.* Isoflurane, a commonly used volatile anesthetic, enhances renal cancer growth and malignant potential *via* the hypoxia-inducible factor cellular signaling pathway *in vitro.* Anesthesiology 2013; 119(3): 593-605. [http://dx.doi.org/10.1097/ALN.0b013e31829e47fd] [PMID: 23774231]

[16] Lai R, Shan W, Zhou D, *et al.* Sevoflurane promotes migration, invasion, and colony-forming ability of human glioblastoma cells possibly *via* increasing the expression of cell surface protein 44. Acta Pharmacol Sin 2019; 40(11): 1424-35. [http://dx.doi.org/10.1038/s41401-019-0221-0] [PMID: 30967592]

[17] Zhou X, Shao Y, Li S, *et al.* An intravenous anesthetic drug-propofol, influences the biological characteristics of malignant tumors and reshapes the tumor microenvironment: A narrative literature review. Front Pharmacol 2022; 13: 1057571. [http://dx.doi.org/10.3389/fphar.2022.1057571] [PMID: 36506511]

[18] Inada T, Kubo K, Kambara T, Koh Shingu. Propofol inhibits cyclo-oxygenase activity in human monocytic THP-1 cells. Canadian Journal of Anesthesia/Journal canadien d anesthésie. 2009 Jan 28;56(3):222–9.

[19] Li X, Li L, Liang F, Liu G, Zhao G. Anesthetic drug propofol inhibits the expression of interleukin-6, interleukin-8 and cyclooxygenase-2, a potential mechanism for propofol in suppressing tumor development and metastasis. Oncol Lett 2018; 15(6): 9523-8. [http://dx.doi.org/10.3892/ol.2018.8515] [PMID: 29805673]

[20] Inada T, Kubo K, Shingu K. Promotion of interferon-gamma production by natural killer cells via suppression of murine peritoneal macrophage prostaglandin E2 production using intravenous anesthetic propofol. Int Immunopharmacol 2010; 10(10): 1200-8. [http://dx.doi.org/10.1016/j.intimp.2010.06.027] [PMID: 20633531]

[21] Yamamoto W, Hamada T, Suzuki J, *et al.* Suppressive effect of the anesthetic propofol on the T cell function and T cell-dependent immune responses. Sci Rep 2024; 14(1): 19337. [http://dx.doi.org/10.1038/s41598-024-69987-z] [PMID: 39164311]

[22] Yuki K, Soriano SG, Shimaoka M. Sedative drug modulates T-cell and lymphocyte function-associated antigen-1 function. Anesth Analg 2011; 112(4): 830-8. [http://dx.doi.org/10.1213/ANE.0b013e31820dcabb] [PMID: 21385989]

[23] Weiser BP, Eckenhoff RG. Propofol inhibits SIRT2 deacetylase through a conformation-specific, allosteric site. J Biol Chem 2015; 290(13): 8559-68. [http://dx.doi.org/10.1074/jbc.M114.620732] [PMID: 25666612]

[24] He GN, Bao NR, Wang S, Xi M, Zhang TH, Chen FS. Ketamine Induces Ferroptosis of Liver Cancer Cells by Targeting lncRNA PVT1/miR-214-3p/GPX4. Drug Des Devel Ther 2021; 15: 3965-78. [http://dx.doi.org/10.2147/DDDT.S332847] [PMID: 34566408]

[25] Hu J, Duan W, Liu Y. Ketamine inhibits aerobic glycolysis in colorectal cancer cells by blocking the NMDA receptor-CaMK II-c-Myc pathway. Clin Exp Pharmacol Physiol 2020; 47(5): 848-56. Available from: https://pubmed.ncbi.nlm.nih.gov/31889340/ [http://dx.doi.org/10.1111/1440-1681.13248] [PMID: 31889340]

[26] Zhou X, Zhang P, Luo W, *et al.* Ketamine induces apoptosis in lung adenocarcinoma cells by regulating the expression of CD 69. Cancer Med 2018; 7(3): 788-95. [http://dx.doi.org/10.1002/cam4.1288] [PMID: 29453833]

[27] Niwa H, Furukawa KI, Seya K, Hirota K. Ketamine suppresses the proliferation of rat C6 glioma cells. Oncol Lett 2017; 14(4): 4911-7. [http://dx.doi.org/10.3892/ol.2017.6806] [PMID: 29085500]

[28] Saito J, Zao H, Wu L, *et al.* "Anti-cancer" effect of ketamine in comparison with MK801 on neuroglioma and lung cancer cells. Eur J Pharmacol 2023; 945: 175580. [http://dx.doi.org/10.1016/j.ejphar.2023.175580] [PMID: 36758782]

[29] Li H, Liu W, Zhang X, Wu F, Sun D, Wang Z. Ketamine suppresses proliferation and induces ferroptosis and apoptosis of breast cancer cells by targeting KAT5/GPX4 axis. Biochem Biophys Res Commun 2021; 585: 111-6. [http://dx.doi.org/10.1016/j.bbrc.2021.11.029] [PMID: 34800882]

[30] Chen LK, Chen SS, Shih CH, Huang ZX, Chen L, Chen KB. Ketamine Promoted Breast Cancer Invasion and Metastasis Through Up-regulating Wnt, BMP, and EGFR Signaling. Anticancer Res 2023; 43(12): 5415-24. [http://dx.doi.org/10.21873/anticanres.16745] [PMID: 38030191]

[31] Rodriguez Arango JA, Zec T, Khalife M. Perioperative Ketamine and Cancer Recurrence: A Comprehensive Review. J Clin Med 2024; 13(7): 1920-0. [http://dx.doi.org/10.3390/jcm13071920] [PMID: 38610685]

[32] Duncan PG, Cullen BF, Rav-Kell L. Thiopental inhibition of tumor immunity. Anesthesiology 1977; 46(2): 97-101. [http://dx.doi.org/10.1097/00000542-197702000-00003] [PMID: 835852]

[33] Lundy J, Lovett EJ III, Conran P. Pulmonary metastases, a potential biologic consequence of anesthetic-induced immunosuppression by thiopental. Surgery 1977; 82(2): 254-6. [PMID: 141748]

[34] Ichiyama T, Nishikawa M, Lipton JM, Matsubara T, Takashi H, Furukawa S. Thiopental inhibits NF-κB activation in human glioma cells and experimental brain inflammation. Brain Res 2001; 911(1): 56-61. [http://dx.doi.org/10.1016/S0006-8993(01)02672-5] [PMID: 11489444]

[35] Keel M, Mica L, Stover J, Stocker R, Trentz O, Härter L. Thiopental-induced apoptosis in lymphocytes is independent of CD95 activation. Anesthesiology 2005; 103(3): 576-84. [http://dx.doi.org/10.1097/00000542-200509000-00021] [PMID: 16129983]

[36] Chen W, Qi Z, Fan P, *et al.* Dexmedetomidine provides type-specific tumour suppression without tumour-enhancing effects in syngeneic murine models. Br J Anaesth 2023; 130(2): 142-53. Available

from: https://pubmed.ncbi.nlm.nih.gov/36494207/
[http://dx.doi.org/10.1016/j.bja.2022.10.036] [PMID: 36494207]

[37] Jun JH, Shim JK, Oh JE, Kim KS, Kwak YL, Soh S. Effects of dexmedetomidine on A549 non-small cell lung cancer growth in a clinically relevant surgical xenograft model. Sci Rep 2023; 13(1): 12471.
[http://dx.doi.org/10.1038/s41598-023-39704-3] [PMID: 37528154]

[38] Cho JS, Seon K, Kim MY, Kim SW, Yoo YC. Effects of Perioperative Dexmedetomidine on Immunomodulation in Uterine Cancer Surgery: A Randomized, Controlled Trial. Front Oncol 2021; 11: 749003.
[http://dx.doi.org/10.3389/fonc.2021.749003] [PMID: 34868950]

[39] Lavon H, Matzner P, Benbenishty A, *et al.* Dexmedetomidine promotes metastasis in rodent models of breast, lung, and colon cancers. Br J Anaesth 2018; 120(1): 188-96.
[http://dx.doi.org/10.1016/j.bja.2017.11.004] [PMID: 29397129]

[40] Adamczyk K, Zuzda K, Jankowski M, *et al.* Effects of Opioids in Cancer Pain: An Interplay Among Genetic Factors, Immune Response, and Clinical Outcomes—A Scoping Review. Cancers (Basel) 2025; 17(5): 863-3.
[http://dx.doi.org/10.3390/cancers17050863] [PMID: 40075716]

[41] Gao L, Yang L, He Y, *et al.* MOR promotes epithelial-mesenchymal transition and proliferation *via* PI3K/AKT signaling pathway in human colorectal cancer. Acta Biochim Biophys Sin (Shanghai) 2022; 55(1): 72-80.
[http://dx.doi.org/10.1093/abbs/gmt118] [PMID: 35983971]

[42] Lennon FE, Mirzapoiazova T, Mambetsariev B, *et al.* The Mu Opioid Receptor Promotes Opioid and Growth Factor-Induced Proliferation, Migration and Epithelial Mesenchymal Transition (EMT) in Human Lung Cancer. de Wever O, editor. PLoS ONE. 2014 Mar 24;9(3):e91577.

[43] Gorur A, Patiño M, Takahashi H, *et al.* Mu-opioid receptor activation promotes *in vitro* and *in vivo* tumor growth in head and neck squamous cell carcinoma. Life Sci 2021; 278: 119541.
[http://dx.doi.org/10.1016/j.lfs.2021.119541] [PMID: 33930368]

[44] Chen DT, Pan JH, Chen YH, *et al.* The mu-opioid receptor is a molecular marker for poor prognosis in hepatocellular carcinoma and represents a potential therapeutic target. Br J Anaesth 2019; 122(6): e157-67.
[http://dx.doi.org/10.1016/j.bja.2018.09.030] [PMID: 30915986]

[45] Maher DP, Walia D, Heller NM. Morphine decreases the function of primary human natural killer cells by both TLR4 and opioid receptor signaling. Brain Behav Immun 2020; 83: 298-302.
[http://dx.doi.org/10.1016/j.bbi.2019.10.011] [PMID: 31626971]

[46] Maher DP, Walia D, Heller NM. Suppression of Human Natural Killer Cells by Different Classes of Opioids. Anesth Analg 2019; 128(5): 1013-21.
[http://dx.doi.org/10.1213/ANE.0000000000004058] [PMID: 30801358]

[47] Bonnet MP, Beloeil H, Benhamou D, Mazoit JX, Asehnoune K. The μ opioid receptor mediates morphine-induced tumor necrosis factor and interleukin-6 inhibition in toll-like receptor 2-stimulated monocytes. Anesth Analg 2008; 106(4): 1142-9.
[http://dx.doi.org/10.1213/ane.0b013e318165de89] [PMID: 18349186]

[48] Bastami S, Norling C, Trinks C, *et al.* Inhibitory effect of opiates on LPS mediated release of TNF and IL-8. Acta Oncol 2013; 52(5): 1022-33.
[http://dx.doi.org/10.3109/0284186X.2012.737932] [PMID: 23145506]

[49] Martin JL, Koodie L, Krishnan AG, Charboneau R, Barke RA, Roy S. Chronic morphine administration delays wound healing by inhibiting immune cell recruitment to the wound site. Am J Pathol 2010; 176(2): 786-99.
[http://dx.doi.org/10.2353/ajpath.2010.090457] [PMID: 20042674]

[50] Xie N, Khabbazi S, Nassar ZD, *et al.* Morphine alters the circulating proteolytic profile in mice:

functional consequences on cellular migration and invasion. FASEB J 2017; 31(12): 5208-16. [http://dx.doi.org/10.1096/fj.201700546R] [PMID: 28784632]

[51] Khabbazi S, Hassanshahi M, Hassanshahi A, Peymanfar Y, Su YW, Xian CJ. Opioids and matrix metalloproteinases: the influence of morphine on MMP-9 production and cancer progression. Naunyn Schmiedebergs Arch Pharmacol 2019; 392(2): 123-33. Available from: https://pubmed.ncbi.nlm.nih.gov/30656360 [http://dx.doi.org/10.1007/s00210-019-01613-6] [PMID: 30656360]

[52] Schoos A, Gabriel C, Knab VM, Fux DA. Activation of HIF-1α by δ-Opioid Receptors Induces COX-2 Expression in Breast Cancer Cells and Leads to Paracrine Activation of Vascular Endothelial Cells. J Pharmacol Exp Ther 2019; 370(3): 480-9. [http://dx.doi.org/10.1124/jpet.119.257501] [PMID: 31300611]

[53] Chang Y-C, Hsu Y-C, Liu C-L, Huang S-Y, Hu M-C, Cheng S-P. Local Anesthetics Induce Apoptosis in Human Thyroid Cancer Cells through the Mitogen-Activated Protein Kinase Pathway. PLoS ONE 2014; 9(2): e89563. [http://dx.doi.org/10.1371/journal.pone.0089563]

[54] Bezu L, Wu Chuang A, Sauvat A, *et al.* Local anesthetics elicit immune-dependent anticancer effects. J Immunother Cancer 2022; 10(4): e004151. [http://dx.doi.org/10.1136/jitc-2021-004151] [PMID: 35483744]

[55] Haraguchi-Suzuki K, Kawabata-Iwakawa R, Suzuki T, Suto T, Takazawa T, Saito S. Local anesthetic lidocaine-inducible gene, growth differentiation factor-15 suppresses the growth of cancer cell lines. Sci Rep 2022; 12(1): 14520. [http://dx.doi.org/10.1038/s41598-022-18572-3] [PMID: 36008442]

[56] Piegeler T, Votta-Velis EG, Liu G, *et al.* Antimetastatic potential of amide-linked local anesthetics: inhibition of lung adenocarcinoma cell migration and inflammatory Src signaling independent of sodium channel blockade. Anesthesiology 2012; 117(3): 548-59. [http://dx.doi.org/10.1097/ALN.0b013e3182661977] [PMID: 22846676]

[57] Keleş D, Sipahi M, İnanç-Sürer Ş, Djamgoz MBA, Oktay G. Tetracaine downregulates matrix metalloproteinase activity and inhibits invasiveness of strongly metastatic MDA-MB-231 human breast cancer cells. Chem Biol Interact 2023; 385: 110730. [http://dx.doi.org/10.1016/j.cbi.2023.110730] [PMID: 37806380]

[58] Lahat A, Horin SB, Lang A, Fudim E, Picard O, Chowers Y. Lidocaine down-regulates nuclear factor-κB signalling and inhibits cytokine production and T cell proliferation. Clin Exp Immunol 2008; 152(2): 320-7. [http://dx.doi.org/10.1111/j.1365-2249.2008.03636.x] [PMID: 18355353]

[59] Ramirez MF, Tran P, Cata JP. The effect of clinically therapeutic plasma concentrations of lidocaine on natural killer cell cytotoxicity. Reg Anesth Pain Med 2015; 40(1): 43-8. [http://dx.doi.org/10.1097/AAP.0000000000000191] [PMID: 25469757]

[60] Krog J, Hokland M, Ahlburg P, Parner E, Tønnesen E. Lipid solubility- and concentration-dependent attenuation of *in vitro* natural killer cell cytotoxicity by local anesthetics. Acta Anaesthesiol Scand 2002; 46(7): 875-81. [http://dx.doi.org/10.1034/j.1399-6576.2002.460719.x] [PMID: 12139545]

[61] Yokoyama M, Nakatsuka H. Yoshitaro Itano, Hirakawa M. Stellate Ganglion Block Modifies the Distribution of Lymphocyte Subsets and Natural-killer Cell Activity. Anesthesiology 2000; 92(1): 109-9. [http://dx.doi.org/10.1097/00000542-200001000-00021] [PMID: 10638906]

[62] Weinschenk S, Weiss C, Benrath J, von Baehr V, Strowitzki T, Feißt M. Anti-Inflammatory Characteristics of Local Anesthetics: Inhibition of TNF-α Secretion of Lipopolysaccharide-Stimulated Leucocytes in Human Blood Samples. Int J Mol Sci 2022; 23(6): 3283. [http://dx.doi.org/10.3390/ijms23063283] [PMID: 35328706]

[63] Van Der Wal S, Vaneker M, Steegers M, *et al.* Lidocaine increases the anti-inflammatory cytokine IL - 10 following mechanical ventilation in healthy mice. Acta Anaesthesiol Scand 2015; 59(1): 47-55. [http://dx.doi.org/10.1111/aas.12417] [PMID: 25312651]

[64] Lang A, Ben Horin S, Picard O, Fudim E, Amariglio N, Chowers Y. Lidocaine inhibits epithelial chemokine secretion via inhibition of nuclear factor κB activation. Immunobiology 2010; 215(4): 304-13.
[http://dx.doi.org/10.1016/j.imbio.2009.05.006] [PMID: 19559500]

[65] Hashemi Goradel N, Najafi M, Salehi E, Farhood B, Mortezaee K. Cyclooxygenase-2 in cancer: A review. J Cell Physiol 2019; 234(5): 5683-99.
[http://dx.doi.org/10.1002/jcp.27411] [PMID: 30341914]

[66] Wang D, Cabalag CS, Clemons NJ, DuBois RN. Cyclooxygenases and Prostaglandins in Tumor Immunology and Microenvironment of Gastrointestinal Cancer. Gastroenterology 2021; 161(6): 1813-29.
[http://dx.doi.org/10.1053/j.gastro.2021.09.059] [PMID: 34606846]

[67] Harris RE. Cyclooxygenase-2 (COX-2) and the Inflammogenesis of Cancer. Sub-cellular biochemistry/Subcellular biochemistry [Internet]. 2007 Jan 1 [cited 2025 Jun 15];93–126.

[68] Li S, Jiang M, Wang L, Yu S. Combined chemotherapy with cyclooxygenase-2 (COX-2) inhibitors in treating human cancers: Recent advancement. Biomedicine & Pharmacotherapy = Biomedecine & Pharmacotherapie [Internet]. 2020 Sep 1 [cited 2023 Jan 2];129:110389.

[69] Majima M, Matsuda Y, Watanabe SI, *et al.* Prostanoids Regulate Angiogenesis and Lymphangiogenesis in Pathological Conditions. Cold Spring Harb Perspect Med 2024; 14(12): a041182.
[http://dx.doi.org/10.1101/cshperspect.a041182] [PMID: 38565267]

[70] Etheridge J, Shah P, Stanworth SJ, *et al.* Association between peri-operative red blood cell transfusion and cancer recurrence in patients undergoing major cancer surgery: an umbrella review. Anaesthesia 2025; 80(S2) (Suppl. 2): 65-74.
[http://dx.doi.org/10.1111/anae.16501] [PMID: 39775775]

[71] Tai YH, Wu HL, Mandell MS, Lin SP, Tsou MY, Chang KY. The association of non–small cell lung cancer recurrence with allogenic blood transfusion after surgical resection: A propensity score analysis of 1,803 patients. Eur J Cancer 2020; 140: 45-54.
[http://dx.doi.org/10.1016/j.ejca.2020.09.004] [PMID: 33039813]

[72] Heppell O, Lopez-Plaza I, Guerra-Londono CE. Perioperative Blood Transfusions and Cancer Progression: A Narrative Review. Curr Oncol Rep 2024; 26(8): 880-9.

[73] Cata JP, Wang H, Gottumukkala V, Reuben J, Sessler DI. Inflammatory response, immunosuppression, and cancer recurrence after perioperative blood transfusions. Br J Anaesth 2013; 110(5): 690-701.
[http://dx.doi.org/10.1093/bja/aet068] [PMID: 23599512]

[74] Deeb AP, Aquina CT, Monson JRT, Blumberg N, Becerra AZ, Fleming FJ. Allogeneic leukocyte-reduced red blood cell transfusion is associated with postoperative infectious complications and cancer recurrence after colon cancer resection. Dig Surg 2020; 37(2): 163-70.
[http://dx.doi.org/10.1159/000498865] [PMID: 30836367]

[75] Nojiri S, Joh T. Albumin suppresses human hepatocellular carcinoma proliferation and the cell cycle. Int J Mol Sci 2014; 15(3): 5163-74.
[http://dx.doi.org/10.3390/ijms15035163] [PMID: 24663086]

[76] Zhu JM, Chen SH, Xu YC, *et al.* ALB inhibits tumor cell proliferation and invasion by regulating immune microenvironment and endoplasmic reticulum stress in clear cell renal cell carcinoma. Biochim Biophys Acta Mol Basis Dis 2025; 1871(3): 167672.
[http://dx.doi.org/10.1016/j.bbadis.2025.167672] [PMID: 39862995]

[77] Jones DT, Ganeshaguru K, Anderson RJ, *et al.* Albumin activates the AKT signaling pathway and protects B-chronic lymphocytic leukemia cells from chlorambucil- and radiation-induced apoptosis. Blood 2003; 101(8): 3174-80.
[http://dx.doi.org/10.1182/blood-2002-07-2143] [PMID: 12480711]

CHAPTER 7

Anesthesia Evaluation of Cancer Patients Prior to Surgery

Michael Schwartz[1,*], **Taylor Tidwell**[1] and **Linh Le**[1]

[1] *Department of Anesthesiology and Perioperative Care, University of California, Irvine Medical Center, Orange, CA, USA*

Abstract: The population of cancer patients and the procedures they undergo have been increasing over the years. Knowing how cancer affects patients is important for perioperative anesthetic management. This chapter will describe the importance of the preoperative evaluation of cancer patients and their perioperative implications. Besides their primary cancers, these patients often have comorbidities, treatment regimens, and side effects that can affect the anesthetic plan. This chapter will explore the different organ systems affected by cancer and the perioperative considerations for the anesthesia provider.

Keywords: Airway assessment, Chemotherapy, ERAS, Frailty, Fibrosis, Hepatotoxicity, Malnutrition, Nutrition, Nephrotoxicity, Paraneoplastic syndrome, Preoperative evaluation, Radiation.

INTRODUCTION

Cancer is the second leading cause of death in the United States, with an estimated incidence of 1,958,310 cases in 2023 [1]. It has a broad clinical presentation, which includes symptoms associated with its location and spread, paraneoplastic syndromes not directly caused by the tumor, and side effects from cancer treatments such as chemotherapy or radiation.

Preoperative evaluation of the cancer patient is a multistep process that allows the anesthesiologist to both gather important medical history and develop a comprehensive intra- and postoperative management plan. Other objectives include conducting a physical exam, obtaining informed consent, and educating the patient or family on the proposed surgery and perioperative care plan [2]. This chapter examines key aspects of the preoperative evaluation of cancer patients and their impacts on anesthesia management.

* **Corresponding author Michael Schwartz:** Department of Anesthesiology and Perioperative Care, University of California, Irvine Medical Center, Orange, CA, USA; E-mail: schwarm2@hs.uci.edu

Bharathi Gourkanti, Irwin Gratz, William Marion, Rajiv Lingaraju & Grace Abramian (Eds.)

Airway Assessment

Cancer patients may have anatomical and physiological changes that complicate airway management. Tumors in the head, neck, or thoracic region can cause obstruction, restricted mouth opening, tracheal deviation, or airway compression. Earlier radiation therapy can lead to fibrosis, increased bleeding, and reduced tissue elasticity, making intubation challenging. Therefore, preoperative airway assessment is a critical component of anesthesia planning, particularly in cancer patients who may present with unique challenges due to tumor-related airway compromise, prior treatments, or anatomical changes. A thorough evaluation allows anesthesiologists to anticipate difficulties, select appropriate airway management strategies, and reduce perioperative risks [2].

Evaluation should begin with a comprehensive history to assess for comorbidities and signs of airway obstruction, including stridor, dyspnea, orthopnea, dysarthria, dysphagia, or voice changes. This should also include a history of prior surgeries, previous radiation or chemotherapy, and alcohol, tobacco, or substance use. If available, reviewing medical records for prior issues with anesthesia or difficult intubation can help guide management [3].

A thorough physical exam should include Mallampati classification, mandibular protrusion, thyromental distance, neck mobility, and auscultation of the neck for stridor. Doctors also inspect the oral cavity for tissue friability, scarring, anatomical irregularities, lesions, burns, excess mucus, or signs of infection. If airway compromise is suspected, reviewing prior imaging studies (CT/MRI) or a flexible nasopharyngoscopy may be needed to evaluate upper airway tumors.

Access/Line Placement

Vascular access is a crucial aspect of perioperative care in cancer patients, who often require long-term intravenous therapy, chemotherapy, and complex surgical procedures. These patients may present with challenges such as difficult peripheral venous access, prior central line placements, and chemotherapy-induced vascular damage [4]. A thorough preoperative vascular access evaluation allows anesthesiologists to anticipate complications, select the most appropriate access method, and optimize patient safety.

Management should be guided by the patient's overall health status, the type and duration of the planned surgery, and ongoing oncologic therapies. Many cancer patients require major procedures that involve significant fluid and electrolyte shifts, blood loss, or intraoperative chemotherapy. Peripheral IV access is the most common first step and may be adequate for minor procedures. Increasing the number or size of peripheral IVs may provide sufficient access for moderately invasive surgeries, depending on the type of procedure and the patient's other comorbidities.

For major surgeries such as those involving the thorax, abdomen, or head and neck, more secure access, such as a central venous line or peripherally inserted central catheter (PICC), may be needed. Central lines such as internal jugular, femoral, or subclavian catheters are ideal options for patients with difficult or limited peripheral access and provide stable access for fluid resuscitation, TPN, vasoactive drug administration, and central venous pressure monitoring [4]. For surgeries with significant anticipated blood loss, prolonged operative times, or patients requiring close hemodynamic monitoring, an arterial line may be indicated. This allows frequent blood sampling and arterial blood gas monitoring to guide intraoperative management.

Overall, vascular access is of critical importance to the successful management of oncology patients during the perioperative period. Access selection must be individualized based on patient history, including previous treatments, type and duration of surgery, and comorbidities.

Nutrition/Fasting/Electrolytes

Nutrition plays a critical role in the anesthetic management of cancer patients. Malnutrition and cachexia are common in this population due to treatment side effects, decreased oral intake, and metabolic demands of the disease itself. Because poor nutritional status is associated with increased morbidity and delayed recovery, it is important to identify malnourished patients and optimize nutrition with a structured preoperative diet, counseling, and supplementation in the perioperative period.

Fasting guidelines must be carefully balanced in cancer patients to reduce the risk of aspiration while minimizing the negative metabolic effects of prolonged fasting. The American Society of Anesthesiologists (ASA) standard preoperative fasting recommendations typically allow clear fluids up to 2 hours before anesthesia and a light meal up to 6 hours prior (Table **1**). However, individualized fasting plans may be necessary in cancer patients, especially those with gastrointestinal tumors, decreased motility, or delayed gastric emptying. For patients receiving enteral nutrition *via* feeding tubes, fasting recommendations should be modified based on the type of formula and the patient's current health status.

Enhanced Recovery After Surgery (ERAS) protocols increasingly advocate for preoperative carbohydrate loading and minimal fasting to preserve lean body mass and improve insulin sensitivity [5]. While this approach is generally safe and effective, it should be used with caution in cancer patients with impaired gastric motility or high risk for aspiration. Close coordination between interdisciplinary teams is essential to creating a safe, individualized fasting and nutrition plan for each cancer patient undergoing anesthesia.

Table 1. American society of anesthesiologists preoperative fasting guidelines [6].

Type of Intake	*Minimum Fasting Duration*
Clear liquids (water, clear tea, fruit juice without pulp, black coffee, carbonated beverages)	2 hours
Breast milk	4 hours
Nonhuman milk, infant formula	6 hours
Light meal, non-clear juice, juice with pulp	6 hours
Heavy meals/fatty foods	8 hours

A majority of cancers occur in the elderly population. This, along with symptoms of anorexia, dysphagia, nausea and vomiting, side effects of chemotherapy such as nephrotoxicity and hepatotoxicity, can lead to malabsorption and malnourishment. Because of this, many patients, especially those with advanced disease, may present with cachexia and frailty. Frailty is a big risk factor in perioperative complications, increased hospitalization, and increased morbidity and mortality [7].

Electrolyte derangements are also very common in cancer patients due to treatment side effects, poor oral intake, malnutrition, and tumor burden. Abnormalities include hyponatremia, hypophosphatemia, hypercalcemia, and hypo or hyperkalemia, with hyponatremia secondary to Syndrome of Inappropriate Antidiuretic Hormone (SIADH) being the most common. In other cases, electrolyte imbalances are due to paraneoplastic syndromes and may be the first presenting sign [8].

Perioperative electrolyte management is essential to prevent cardiac arrhythmias, ensure hemodynamic stability, and reduce postoperative complications. A thorough preoperative evaluation includes assessing serum electrolytes, especially in patients with significant comorbidities such as end-stage renal failure on dialysis. Other significant risk factors include malignancy, endocrine disorders, malabsorption, or those taking medications such as diuretics, chemotherapy, total parenteral nutrition, laxatives, or antidopaminergic agents [8]. Severe electrolyte derangements should be optimized preoperatively and closely managed intraoperatively for emergent or urgent procedures. Elective cases may be delayed until the patient is stable and serum electrolytes are optimized.

Toxicities from Chemotherapeutics and Radiation

All cancer patients should undergo a thorough review of current treatments preoperatively. Chemotherapy can have profound effects on several organ systems with multiple toxicity-related side effects. Toxicity levels depend on the duration of treatment, dosage, and type of agent used [2] and can be seen in Tables **2** and **3**. For more detailed information, read chapters 3, 4, and 5.

Table 2. Common chemotherapeutics and side effects.

Drug Class	Major Toxicities	Anesthesia Considerations
Platinum Agents -Cisplatin -Carboplatin	Nephrotoxicity Ototoxicity	-Renally dose medications -Avoid nephrotoxic agents -Monitor renal function
Alkylating agents -Cyclophosphamide -Ifosfamide	Hemorrhagic cystitis	-Monitor renal function, urine output, and hemoglobin.
Antimetabolites -Methotrexate -Gemcitabine -5-fluorouracil	Hepatotoxicity	-Monitor liver enzymes and coagulation factors.
Antimicrotubule Agents -Vinca Alkaloids (vincristine, vinblastine) -Taxanes (paclitaxel, docetaxel)	Peripheral neuropathy	-Careful positioning to prevent nerve injury.
Antitumor Antibiotics -Doxorubicin -Mitomycin C -Bleomycin -Busulfan	Cardiotoxicity (Doxorubicin) Pulmonary fibrosis (Bleyomycin, Busulfan)	-Preoperative cardiac evaluation. -Consider echocardiogram, stress testing, and electrocardiogram. -Avoid high FiO_2, use lung protective ventilation.
Nitrosoureas -Lomustine -Carmustine	Neurotoxicity	-Consider intraoperative nerve monitoring. -Carefully assess neurologic baseline preoperatively.

Table 3. Radiation therapy and side effects.

Organ System	Acute (up to 4 Weeks)	Intermediate (1-3 Months)	Late (Several Months to Years)
Cardiac	Pericarditis, pericardial effusion, fibrosis	-	-
Pulmonary	Exudative phase	Latent phase	Pleural effusions, pulmonary fibrosis, pneumonitis, esophagotracheal fistula

(Table 3) cont.....

Organ System	Acute (up to 4 Weeks)	Intermediate (1-3 Months)	Late (Several Months to Years)
Gastrointestinal	Malnutrition, anorexia, nausea, emesis, esophagitis, gastroenteritis, dehydration	Bowel adhesion and obstruction, enteric fistula	Malabsorption
Dermatologic	Erythema, rash, hair loss	-	-
Hematologic	Bone marrow depression	-	-
Miscellaneous	Electrolyte abnormalities	Ascites	-

Pain Management

Cancer patients often have significant chronic pain and nausea that require careful assessment in the perioperative period. Generally, most baseline medications such as antidepressants, anxiolytics, and opiates such as methadone or buprenorphine should be continued preoperatively. Reducing or holding these medications may result in acute withdrawal, hemodynamic instability, and poorly controlled pain intraoperatively. Oncologic pain should be managed with multimodal analgesia (opioids, acetaminophen, NSAIDs, gabapentinoids) to maximize comfort while also decreasing the risk of opioid dependence [9]. Other nonopioid analgesics include ketamine (bolus or drip) or tricyclic antidepressants for neuropathic pain. For major surgeries or opiate tolerant patients, methods such as intravenous patient-controlled analgesia (PCA) or regional anesthesia should be considered. Escalation of therapy should follow the World Health Organization's (WHO) Analgesic Ladder (Fig. **1**) [10] and be individualized based on patient tolerance, current pain regimen, risk of dependence, and type of surgery.

End-of-Life Care/Psychological Evaluation

Preoperative assessment of cancer patients should include the goal of care discussion, especially in patients with severe disease undergoing major surgery. In patients with terminal disease, it is imperative to have a thorough interdisciplinary discussion with the patient and their caregivers to ensure that the benefits of surgery outweigh the risks. The next step is clarifying perioperative code status with the patient, their caregivers, and the surgical care team.

Throughout this process, it is important to consider the emotional state of the patient. Cancer patients have significantly increased rates of psychological distress, with a prevalence of 5-50% (depressive disorders between 0-46%, anxiety disorders between 1-49%) [11]. These conditions are associated with poorer surgical outcomes, including increased postoperative pain, impaired wound healing, and a longer hospital stay. Referral for psychiatric evaluation and cognitive behavioral therapy may be beneficial in the weeks leading up to surgery to optimize emotional health preoperatively [12]. Providing reassurance through education about the proposed anesthetic pain, surgery, and pain management plan is an integral part of the preoperative evaluation, which may also help alleviate patient anxiety. Although often overlooked, addressing the psychosocial and emotional needs of cancer patients can significantly impact the quality of care and improve the perioperative experience.

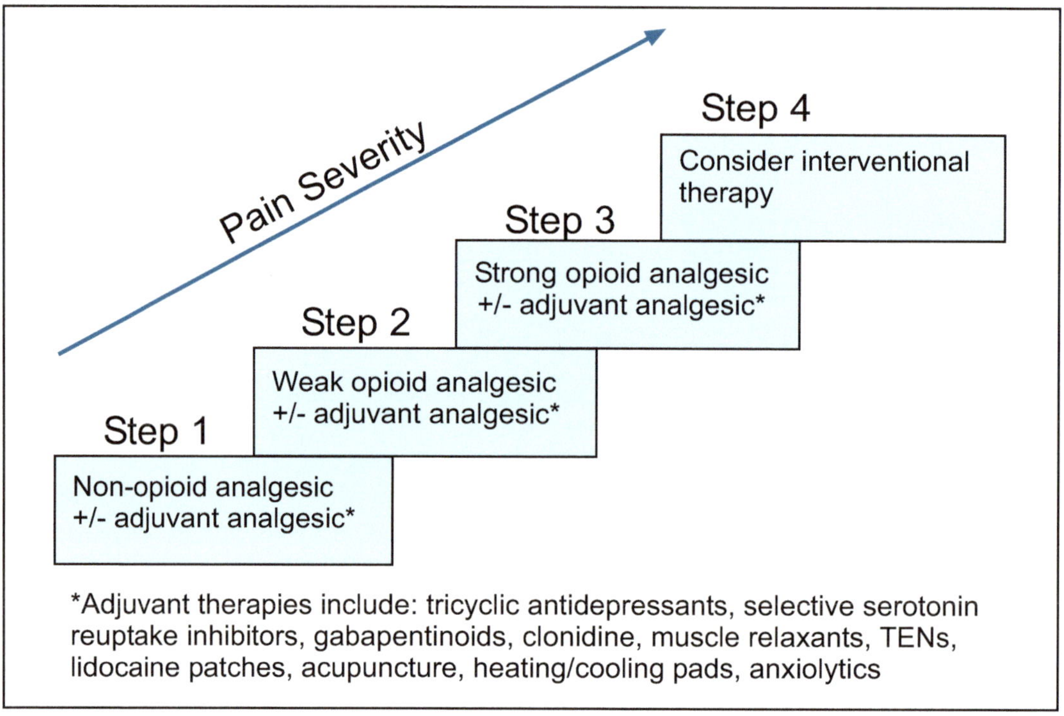

Fig. (1). WHO analgesic ladder.

Patients with terminal cancers often have "do not resuscitate and/or do not intubate (DNR/DNI)" orders in their advance directives. Decisions about suspending or withdrawing DNR/DNI orders should be discussed with patients or power of attorneys prior to any surgical procedures. Details on how the DNR/DNI will be managed in the perioperative period should be documented.

Musculoskeletal

Malignant primary bone cancers comprise only 0.2% of all neoplasms, with an estimated 3970 new cases diagnosed in 2024 [13]. Bone tumors include chondrosarcoma (30%), osteosarcoma (35%), malignant giant cell tumor of bone

(<5%), Ewing sarcoma (16%), and chondromas (<5%). Metastatic bone tumors occur more frequently than primary tumors, with breast and prostate cancers being the most common [13]. Primary bone tumors are aggressive and may damage surrounding soft tissue, muscle, and neurovascular structures. Patients who undergo bone tumor excision have often received multiple other treatments, including chemotherapy and radiation, and may require extensive optimization before surgery. For patients with severe anemia or thrombocytopenia, preoperative erythropoietin administration and transfusion of packed red blood cells or platelet transfusion may be beneficial. If significant blood loss is expected from a highly vascular tumor, preoperative embolization may be beneficial to reduce intraoperative bleeding and should be considered. Communication with the surgeon is essential to determine an appropriate anesthetic plan for intraoperative monitoring, pain management, access, and expected blood loss [14].

There are many types of surgeries performed by orthopedic oncology surgeons, many of which require unique positioning. Patients must be placed in anatomic positions with pressure points padded to reduce the risk of compression injury. Considerations for intraoperative management in the most common positions are summarized in Table **4**.

Table 4. Special considerations for positioning in cancer patients.

Position	Anesthetic Considerations
Supine	-Upper extremities should be padded, supinated, and abducted at < 90 degrees. -Head in neutral position with gel pad or donut with occasional readjustment to prevent pressure injury.
Lateral Decubitus	-Well-padded operating table. -Head and neck in neutral and midline position with no excessive pressure on the dependent ear or eyes. -Axillary roll to enable blood flow to the dependent arm and head and prevent neurovascular injury.
Prone	-Head and neck in neutral position during and after positioning to decrease risk of spinal cord/brachial plexus injury. -Eyes should be checked routinely to avoid pressure injury and decrease the risk of postoperative vision loss. -Arms up and adjacent to the head with elbows flexed or adducted alongside the patient with padding. -Avoid excessive pressure on the breasts and abdomen with chest roll.

Neurologic

Malignancies can affect the nervous system in multiple ways: through direct tumor involvement (primary or metastatic lesions), paraneoplastic syndromes, and toxicities or side effects from cancer treatments. A thorough neurologic evaluation is, therefore, critical to identify existing deficits or neurologic diseases, anticipate potential complications, and plan perioperative management. The goals are to document baseline neurologic function, optimize any neurologic condition (*e.g.*, controlling seizures or intracranial pressure), and tailor the anesthetic plan to the patient's neurologic status. This ensures patient safety and helps prevent postoperative neurologic deterioration.

Assessment of Existing Neurologic Conditions

Cancers frequently involve the central nervous system (CNS) either as primary tumors (*e.g.*, gliomas, meningiomas) or as metastatic disease (common with lung, breast, melanoma, and others). Preoperative evaluation focuses on the neurologic exam and intracranial pressure status. It is essential to identify and document all baseline neurologic deficits – focal weakness, cranial nerve palsies, visual field cuts, cognitive changes – prior to surgery. This documentation serves two purposes: planning perioperative management (*e.g.*, positioning to protect a weak limb, avoiding hypotension in those with a history of ischemic stroke) and providing a comparison for postoperative neurologic assessments.

Many patients may have unrelated neurological comorbidities (such as prior stroke, seizure disorders, or neurodegenerative diseases) or neurologic complications from cancer therapy. Any history of cerebrovascular accident or transient ischemic attack should be noted, as prior stroke increases the risk of perioperative stroke and may necessitate optimized blood pressure and antiplatelet management. Close blood pressure control is vital as both hypotension (risking ischemia) and HTN (risking hemorrhage or edema) can be detrimental. Seizure disorders require confirmation of medication compliance, and anti-epileptic drugs should be continued during the perioperative period.

Importantly, cancer therapies themselves can cause persistent neurologic deficits. A common example is chemotherapy-induced peripheral neuropathy (CIPN) from agents like platinum compounds, taxanes, or vinca alkaloids. These neuropathies are often sensory, causing numbness, tingling, and gait instability in a stocking-glove distribution. CIPN is reported in a large fraction of patients; taxane-based chemotherapy leads to neuropathy that can persist for years in roughly 30% of patients [15].

Other treatment-related neurological issues include chemotherapy-related ototoxicity and cognitive changes, which manifest as mild cognitive impairment. Patients with baseline cognitive dysfunction or prior cranial irradiation may be at higher risk of postoperative delirium. In patients with cognitive impairment or baseline confusion, sedative premedication is often avoided, as it can precipitate delirium or further cloud the neurologic exam. Instead, non-pharmacological comfort measures or very low-dose short-acting anxiolytics are used if necessary.

Paraneoplastic Neurologic Syndromes

Paraneoplastic neurologic syndromes are remote effects of cancer whereby an immune-mediated process impairs neurologic function. Although relatively rare, they are crucial to identify because they can significantly alter anesthetic management. Common paraneoplastic neurologic syndromes include Lambert-Eaton myasthenic syndrome (LEMS) and myasthenia gravis (MG).

LEMS is classically associated with small-cell lung carcinoma and leads to proximal muscle weakness, autonomic dysfunction, and reduced reflexes [16]. It is characterized by an autoimmune attack on presynaptic calcium channels at the neuromuscular junction. LEMS is especially important because it causes marked sensitivity to neuromuscular blocking drugs [17]. Patients with LEMS can have an exaggerated response to both depolarizing and nondepolarizing muscle relaxants, increasing the risk of prolonged paralysis and postoperative respiratory failure. Therefore, the preoperative evaluation must uncover subtle signs of LEMS so that the anesthetic plan can be adjusted – minimizing or avoiding muscle relaxants, using lower doses with close neuromuscular monitoring, and preparing for postoperative ventilation if needed.

Another important tumor-associated neurologic disorder is myasthenia gravis (MG) in the context of thymoma. Approximately 30–40% of thymoma patients have overt MG symptoms [18]. MG causes fatigable skeletal muscle weakness due to autoantibodies against postsynaptic acetylcholine receptors. In a preoperative assessment, any history of fluctuating muscle weakness or ptosis should prompt evaluation for MG, especially if a thymic mass is present. Known MG patients must be optimized before surgery – cholinesterase inhibitors, immunosuppressants, or IVIG/plasmapheresis for severe cases. Importantly, MG patients are highly sensitive to nondepolarizing neuromuscular blockers and relatively resistant to succinylcholine [19]. They also have reduced respiratory muscle reserve and have a high aspiration risk due to bulbar weakness. Thus, preoperative planning includes scheduling surgery at a time of day when strength is maximal (often morning), continuing anticholinesterase medications, and formulating an anesthetic plan that avoids muscle relaxants or uses short-acting agents with readiness to support ventilation.

Beyond myasthenic syndromes, other paraneoplastic neurologic disorders include paraneoplastic encephalitis (limbic encephalitis associated with small-cell lung cancer or ovarian teratomas), which can cause seizures, memory loss, and psychiatric symptoms; and paraneoplastic autonomic neuropathy, which can lead to severe blood pressure fluctuations and arrhythmias. Paraneoplastic cerebellar degeneration, often associated with breast, gynecologic, or lung cancer, causes ataxia, dysarthria, and nystagmus. These patients are at risk for aspiration due to incoordination of swallowing and falls.

CNS Involvement

Part of the CNS involvement assessment involves reviewing any prior treatments for CNS disease. Patients might have had surgeries, whole-brain radiation, or radiosurgery for metastases. Prior neurosurgical interventions can leave shunts or Ommaya reservoirs in place; the patency of a shunt should be confirmed, and if the patient has a programmable shunt valve, the setting should be noted.

Any symptoms associated with an intracranial tumor must be noted, including headaches, vomiting, seizures, or changes in mental status. These findings may indicate that the patient has increased ICP and is at risk of herniation or hemodynamic instability with abrupt changes in ICP. Measures can be taken preoperatively to control intracranial hypertension (HTN): corticosteroids are often continued (or initiated) to reduce peritumoral edema, which can markedly relieve symptoms and improve neurologic function [20]. Dexamethasone administration in the days leading up to surgery has been shown to decrease intracranial pressure and improve alertness in patients with brain tumors, albeit at the cost of inducing hyperglycemia – requiring blood glucose monitoring and management [21].

If a patient is at risk for increased ICP but is also anxious, judicious use of an anxiolytic is balanced against the need to prevent hypercapnia. Induction of anesthesia is performed with strategies to blunt any rise in intracranial pressure. This often means using an opioid and lidocaine to attenuate the response to laryngoscopy and avoiding drugs that might drastically raise cerebral blood flow. Hyperventilation after induction may be used briefly to lower $PaCO_2$ and ICP before surgical opening. Patients with brain tumors should be positioned with the head elevated and neck veins unobstructed to facilitate venous drainage.

In addition, patients with brain tumors may receive anticonvulsants if they have had seizures or if the tumor location confers high seizure risk; these medications should be maintained through the perioperative period. The anesthesiologist should verify that serum anticonvulsant levels are therapeutic and be prepared to treat intraoperative seizures if they occur.

When malignancy involves the spinal cord, signs of spinal cord compression (limb weakness, sensory level, incontinence) should be recognized early, as this often constitutes a surgical emergency. Although controversial due to varying results, high-dose corticosteroids are often started to reduce spinal cord edema and prevent worsening of neurologic function [22]. The anesthesiologist must handle such patients with extreme care during positioning and intubation to avoid exacerbating cord compression. For instance, in cervical spinal cord compression, neck manipulation is minimized, and manual in-line stabilization is used if intubation is required. If a patient has a chronic spinal cord injury, autonomic dysreflexia (especially with lesions above T6) and abnormal hemodynamic responses must be anticipated [23].

In any patient with a known CNS tumor or metastasis, neuraxial anesthesia may be contraindicated if there is elevated intracranial pressure or risk of herniation. This consideration typically favors general anesthesia for cases involving intracranial pathology, unless the surgery specifically requires an awake technique.

Cardiac

Many malignancies and their treatments have direct or indirect cardiac implications that influence perioperative outcomes. Consequently, the preoperative cardiac evaluation of a cancer patient must be meticulous, accounting for baseline cardiac function, cardiotoxicities of prior therapies, tumor-related cardiac complications, and the anticipated physiologic stress of surgery. The primary goals are to stratify risk, optimize cardiovascular status, and design a perioperative plan that reduces morbidity and mortality while accommodating the urgency and goals of cancer treatment.

A comprehensive cardiac evaluation begins with a detailed history and physical examination. Traditional cardiovascular risk factors—HTN, diabetes mellitus (DM), coronary artery disease (CAD), prior myocardial infarction (MI), heart failure, and arrhythmias—must be assessed, as in any general surgical patient. Additionally, cancer itself is a pro-inflammatory and hypercoagulable state, increasing the risk of arterial and venous thromboembolism (VTE), myocardial injury, and stroke [24]. Furthermore, patients with cancer often experience deconditioning, anemia, cachexia, and chronic inflammation, all of which can impair cardiac reserve. Functional capacity, often estimated in metabolic equivalents (METs), serves as a crucial metric; patients unable to perform activities such as climbing a flight of stairs or walking several blocks may warrant further cardiac testing, including stress imaging or echocardiography.

One of the most significant contributors to cardiac risk in cancer patients is prior exposure to cardiotoxic cancer therapies. Anthracyclines (*e.g.*, doxorubicin), HER2-targeted agents (*e.g.*, trastuzumab), and certain tyrosine kinase inhibitors are well-established culprits in causing cardiomyopathy [24]. Anthracyclines, for instance, are dose-dependent in their cardiac effects and can lead to irreversible dilated cardiomyopathy years after administration. Trastuzumab-induced dysfunction, while often reversible, still necessitates careful surveillance. Radiation therapy involving the thorax (especially when targeting left-sided breast cancer, lymphoma, or mediastinal tumors) can result in pericarditis, accelerated CAD, valvular fibrosis, and restrictive cardiomyopathy [25]. These sequelae may not manifest until years after exposure. Therefore, patients with a history of such treatments must undergo cardiac screening with at a minimum a transthoracic echocardiogram to assess ejection fraction, wall motion abnormalities, and valvular function. In some cases, additional testing, such as natriuretic peptides or cardiac MRI, may be indicated to detect subclinical myocardial injury.

Beyond treatment-induced cardiomyopathy, cancer patients are also at risk for tumor-related cardiac complications, including pericardial effusion, tamponade, or direct tumor invasion of cardiac structures [26]. Lung and breast cancers can metastasize to the pericardium, while renal cell carcinoma is notorious for tumor thrombus extending into the inferior vena cava and occasionally into the right atrium. These conditions may present subtly or be discovered incidentally on preoperative imaging, but they can have critical intraoperative implications. A pericardial effusion, even if asymptomatic, could precipitate hemodynamic collapse under general anesthesia due to decreased preload and impaired cardiac output. Therefore, if pericardial disease is suspected or known, an echocardiogram is essential. For patients with known cardiac metastases, the anesthetic plan must be tailored to avoid sudden shifts in preload or afterload and to ensure the availability of vasopressors and volume resuscitation as needed.

A key component of preoperative assessment is determining whether the cancer patient has adequate hemodynamic reserve to tolerate the surgical procedure. This is particularly relevant in high-risk or emergent surgeries or in patients with concurrent systemic illness. For patients with signs or symptoms of congestive heart failure (CHF), brain natriuretic peptide (BNP) or N-terminal pro-BNP levels can help guide further evaluation [27]. Elevated levels suggest volume overload or myocardial stress and may prompt optimization with diuretics or delay of elective surgery for cardiac workup. Similarly, patients with known CAD or unexplained angina should be considered for functional testing or coronary angiography if the surgery is high-risk. However, clinicians must balance the urgency of cancer resection with the risks of delaying surgery for cardiac testing, particularly when survival or symptom control hinges on prompt oncologic intervention.

Finally, the implications of cardiac findings on anesthesia management are significant. Patients with heart failure or valvular disease may require advanced monitoring intraoperatively, including arterial lines or central venous access. Those with arrhythmias or conduction abnormalities—especially if pacemakers or defibrillators are present—require interrogation of the device preoperatively and perioperative planning to manage electromagnetic interference. Hemodynamic goals during anesthesia should aim to maintain perfusion while avoiding volume overload, myocardial ischemia, or exacerbation of heart failure. Postoperatively, patients with borderline cardiac function may benefit from telemetry monitoring or even ICU-level care for early detection of MI, arrhythmias, or fluid shifts.

Hematologic

The hematologic system plays a central role in the perioperative care of cancer patients, given the frequent interplay between malignancy, its treatment, and hemostasis. Cancer patients often present with complex hematologic profiles due to tumor-related marrow suppression, paraneoplastic phenomena, chemotherapy-induced cytopenias, or underlying hematologic malignancies. As a result, a thorough preoperative evaluation of the hematologic system is critical to identify and address coagulopathies, anemia, thrombocytopenia, and thromboembolic risks, thereby reducing perioperative complications.

An important consideration in the preoperative period is thromboembolic risk and anticoagulation. Cancer patients have a significantly elevated baseline risk of venous thromboembolism (VTE), and those undergoing major surgery are at even greater risk. Some patients may already be on anticoagulation for prior deep vein thrombosis (DVT), pulmonary embolism (PE), or atrial fibrillation (AF). In such cases, coordination with cardiology and/or hematology is often needed to determine whether bridging with low-molecular-weight heparin (LMWH) is appropriate or whether anticoagulation can be safely held. The prothrombotic and hemorrhagic risks must be balanced, especially in patients with thrombocytopenia from chemotherapy or bone marrow involvement.

Coagulopathy is frequently encountered in cancer patients due to liver dysfunction, disseminated intravascular coagulation (DIC), vitamin K deficiency, or the presence of circulating anticoagulants. DIC, in particular, is a life-threatening condition seen in association with aggressive malignancies such as acute promyelocytic leukemia (APL), pancreatic cancer, and mucin-producing adenocarcinomas [28]. It is characterized by widespread activation of clotting cascades leading to both thrombosis and bleeding. Preoperative evaluation includes measurement of prothrombin time (PT), activated partial thromboplastin time (aPTT), fibrinogen, and D-dimer. Correction of coagulopathy, if feasible, should be attempted with fresh frozen plasma, cryoprecipitate, or vitamin K prior to surgery. For patients on therapeutic anticoagulation for prior DVT/VTE or AF, the decision to reverse or bridge therapy depends on thrombotic risk, bleeding risk, and surgical urgency. LMWH is commonly used as a bridging agent; however, careful timing around the procedure is essential to avoid bleeding complications.

On the other hand, hypercoagulability is also one of the most pervasive hematologic complications in cancer patients [29]. Malignancy creates a prothrombotic environment through multiple mechanisms, including tumor cell expression of tissue factor, cytokine release, and immobility [30]. This places cancer patients at increased risk of DVT, PE, and arterial thrombosis. Surgery further amplifies this risk. Preoperative evaluation must assess for prior thrombotic events, current anticoagulation use, and risk factors such as central venous catheters, chemotherapy, or immobility. Venous duplex ultrasonography may be indicated in patients with limb swelling or a history of DVT. Perioperative prophylaxis with pharmacologic (*e.g.*, low-dose enoxaparin) or mechanical (*e.g.*, intermittent pneumatic compression) measures should be planned for all patients unless contraindicated by active bleeding or severe thrombocytopenia.

One of the most common hematologic abnormalities encountered in cancer patients is anemia, which may arise from chronic disease, nutritional deficiencies, bone marrow infiltration, chemotherapy, or blood loss. Anemia is a well-established predictor of increased perioperative morbidity and mortality. Even mild reductions in hemoglobin can impair oxygen delivery and increase the risk of intraoperative hypotension, myocardial ischemia, and delayed recovery. Therefore, preoperative screening with a complete blood count (CBC) is standard, and further investigation may be needed to identify the etiology. Iron studies, vitamin B12, folate levels, and reticulocyte count can be helpful in distinguishing between iron-deficiency anemia, anemia of chronic disease, and myelodysplastic syndromes [31]. In patients with symptomatic anemia or hemoglobin levels below surgical thresholds, transfusion or erythropoiesis-stimulating agents may be considered. However, transfusion must be balanced with potential risks, including immunomodulation and volume overload.

Thrombocytopenia is another critical consideration, especially in patients with hematologic malignancies, bone marrow involvement, or those receiving myelosuppressive therapy. Platelet counts below 100,000/μL warrant caution, while counts below 50,000/μL are generally considered unsafe for major surgery [31]. Spontaneous bleeding becomes a risk at counts under 20,000/μL. Preoperative evaluation should include not only platelet count but also an assessment of platelet function, especially if the patient has been exposed to antiplatelet agents, uremia, or sepsis. If platelet transfusion is indicated, timing is crucial, as the transfused platelets may have a limited lifespan, particularly in patients with immune-mediated destruction or splenomegaly. Coordination with hematology is often necessary to guide perioperative transfusion strategies and manage cases with refractory thrombocytopenia or ongoing platelet consumption.

Patients with hematologic malignancies such as leukemia, lymphoma, or multiple myeloma pose additional perioperative challenges. These conditions often involve profound cytopenias, impaired immunity, and systemic involvement. Preoperative assessment in such patients must include a review of recent chemotherapy or bone marrow transplant status, immunosuppressive regimens, and infectious risk. Absolute neutrophil count (ANC) is essential in assessing the risk of perioperative infection. Elective surgeries are typically deferred if the ANC is below 1000/μL, unless the procedure is urgent [30]. Prophylactic antibiotics, granulocyte colony-stimulating factor (G-CSF), or growth factors may be necessary in neutropenic patients undergoing surgery.

Transfusion history is another important consideration in cancer patients, especially those who have received multiple blood products. Alloimmunization can complicate crossmatching and delay transfusions. A type and screen or type and cross, and in some cases, extended red blood cell antigen matching, should be done well in advance. Additionally, a history of transfusion-related reactions or graft-versus-host disease in immunocompromised patients may necessitate irradiated blood products to prevent life-threatening complications.

Endocrine

Malignancies—particularly endocrine tumors and cancers treated with systemic therapies—can disrupt hormonal balance, precipitate metabolic crises, and alter stress responses. Additionally, pituitary, adrenal, and thyroid axes may be affected by tumor burden or therapeutic interventions, all of which have direct implications for anesthetic and perioperative management [32]. A comprehensive evaluation of endocrine function is therefore essential to prevent intraoperative instability, delayed recovery, and postoperative complications.

Endocrine dysfunction may arise due to primary tumors of endocrine glands, metastatic infiltration, paraneoplastic syndromes, or treatment-related injury. Common malignancies with direct endocrine implications include thyroid cancer, adrenal tumors, pancreatic neuroendocrine tumors, and pituitary adenomas. These tumors may be functional (hormone-secreting) or non-functional but locally compressive. For example, pheochromocytomas, paragangliomas, and functioning adrenocortical carcinomas can secrete excess catecholamines or cortisol, leading to life-threatening HTN, arrhythmias, or Cushingoid features. In such cases, preoperative endocrine control is lifesaving. Pheochromocytomas must be adequately treated with alpha-adrenergic blockade followed by beta-blockade only after alpha-blockade is established. Inadequate preparation can result in hypertensive crises during induction, tumor manipulation, or extubation [33]. Similarly, patients with cortisol-secreting tumors require steroid tapering or pharmacologic suppression with agents like ketoconazole prior to resection.

Thyroid function is another critical component of preoperative endocrine evaluation [34]. While thyroid cancer itself may not always result in functional hormone excess or deficiency, surgical treatment and radiation therapy can impair thyroid status. Hypothyroidism may present subtly but has profound perioperative consequences, including delayed drug metabolism, hypoventilation, bradycardia, and impaired thermoregulation. Severe hypothyroidism (myxedema) poses a high surgical risk and must be corrected before elective procedures. Conversely, hyperthyroidism—whether due to thyroid cancer or iatrogenic causes—can precipitate thyroid storm under the stress of surgery, characterized by fever, tachycardia, HTN, and altered mental status. Patients with suspected thyrotoxicosis should have thyroid function tests (TFT) checked, and if positive, should be treated with beta-blockers, thionamides (*e.g.*, methimazole), and possibly steroids prior to any non-emergent surgery.

Pituitary dysfunction is particularly relevant in patients with sellar masses, prior pituitary surgery, or cranial radiation. Hypopituitarism may result in adrenal insufficiency, hypothyroidism, hypogonadism, or diabetes insipidus (DI)—any of which can pose significant perioperative risks if unrecognized. Adrenal insufficiency is the most acutely dangerous, as it can lead to refractory hypotension, hyponatremia, and cardiovascular collapse under surgical stress. Preoperative screening for adrenal insufficiency involves morning serum cortisol levels or stimulation tests if suspicion is high. Patients on chronic corticosteroids or those with prior pituitary interventions often require stress-dose steroids during surgery to prevent adrenal crisis [35]. This typically involves hydrocortisone boluses or continuous infusion and tapering in the postoperative period. Similarly, patients with DI may require careful perioperative monitoring of fluid status and sodium levels, with desmopressin administered as needed to prevent hypernatremia and volume depletion.

Metabolic complications related to endocrine malignancies or therapies must also be considered. Hypercalcemia is a common metabolic emergency, often seen in cancers such as multiple myeloma, breast, and lung cancers, or in paraneoplastic syndromes due to parathyroid hormone-related protein (PTHrP) secretion. Hypercalcemia may cause arrhythmias, altered mental status, and dehydration. Preoperative optimization includes aggressive IV hydration, bisphosphonates, and correction of electrolytes. Similarly, hypoglycemia can occur in patients with insulin-secreting tumors or advanced liver disease. On the other hand, steroid-induced or diabetes-related hyperglycemia is common and must be controlled preoperatively, as poor glycemic control is associated with increased infection rates, impaired wound healing, and perioperative morbidity. Blood glucose targets are typically maintained between 140–180 mg/dL in the perioperative period to avoid both hypo- and hyperglycemia [35].

Pulmonary

When evaluating patients with lung cancer, the anesthesiologist should focus on underlying lung disease and associated symptoms as well as comorbid conditions. This assessment should focus on a history and physical, cardiopulmonary evaluation, labs, imaging, and airway assessment. Preoperative history should include smoking history, symptoms, functional status, and comorbidities. One of the biggest risk factors for lung cancer is cigarette smoking [36]. Patient's smoking should be documented, including pack history, current status, and cessation attempts. Oftentimes, patients with lung cancer continue smoking despite their diagnosis and prognosis. Prior to surgery and anesthesia, it is recommended that patients abstain from cigarette smoking. Cigarette smoking may lead to increased cardiopulmonary complications, increased hospital stay, and increased morbidity, with timely cessation reducing these events and possibly helping with wound healing [36] [37]. Patients should be encouraged to stop smoking prior to surgical interventions.

Common symptoms of lung cancer may include dyspnea, cough, hemoptysis, wheezing, weight loss, and fatigue [38]. If the tumor is large enough or lymphadenopathy is severe, patients may experience upper extremity and/or facial edema due to obstruction of the superior vena cava. If the tumor grows, it may also cause shoulder and arm pain and neuropathy. Spread of the tumor into the pleura may also cause pleuritic chest pain. Anesthesiologists should document the severity of symptoms as well as determine baseline functional status. Lung cancers can lead to paraneoplastic syndromes, as mentioned in the endocrine section. These can manifest in a variety of ways, such as hypercalcemia, hypoglycemia, SIADH, hyperthyroidism, and Cushing's syndrome [39]. Baseline basic metabolic panel (BMP) and TFTs should be obtained on lung cancer patients and monitored as needed.

Patients with lung cancer often have other comorbidities, including underlying lung disease, such as chronic obstructive pulmonary disease (COPD), asthma, and interstitial lung disease (ILD). Cardiac disease, including HTN, CAD, and CHF, as well as neurovascular disease, including strokes and VTE, are also often present due to smoking history. These comorbidities should be optimized prior to surgery, and patients will often be referred to specialists for management.

Based on the severity and size of the tumor, imaging studies are obtained preoperatively. These studies may include plain chest x-ray (CXR), CT, and PET scans. Bronchoscopy may also be performed beforehand, which may determine the surgical approach, degree of obstruction, need for specialized airway equipment, and ability to ventilate and/or intubate a patient with a possible difficult airway. These images should be reviewed and discussed with the surgeon prior to the procedure. The size and location of the tumor may also affect airway management, including the need for a double lumen tube (DLT) or bronchial placement, as well as the need for vascular access, including large bore IV or arterial line placement. Due to the risk of bleeding, a CBC and T+C should be obtained.

Besides primary lung tumors, cancers from other organ systems and their treatment can have pulmonary effects. These may include metastasis, pleural effusions, and treatment-related pulmonary toxicity. Malignant pleural effusions (MPE) can occur in up to 15% of patients with cancer. Several studies have shown lung cancer has the highest incidence of MPE, followed by breast, lymphomas, ovarian, gastrointestinal, and then all other types of cancers [40] [41]. The approximate percentage of MPE cases by cancer type is shown in Table **5**. Patients presenting with effusions should be evaluated for their size and clinical manifestations such as dyspnea and hypoxia. Usually, effusions are associated with advanced disease and have a poor prognosis. If effusions are large, preoperative thoracentesis may be warranted to alleviate symptoms.

Radiation-induced lung injury can occur during the treatment of both lung cancer and other localized cancers, including those of the esophagus, breast, thyroid, and hematologic systems. Radiation can lead to both pulmonary pneumonitis and fibrosis. After radiation therapy, lungs can go through stages of injury, which include immediate, latent, acute exudative, intermediate, and fibrosis stages. These stages usually follow a time course and progress from patients being asymptomatic to developing cough, fevers, dyspnea, pleuritic chest pain, and malaise. Symptoms may resolve or diminish during the intermediate phase; however, they may return during the fibrosis stage, presenting as cough, dyspnea, and decreased lung volumes due to fibrosis of the lung tissue. Chemotherapy agents, such as bleomycin, have been associated with an increased risk of causing pulmonary fibrosis due to DNA reaction and the production of chain scission [42]. Patients with pulmonary fibrosis have a high risk of morbidity and mortality when mechanical ventilation is indicated, and no specific evidence has shown any ventilation techniques to be superior in improving outcomes [43].

Table 5. Incidence of malignant pleural effusions by cancer type.

Cancer Type	Approximate Percent of MPE Cases
Lung	30-40%
Breast	20-35%
Lymphoma	10-15%
Ovarian	5-10%
Gastrointestinal	5-10%
Other Cancers	<5%

Ears, Nose, and Throat (ENT)

Thyroid Cancer

The two most common types of thyroid cancer are papillary (84%) and follicular (9%) cancers [44]. The remaining types include medullary and anaplastic, which are less common but tend to be more aggressive with a worse prognosis. Patients with primary thyroid cancer are often diagnosed incidentally and are often asymptomatic. However, they can present with painless or sometimes painful lumps or nodules, but larger tumors can cause obstructive symptoms due to compression of airway structures and the esophagus. These symptoms can appear as hoarseness, voice changes, persistent cough, and difficulty with swallowing or breathing. Metastatic thyroid cancer can present with more constitutional symptoms, while medullary thyroid cancer can cause gastrointestinal symptoms.

Most primary thyroid cancers do not cause thyroid dysfunction, so thyroid function tests are usually within normal limits. However, TFTs are often obtained to monitor cancer progression and postoperative evaluation. If the parathyroids are believed to be involved, then calcium and parathyroid hormone (PTH) may also be obtained. Patients with other cancers on chemotherapeutics or who have received radiation may present with thyroid dysfunction. Specific therapeutics, including tyrosine kinase inhibitors (TKI) (sunitinib), cytokines (interferon-alpha), monoclonal antibodies (ipilimumab), as well as radiation therapy, can lead to hypothyroidism [45]. Patients on these treatments should have TFTs assessed and should be euthyroid prior to surgery.

Due to concerns about airway compromise, it is imperative to conduct a thorough preoperative airway evaluation prior to administering anesthesia. Routine imaging is usually not performed and is reserved for patients with obstructive symptoms. Imaging to evaluate the tumor and any mass effect may include CT scan, MRI, and fiberoptic laryngoscopy. If imaging is obtained, it should be reviewed, and airway management should be discussed with the ENT surgeon prior to the procedure and induction of anesthesia. Physical exam should include a standard airway exam and should note the patient's ability to talk, swallow, neck mobility, tracheal deviation, and ability to lie flat. Large tumors that obstruct the esophagus may also increase the risk of aspiration, so rapid sequence induction (RSI) and intubation may be indicated. Concerns for a difficult airway should prompt the anesthesia provider to have all necessary difficult airway equipment available. If necessary, an awake fiberoptic intubation may be performed to avoid trouble with ventilating patients after induction. If the patient has a large mass, an emergent or even planned awake tracheostomy may be difficult due to distorted anatomy. However, emergent tracheostomy supplies should be available, and ENT surgery should be readily available during induction and intubation. Decisions regarding airway management during the procedure should be discussed; however, in most cases, a specialized nerve integrity monitor (NIM) tube is used due to the increased risk of injury to branches of the superior laryngeal nerve. If a NIM tube is used, anesthesiologists should avoid using long-acting neuromuscular blocking agents unless sugammadex is readily available for reversal prior to nerve monitoring begins. Finally, plans for extubation should be discussed at the start of the case. Concerns for swelling, edema, anatomical changes due to surgery, bleeding, and vocal cord injury can lead to difficult airway management after extubation, and again, ENT surgery should be present on emergence.

Laryngeal and Oropharyngeal Cancer

Similar to thyroid cancer surgery, preoperative evaluation for these cancers should focus on airway evaluation. Patients may present with symptoms such as pain, dysphagia, dysphonia, stridor, difficulty breathing, nasal obstruction, and lymphadenopathy. Depending on the severity of the disease, patients may have more constitutional symptoms, and if they have difficulty eating, they may have cachexia and be malnourished. It is important to assess prior treatments, including the use of chemotherapy and radiation, which are often used prior to surgical excision. As mentioned in prior sections, chemotherapies may affect other organ systems, so a full history and PE are necessary. Direct radiation can cause fibrosis, necrosis, changes in airway anatomy, thyroid changes, and vascular damage. Malnutrition from decreased oral intake may also be present, so electrolyte derangements may be common. Since there is a high incidence of alcohol and smoking abuse with these cancers, concomitant cardiopulmonary, hematologic and hepatic disease may be present. Because of these concerns, labs including CBC, CMP, TFTs, and coagulation profiles are usually obtained.

When performing an airway evaluation, focus should be on signs of obstruction, which may occur anywhere along the respiratory tract. Stridor, wheezing, and decreased breath sounds may be heard on auscultation. Radiation-induced fibrosis may cause limited neck mobility as well as trismus. Prior head and neck surgeries may cause scarring and distorted anatomy, which may make ventilation, intubation, and even surgical airways difficult. Prior to surgery, direct laryngoscopy as well as imaging, including X-rays, CTs, and MRIs, should be evaluated and discussed with the ENT surgeon to develop a plan for airway management. Need for fiberoptic intubation, awake intubation, or awake tracheostomy should be discussed.

Decisions for airway management, the type of endotracheal tube, and the need for a shared airway should be discussed prior to surgery. A NIMs tube may be required for nerve monitoring. Depending on the type and location of the tumor, rigid bronchoscopy or jet ventilation may need to be used or be available. As with thyroid cancer, patients may be at increased risk for aspiration due to compression/obstruction of the esophagus, so RSI may be indicated.

Gastrointestinal

Esophageal Cancer

Esophageal cancer patients often present with malnutrition, nausea and vomiting, dysphagia, and weight loss. Patients often have reflux and may have an increased risk for aspiration. Larger tumors may cause tracheal deviation and respiratory compromise, which may cause difficulty with intubation and ventilation. Patients with esophageal cancer often undergo radiation therapy, which can lead to both local and pulmonary fibrosis [46]. There is an increased incidence of esophageal cancer in patients who use alcohol and tobacco, so comorbidities associated with those conditions should be evaluated [47].

Prior to surgery, patients should have a thorough airway evaluation performed. Depending on symptoms and documented imaging, anesthesiologists may need to plan for difficult airway management, including RSI or awake intubation with a fiberoptic scope. Lung isolation may be required for the surgical approach, so one lung ventilation with either a double lumen tube (DLT) or bronchial blockers may be indicated. Labs should be obtained focusing on increased risk for anemia, electrolyte derangements, and liver dysfunction, including CBC, BMP, LFT, and coagulation profile. Due to risk for surgical bleeding and proximity of vascular structures during surgery, an active type and cross as well as placement of large bore IV access, central lines, and arterial lines may be indicated.

Patients often have postoperative pulmonary complications due to atelectasis, aspiration, and pneumonia, which may require postoperative mechanical ventilation [48]. Preoperative assessment should focus on efforts to reduce these pulmonary complications. Preoperative thoracic epidural or regional nerve block placement may be indicated for postoperative pain management to improve respiratory status [49]. Conservative fluid management may be indicated to reduce the risk of pulmonary edema postoperatively [50]. Overall, esophagectomy has a high surgical risk withan expected 30-day cardiovascular death or MI risk >5% according to the 2014 European Society of Cardiology and European Society of Anesthesiology (ESC/ESA) guidelines on noncardiac surgery [26]. Patients at increased risk usually have severe comorbidities, malnutrition, poor functional status, and tumors located in the cervical esophagus due to the risk for airway compromise.

Colon, Rectum, and Anal Cancers

Patients often present with rectal bleeding. Bleeding can cause severe anemia, leading to dyspnea and fatigue. With large tumors, signs of obstruction may be present, including constipation, abdominal distention, and vomiting. Progressive disease can lead to decreased absorption, malnutrition and weight loss [51].

Preoperatively, baseline BMP, CBC, LFTs, and coagulation panels should be obtained. Depending on the amount of bleeding and degree of anemia, patients may require preoperative transfusion or have an active type and cross for surgery. Bowel preparation regimen prior to surgical procedures can lead to dehydration and electrolyte derangements. Electrolytes should be replaced as indicated, especially if patients are symptomatic, and patients are encouraged to maintain oral intake of liquids as close to the procedure to remain euvolemic. Depending on the type of procedure and approach, large volume and blood loss may be expected, so large-bore IV access should be obtained. Discussion with surgeons for pain management should be discussed, and if an open procedure is planned or anticipated, a decision for pain control, including epidural placement or regional block, may be performed [52]. Finally, patients may be at increased risk for aspiration due to obstruction. RSI may be indicated, and some patients may benefit from preoperative gastric decompression.

Gastric Cancer

The preoperative approach to gastrectomy is similar to other GI surgeries. As with other GI cancers, preoperative optimization can help reduce postoperative complications [53]. Preoperative evaluation should focus on symptoms of fatigue, weight loss, gastrointestinal obstruction, vomiting, and dehydration. Volume and electrolyte status should be assessed. Prior treatments, including radiation and chemotherapy, and their effects should be determined. Aspiration precautions should be observed especially in patients with gastric outlet obstruction. Patients may arrive for surgery with nasogastric tubes already present for gastric decompression. RSI or awake fiberoptic intubation may be indicated. Again, regional techniques may be beneficial for pain management and reduce the risk of pulmonary complications [52].

Hepatic Carcinoma

The estimated incidence of new liver, intrahepatic bile duct, and gallbladder cancer cases in the United States in 2025 will be about 55,000 [54]. However, liver resection is also performed due to liver metastasis from other cancers. Patients often present asymptomatically, but may have symptoms of weight loss, fatigue, anorexia, abdominal pain or fullness, fevers, and palpable mass with advanced disease. Signs of liver dysfunction may include jaundice, increased bleeding, pruritus, changes in bowel and urine, peripheral edema, cirrhosis and ascites, with more severe cases resulting in portal HTN, splenomegaly, caput medusae, gastric or esophageal varices, and encephalopathy. Although less common, paraneoplastic syndromes from liver cancer can lead to hypoglycemia, hypercalcemia, hypercholesterolemia, and erythrocytosis [55]. Liver function and severity of disease should be evaluated with BMP, LFT, CBC, and coagulation studies. The Child-Pugh clinical scoring system (Table **6**) is one assessment tool that can be used to determine the severity of liver disease, which can indicate patient risk for surgery [56]. Based on the criteria, the Child-Pugh score is calculated from 5 to 15 points. Higher scores are associated with more severe disease and worse prognosis. Due to associated comorbidities, preoperative EKG and ECHO may be indicated prior to surgeries.

Table 6. Child-pugh scoring system.

Points	**1**	**2**	**3**
Ascites	None	Small or diuretic-controlled	Moderate
Encephalopathy	Absent	Mild	Significant
Albumin (g/dL)	>3.5	2.8-3.5	<2.8
Total Bilirubin (mg/dL)	<2	2-3	>3
PT sec >control or INR	<4 or <1.7	4-6 or 1.7-2.3	>6 or >2.3
Score	Class A: 5-6 points, 10% perioperative mortality	Class B:7–9 points, 30% perioperative mortality	Class C:10-15 points, 85% perioperative mortality

Although surgical techniques, including the Pringle maneuver, have reduced bleeding risks during hepatectomies [57], patients should still have an active type and cross as well as appropriate large-bore IV access and arterial line placement as indicated before major liver resection. As with other major GI surgeries, risks for aspiration and the need for adequate pain management, including the use of regional techniques, should be anticipated.

Besides primary liver cancer, hepatic injury can occur due to chemotherapeutics from other cancer treatments. Liver function can be affected by cytotoxic, molecularly targeted, and immunotherapeutic agents. These agents can cause direct or indirect hepatotoxicity. Effects of drugs on the liver may include hepatocellular injury, inflammation, cholestasis, endothelial injury, and thrombosis. Some chemotherapies associated with increased risk of hepatotoxicity include methotrexate, oxaliplatin, and irinotecan, but a comprehensive and updated list can be found at the NIH's LiverTox website [58]. Use of chemotherapeutics can also increase the incidence of hepatitis B and C infection, so patients are often prophylactically treated when undergoing chemotherapy. Hepatitis reactivation may initially be asymptomatic but may progress to jaundice and liver failure [59]. Doses and regimens may need to be adjusted based on LFTs.

Pancreatic Cancer

Patients with pancreatic cancer can present with weight loss, anorexia, obstructive jaundice (usually painless), abdominal and/or back pain, nausea and vomiting from duodenal obstruction, fatigue, malaise, and new-onset DM. Physical examination may reveal weight loss, abdominal tenderness, palpable gallbladder known as Courvoisier's sign, and signs of jaundice, including scleral icterus and pruritus. As with other major abdominal procedures, anesthesiologists should focus on aspiration risk, fluid and blood loss, and pain management when preparing for pancreatic surgery. There is a high incidence of DM with pancreatic cancer, with up to 80% of patients having DM or glucose intolerance [60]. Preparation for tight glucose management due to the effects of pancreatic cancer on insulin production is also vital to prevent postoperative complications. Glucose management should be optimized prior to surgery and tightly managed intraoperatively.

Renal, Genitourinary, Gynecologic Cancer

Renal Cancer

Patients with renal cancer often present with hematuria, pain, and obstructive symptoms [61]. There are numerous risk factors contributing to the development of renal cancer, including but not limited to smoking, obesity, HTN, occupational exposures, and a history of kidney stones.

Along with primary renal cancers, patients being treated with chemotherapeutic agents for other cancers may develop nephrotoxicity and kidney injury. Nephrotoxic drugs may cause either acute or chronic renal injury. The mechanism of action is variable but may include oxidative stress, inflammation, direct tubular toxicity, and crystallization, which may affect any part of the kidney, including the glomeruli, tubules, interstitium, and renal vasculature [62]. These effects may lead to acute kidney injury, which, over time, can cause chronic kidney damage and eventually renal failure. This can result in electrolyte disorders, including hypomagnesemia, and delayed drug clearance, which can lead to increased systemic toxicity. Patients may develop Fanconi-like syndrome, which, like the inherited version, causes impairment of the reabsorption at the proximal renal tubules [63]. This can lead to glycosuria, hypophosphatemia, hypokalemia, hyponatremia, hypouricemia, aminoaciduria, and type 2 renal tubular acidosis. Patients with Fanconi-like syndrome may present with dehydration, polyuria, polydipsia, electrolyte abnormalities, weakness, bone pain, growth retardation, and metabolic acidosis. Direct vascular injury can lead to cystitis and hemolytic uremic syndrome (HUS). Refer back to Table **2** for a list of common chemotherapeutic drugs, including their mechanism of action and side effects [2].

When evaluating patients with renal cancer or therapeutics that may cause nephrotoxicity, practitioners should be cognizant of symptoms resulting from severe electrolyte abnormalities and acidosis. Depending on the severity of renal involvement, BMP should be obtained to assess renal function. In cases of severe renal dysfunction or end-stage renal disease (ESRD) requiring dialysis, patients should be asked when their last dialysis session occurred, have their volume status assessed, and baseline potassium, as well as possible arterial blood gas, should be obtained. Anesthetic management of patients should be tailored based on preoperative findings. Patients may require volume optimization, dialysis, and electrolyte replacement as indicated.

The type of surgery and severity of renal cancer and concomitant comorbidities will determine the preoperative anesthetic plan. Nephrectomies can be performed laparoscopically or open, and can either be radical or partial (nephron-sparing). For larger cases, anesthesiologists should plan for appropriate IV access with possible central and arterial line placement due to concerns for bleeding (especially with partial nephrectomies). Patients should have preoperative labs optimized and tailored to disease severity as well as associated comorbidities. BMP, CBC, and coagulation studies are usually standard with other labs and imaging studies obtained based on individual patients. If patients have ESRD, they should continue on their dialysis schedule, and our institution's policy is to have a potassium level checked by the laboratory or through point-of-care testing the day of surgery.

Prostate and Bladder Cancer

Patients with prostate cancer present with urinary symptoms, hematuria, weight loss, and fatigue. In advanced disease, patients may present with bone pain from metastasis. Frailty is common since a majority of prostate cancer occurs in elderly men, which can lead to an increase in postoperative morbidity and mortality [7]. Bladder cancer presents with gross hematuria, pain, and occasionally with ureteral obstruction from the tumor. Both can metastasize to the liver, lungs, and bone with associated clinical abnormalities. Constitutional symptoms usually indicate advanced disease or metastasis and often have a poor prognosis.

Preoperative assessment should focus on optimizing comorbid conditions and improving nutrition to reduce postoperative complications. Preoperative labs should include CBC to assess anemia, BMP to assess kidney function due to risk of obstructive uropathy, and baseline sodium, as intraoperative hyponatremia during TURP can occur, and a coagulation panel if the neuraxial technique is to be performed. Other labs and studies should be based on co-existing comorbidities and their severity. Preoperative stenting may be required to relieve obstruction and improve kidney function.

Prostate surgeries include radical prostatectomies (which can be performed as laparoscopic, robotic-assisted, or open) as well as transurethral resection of the prostate (TURP). Bladder surgeries usually include transurethral resection of bladder tumor (TURBT) for smaller non-invasive tumors and radical cystectomies for larger tumors that have invaded the muscle. Standard ASA monitoring may be appropriate, but the need for additional central venous access and arterial line placement with close hemodynamic monitoring should again be based on the severity of comorbidities.

Gynecologic Cancers

Gynecological cancers can present with a variety of symptoms, but may include abnormal uterine/vaginal bleeding, pelvic and abdominal pain, abdominal distention, fatigue, weight loss, ascites, and bowel and bladder obstruction with advanced disease. A wide variety of procedures can be performed for gynecologic cancers, ranging from simple hysteroscopies to diagnostic laparoscopies and exploratory laparotomies.

Preoperative assessment should focus on aspiration risks due to abdominal distention and ascites, as well as a lung exam to evaluate for pleural effusions, which are common, especially in ovarian cancer [64]. Preoperative labs and imaging depend on the type and severity of cancer as well as concomitant comorbidities and their severity. Smaller procedures may only require standard monitors and labs, while larger procedures may require further workup, monitoring, vascular access, and pain management strategies, depending on associated comorbidities. If abdominal distention or large-volume ascites are present, aspiration precautions with RSI should be performed.

CONCLUSION

In summary, a thorough preoperative assessment is vital for cancer patients to ensure optimal perioperative management and improve overall surgical outcomes. Given the complexity of cancer and its associated comorbidities, it is important to understand how different types of malignancy and chemotherapies can impact physiology, drug metabolism, and airway patency. Conducting a detailed evaluation allows anesthesiologists to identify potential risks, optimize intraoperative management, and minimize postoperative complications.

REFERENCES

[1] Siegel RL, Miller KD, Wagle NS, Jemal A. Cancer statistics, 2023. CA Cancer J Clin 2023; 73(1): 17-48.
[http://dx.doi.org/10.3322/caac.21763] [PMID: 36633525]

[2] Fischer SP. Preoperative Evaluation of the Cancer Patient. Anesthesiol Clin North America 1998; 16(3): 533-46. Available from: https://www.sciencedirect.com/science/article/pii/S0889853705700419
[http://dx.doi.org/10.1016/S0889-8537(05)70041-9]

[3] Zambouri A. Preoperative evaluation and preparation for anesthesia and surgery. Hippokratia 2007; 11(1): 13-21.
[PMID: 19582171]

[4] Gallieni M, Pittiruti M, Biffi R. Vascular access in oncology patients. CA Cancer J Clin 2008; 58(6): 323-46.
[http://dx.doi.org/10.3322/CA.2008.0015] [PMID: 18971486]

[5] Melnyk M, Casey RG, Black P, Koupparis AJ. Enhanced recovery after surgery (ERAS) protocols: Time to change practice? Can Urol Assoc J 2013; 5(5): 342-8. Available from: https://www.ncbi.nlm.nih.gov/pmc/articles/PMC3202008/
[http://dx.doi.org/10.5489/cuaj.693] [PMID: 22031616]

[6] Practice guidelines for preoperative fasting and the use of pharmacologic agents to reduce the risk of pulmonary aspiration: application to healthy patients undergoing elective procedures. Anesthesiology 2017; 126(3): 376-93.
[http://dx.doi.org/10.1097/ALN.0000000000001452] [PMID: 28045707]

[7] George EL, Hall DE, Youk A, *et al.* Association between patient frailty and postoperative mortality across multiple noncardiac surgical specialties. JAMA Surg 2021; 156(1): e205152. Available from: https://pubmed.ncbi.nlm.nih.gov/33206156/
[PMID: 33206156]

[8] Rosner MH, Dalkin AC. Electrolyte disorders associated with cancer. Adv Chronic Kidney Dis 2014; 21(1): 7-17. Available from: https://www.akdh.org/article/s1548-5595(13)00077-3/fulltext#:~:text=Patients%20with%20malignancies%20commonly%20experience,unique%20to%20the%20underlying%20cancer
[http://dx.doi.org/10.1053/j.ackd.2013.05.005] [PMID: 24359982]

[9] Kianian S, Bansal J, Lee C, Zhang K, Bergese SD. Perioperative multimodal analgesia: a review of efficacy and safety of the treatment options. APS 2024; 2(9).

[http://dx.doi.org/10.1007/s44254-023-00043-1]

[10] Anekar AA, Hendrix JM, Cascella M. WHO Analgesic Ladder.StatPearls. Treasure Island, FL: StatPearls Publishing 2025. Updated 2023 Apr 23 Internet Available from: https://www.ncbi.nlm.nih.gov/books/NBK554435/

[11] Herschbach P, Keller M, Knight L, *et al.* Psychological problems of cancer patients: a cancer distress screening with a cancer-specific questionnaire. Br J Cancer 2004; 91(3): 504-11. Available from: https://www.nature.com/articles/6601986#citeas [http://dx.doi.org/10.1038/sj.bjc.6601986] [PMID: 15238979]

[12] Huang J, Irvine D. Anesthesia Pain and Safety Considerations in Cancer Patients [Internet]. Anesthesia Patient Safety Foundation. 2022 [cited 2025 Mar 7]. Available from: https://www.apsf.org/article/anesthesia-pain-and-safety-considerations-in-cancer-patients/

[13] Yang J, Lou S, Yao T. Trends in primary malignant bone cancer incidence and mortality in the United States, 2000–2017: A population-based study. J Bone Oncol 2024; 46: 100607-7. Available from: https://pubmed.ncbi.nlm.nih.gov/38778835/ [http://dx.doi.org/10.1016/j.jbo.2024.100607] [PMID: 38778835]

[14] Anderson MR, Jeng CL, Wittig JC, Rosenblatt MA. Anesthesia for patients undergoing orthopedic oncologic surgeries. J Clin Anesth 2010; 22(7): 565-72. Available from: https://tumorsurgery.org/Portals/0/Anesthesis%20for%20patients%20undergoing%20ortho%20oncol%20surg.pdf [http://dx.doi.org/10.1016/j.jclinane.2010.02.011] [PMID: 21056818]

[15] Ewertz M, Qvortrup C, Eckhoff L. Chemotherapy-induced peripheral neuropathy in patients treated with taxanes and platinum derivatives. Acta Oncol 2015; 54(5): 587-91. Available from: https://www.ncbi.nlm.nih.gov/pubmed/25751757 [http://dx.doi.org/10.3109/0284186X.2014.995775] [PMID: 25751757]

[16] Al Jahdali H. Evaluation of the patient with lung cancer. Ann Thorac Med 2008; 3(6) (Suppl. 2): 74. [http://dx.doi.org/10.4103/1817-1737.43108]

[17] Weingarten TN, Araka CN, Mogensen ME, *et al.* Lambert-Eaton myasthenic syndrome during anesthesia: a report of 37 patients. J Clin Anesth 2014; 26(8): 648-53. [http://dx.doi.org/10.1016/j.jclinane.2014.09.009] [PMID: 25468580]

[18] Robinson SP, Akhondi H. Thymoma [Internet]. PubMed. Treasure Island (FL): StatPearls Publishing; 2021. Available from: https://www.ncbi.nlm.nih.gov/books/NBK559291/

[19] Neuman A, Granlund B. Anesthesia For Patients With Myasthenia Gravis [Internet]. PubMed. Treasure Island (FL): StatPearls Publishing; 2021. Available from: https://www.ncbi.nlm.nih.gov/books/NBK572091/

[20] Dang AQ, Raty SR. Perioperative Care of the Surgical Patient: Brain. Elsevier eBooks. 2022 Jul 15;210–23.

[21] Sivanaser V, Manninen P. Preoperative Assessment of Adult Patients for Intracranial Surgery. Anesthesiology Research and Practice [Internet]. 2010 [cited 2020 Feb 1];2010:1–11. Available from: https://www.ncbi.nlm.nih.gov/pmc/articles/PMC2911602/ [http://dx.doi.org/10.1155/2010/241307]

[22] Lee BJ, Jeong JH. Review: Steroid Use in Patients With Acute Spinal Cord Injury and Guideline Update. Korean J Neurotrauma 2022; 18(1): 22-30. [http://dx.doi.org/10.13004/kjnt.2022.18.e21] [PMID: 35557630]

[23] Eldahan KC, Rabchevsky AG. Autonomic dysreflexia after spinal cord injury: Systemic pathophysiology and methods of management. Auton Neurosci 2018; 209: 59-70. Available from: https://www.ncbi.nlm.nih.gov/pmc/articles/PMC5677594/ [http://dx.doi.org/10.1016/j.autneu.2017.05.002] [PMID: 28506502]

[24] Carver JR, Shapiro CL, Ng A, *et al.* American Society of Clinical Oncology clinical evidence review on the ongoing care of adult cancer survivors: cardiac and pulmonary late effects. J Clin Oncol 2007;

25(25): 3991-4008.
[http://dx.doi.org/10.1200/JCO.2007.10.9777] [PMID: 17577017]

[25] Yusuf SW, Sami S, Daher IN. Radiation-Induced Heart Disease: A Clinical Update. Cardiology Research and Practice [Internet]. 2011 [cited 2020 Jan 20];2011:1–9. Available from: https://www.hindawi.com/journals/crp/2011/317659/citations/
[http://dx.doi.org/10.4061/2011/317659]

[26] Kristensen SD, Knuuti J, Saraste A, *et al.* 2014 ESC/ESA Guidelines on non-cardiac surgery: cardiovascular assessment and management. Eur Heart J 2014; 35(35): 2383-431.
[http://dx.doi.org/10.1093/eurheartj/ehu282] [PMID: 25086026]

[27] Jaffe AS, Babuin L, Apple FS. Biomarkers in acute cardiac disease: the present and the future. J Am Coll Cardiol 2006; 48(1): 1-11. Available from: https://mayoclinic.pure.elsevier.com/en/publications/biomarkers-in-acute-cardiac-disease-the-present-and-the-future
[http://dx.doi.org/10.1016/j.jacc.2006.02.056] [PMID: 16814641]

[28] Levi M, Scully M. How I treat disseminated intravascular coagulation. Blood 2018; 131(8): 845-54. Available from: https://ashpublications.org/blood/article/131/8/845/104418/How-I-treat-dissemina-ed-intravascular-coagulation
[http://dx.doi.org/10.1182/blood-2017-10-804096] [PMID: 29255070]

[29] Key NS, Khorana AA, Kuderer NM, *et al.* Venous thromboembolism prophylaxis and treatment in patients with cancer: asco clinical practice guideline update. J Clin Oncol 2020; 38(5): 496-520.
[http://dx.doi.org/10.1200/JCO.19.01461] [PMID: 31381464]

[30] Falanga A, Russo L, Milesi V, Vignoli A. Mechanisms and risk factors of thrombosis in cancer. Crit Rev Oncol Hematol 2017; 118: 79-83.
[http://dx.doi.org/10.1016/j.critrevonc.2017.08.003] [PMID: 28917273]

[31] Gómez-Ramírez S, Bisbe E, Shander A, Spahn DR, Muñoz M. Management of Perioperative Iron Deficiency Anemia. Acta Haematol 2019; 142(1): 21-9. Available from: https://www.karger.com/Article/Abstract/496965
[http://dx.doi.org/10.1159/000496965] [PMID: 30970362]

[32] Kotwal A, Gustafson MP, Bornschlegl S, *et al.* Immune Checkpoint Inhibitor-Induced Thyroiditis Is Associated with Increased Intrathyroidal T Lymphocyte Subpopulations. Thyroid 2020; 30(10): 1440-50.
[http://dx.doi.org/10.1089/thy.2020.0075] [PMID: 32323619]

[33] Thompson GB, Young WF Jr. Adrenal incidentaloma. Curr Opin Oncol 2003; 15(1): 84-90.
[http://dx.doi.org/10.1097/00001622-200301000-00013] [PMID: 12490767]

[34] Franklyn J, Shephard M. Evaluation of Thyroid Function in Health and Disease. In: Feingold KR, Ahmed SF, Anawalt B, et al., editors. Endotext [Internet]. South Dartmouth (MA): MDText.com, Inc.; 2000. Available from: https://www.ncbi.nlm.nih.gov/books/NBK285546/

[35] Dineen R, Thompson CJ, Sherlock M. Adrenal crisis: prevention and management in adult patients. Ther Adv Endocrinol Metab 2019; 10(1): 2042018819848218. Available from: https://journals.sagepub.com/doi/full/10.1177/2042018819848218
[http://dx.doi.org/10.1177/2042018819848218] [PMID: 31223468]

[36] Lederman D, Easwar J, Feldman J, Shapiro V. Anesthetic considerations for lung resection: preoperative assessment, intraoperative challenges and postoperative analgesia. Ann Transl Med 2019; 7(15): 356-6.
[http://dx.doi.org/10.21037/atm.2019.03.67] [PMID: 31516902]

[37] Vu JV, Lussiez A. Smoking Cessation for Preoperative Optimization. Clin Colon Rectal Surg 2023; 36(3): 175-83.
[http://dx.doi.org/10.1055/s-0043-1760870] [PMID: 37113283]

[38] Roy P. Preoperative pulmonary evaluation for lung resection. J Anaesthesiol Clin Pharmacol 2018;

34(3): 296-300. Available from: https://www.ncbi.nlm.nih.gov/pmc/articles/PMC6194844/ [http://dx.doi.org/10.4103/joacp.JOACP_89_17] [PMID: 30386009]

[39] Kanaji N, Watanabe N, Kita N, *et al.* Paraneoplastic syndromes associated with lung cancer. World J Clin Oncol 2014; 5(3): 197-223. Available from: https://www.ncbi.nlm.nih.gov/pmc/articles/PMC4127595/
[http://dx.doi.org/10.5306/wjco.v5.i3.197] [PMID: 25114839]

[40] Ferreiro L, Suárez-Antelo J, Álvarez-Dobaño JM, Toubes ME, Riveiro V, Valdés L. Malignant Pleural Effusion: Diagnosis and Management. Can Respir J 2020; 2020: 1-11.
[http://dx.doi.org/10.1155/2020/2950751] [PMID: 33273991]

[41] Skok K, Hladnik G, Grm A, Crnjac A. Malignant Pleural Effusion and Its Current Management: A Review. Medicina (Kaunas) 2019; 55(8): 490.
[http://dx.doi.org/10.3390/medicina55080490] [PMID: 31443309]

[42] Libura J, Bettens F, Radkowski A, Tiercy JM, Piguet PF. Risk of chemotherapy-induced pulmonary fibrosis is associated with polymorphic tumour necrosis factor-a2 gene. Eur Respir J 2002; 19(5): 912-8.
[http://dx.doi.org/10.1183/09031936.02.00238102] [PMID: 12030733]

[43] Marchioni A, Tonelli R, Rossi G, *et al.* Ventilatory support and mechanical properties of the fibrotic lung acting as a "squishy ball". Ann Intensive Care 2020; 10(1): 13.
[http://dx.doi.org/10.1186/s13613-020-0632-6] [PMID: 32020548]

[44] Boucai L, Zafereo M, Cabanillas ME. Thyroid Cancer. JAMA 2024; 331(5): 425-35. Available from: https://jamanetwork.com/journals/jama/article-abstract/2814532
[http://dx.doi.org/10.1001/jama.2023.26348] [PMID: 38319329]

[45] Hartmann K. Thyroid Disorders in the Oncology Patient. J Adv Pract Oncol 2015; 6(2): 99-106.
[PMID: 26649243]

[46] Jarzebska N, Karetnikova ES, Markov AG, Kasper M, Rodionov RN, Spieth PM. Scarred Lung. An Update on Radiation-Induced Pulmonary Fibrosis. Front Med (Lausanne) 2021; 7: 585756.
[http://dx.doi.org/10.3389/fmed.2020.585756] [PMID: 33521012]

[47] Abbas G, Krasna M. Overview of esophageal cancer. Ann Cardiothorac Surg 2017; 6(2): 131-6. Available from: https://www.ncbi.nlm.nih.gov/pmc/articles/PMC5387155/
[http://dx.doi.org/10.21037/acs.2017.03.03] [PMID: 28447001]

[48] Mboumi IW, Reddy S, Lidor AO. Complications after Esophagectomy. Surg Clin North Am 2019; 99(3): 501-10.
[http://dx.doi.org/10.1016/j.suc.2019.02.011] [PMID: 31047038]

[49] Feenstra ML, van Berge Henegouwen MI, Hollmann MW, Hermanides J, Eshuis WJ. Analgesia in esophagectomy: a narrative review. J Thorac Dis 2023; 15(9): 5099-111. Available from: https://www.ncbi.nlm.nih.gov/pmc/articles/PMC10586998/
[http://dx.doi.org/10.21037/jtd-23-241] [PMID: 37868851]

[50] Abulfazl Shirinzadeh, Talebi Y. Pulmonary Complications due to Esophagectomy. DOAJ (DOAJ: Directory of Open Access Journals). 2011 Jan 1; (3), 93–96.

[51] Patel S, Lutz J, Panchagnula U, Bansal S. Anesthesia and perioperative management of colorectal surgical patients - specific issues (part 2). J Anaesthesiol Clin Pharmacol 2012; 28(3): 304-13. Available from: https://www.ncbi.nlm.nih.gov/pmc/articles/PMC3409937/
[http://dx.doi.org/10.4103/0970-9185.98321] [PMID: 22869934]

[52] Desai N, El-Boghdadly K, Albrecht E. Epidural *vs.* transversus abdominis plane block for abdominal surgery – a systematic review, meta□analysis and trial sequential analysis. Anaesthesia 2021; 76(1): 101-17.
[http://dx.doi.org/10.1111/anae.15068] [PMID: 32385856]

[53] Allum WH, Blazeby JM, Griffin SM, Cunningham D, Jankowski JA, Wong R. Guidelines for the

management of oesophageal and gastric cancer. Gut 2011; 60(11): 1449-72. Available from: https://gut.bmj.com/content/60/11/1449
[http://dx.doi.org/10.1136/gut.2010.228254] [PMID: 21705456]

[54] American Cancer Society. American Cancer Society | Cancer Facts & Statistics [Internet]. American Cancer Society | Cancer Facts & Statistics. 2019. Available from: https://cancerstatisticscenter.cancer.org/

[55] Burciu C, Sirli R, Bende R, *et al.* Paraneoplastic Syndromes in Hepatocellular Carcinoma, Epidemiology, and Survival: A Retrospective Seven Years Study. Medicina [Internet]. 2024 Apr 1;60(4):552. Available from: https://www.mdpi.com/1648-9144/60/4/552

[56] Wan SZ, Nie Y, Zhang Y, Liu C, Zhu X. Assessing the Prognostic Performance of the Child-Pugh, Model for End-Stage Liver Disease, and Albumin-Bilirubin Scores in Patients with Decompensated Cirrhosis: A Large Asian Cohort from Gastroenterology Department. Dis Markers 2020; 2020: 1-9.
[http://dx.doi.org/10.1155/2020/5193028] [PMID: 32148566]

[57] Hartog A, Mills G. Anaesthesia for hepatic resection surgery. Contin Educ Anaesth Crit Care Pain 2009; 9(1): 1-5.
[http://dx.doi.org/10.1093/bjaceaccp/mkn050]

[58] Bethesda. LiverTox: Clinical and Research Information on Drug-Induced Liver Injury [Internet]. PubMed. Bethesda (MD): National Institute of Diabetes and Digestive and Kidney Diseases; 2012. Available from: https://www.ncbi.nlm.nih.gov/books/NBK547852/

[59] Torres HA, Davila M. Reactivation of hepatitis B virus and hepatitis C virus in patients with cancer. Nat Rev Clin Oncol 2012; 9(3): 156-66. Available from: https://www.nature.com/articles/nrclinonc.2012.1
[http://dx.doi.org/10.1038/nrclinonc.2012.1] [PMID: 22271089]

[60] Wang F, Herrington M, Larsson J, Permert J. The relationship between diabetes and pancreatic cancer. Mol Cancer 2003; 2(1): 4. Available from: https://www.ncbi.nlm.nih.gov/pmc/articles/PMC149418/
[http://dx.doi.org/10.1186/1476-4598-2-4] [PMID: 12556242]

[61] Scelo G, Larose TL. Epidemiology and Risk Factors for Kidney Cancer. J Clin Oncol 2018; 36(36): 3574-81. Available from: https://www.ncbi.nlm.nih.gov/pubmed/30372394
[http://dx.doi.org/10.1200/JCO.2018.79.1905] [PMID: 30372394]

[62] Santos MLC, Brito BB, Silva FAF, Botelho ACS, Melo FF. Nephrotoxicity in cancer treatment: An overview. World J Clin Oncol 2020; 11(4): 190-204.
[http://dx.doi.org/10.5306/wjco.v11.i4.190] [PMID: 32355641]

[63] Alhaqas G, Ahmed F, Taha S, Akl A, Abdullah S. SAT-027 Cisplatin Nephrotoxicity in a Patient with Cervical Cancer with Acquired Type 2 Renal Tubular Acidosis: Review of Literature and Case Report. Kidney Int Rep 2020; 5(3): S13-3.
[http://dx.doi.org/10.1016/j.ekir.2020.02.032]

[64] Miyoshi A, Miyatake T, Hara T, Tanaka A, Naoko Komura, Shinnosuke Komiya, et al. Etiology of Ascites and Pleural Effusion Associated with Ovarian Tumors: Literature Review and Case Reports of Three Ovarian Tumors Presenting with Massive Ascites, but without Peritoneal Dissemination. Case Reports in Obstetrics and Gynecology [Internet]. 2015 Jan 1 [cited 2025 Feb 4];2015:1–5. Available from: https://pmc.ncbi.nlm.nih.gov/articles/PMC4697079/

CHAPTER 8

Unique Anesthetic Considerations in Cancer Patients

Mia Ye[1] and **Mina Ghaly**[1,*]

[1] *Department of Anesthesiology, George Washington School of Medicine and Health Sciences, Washington, DC, USA*

Abstract: In this chapter, we examine how unique situations arise in cancer patients and how they affect anesthetic management. The conditions include septic and obese patients, cancer-causing paraneoplastic syndromes such as Cushing's and Lambert-Eaton Syndromes or tumor compression causing mesenteric ischemia. Finally, we examine anesthetic options for patients undergoing stem cell transplantation.

Keywords: Cushing's syndrome, Lambert-Eaton myasthenic syndrome, Mesenteric ischemia, Obese patient, Paraneoplastic syndromes, Stem cell treatment, Sepsis, Tumor compression, Unique anesthesia consideration.

INTRODUCTION

The anesthetic management of cancer patients is a complex challenge that requires an understanding of the relationship between malignancy, comorbid conditions, and the body's response to surgical stress and anesthetic agents. Cancer, along with the associated treatments, can significantly alter physiological systems requiring specialized and individualized anesthesia techniques. This chapter explores the unique anesthetic considerations involved in caring for cancer patients, with a focus on systemic and comorbid conditions, tumor compression, paraneoplastic syndromes, and specialized anesthetic management techniques.

Systemic and comorbid conditions, such as sepsis and obesity, are common among cancer patients and pose significant challenges to anesthesiologists. Sepsis, a critical and often life-threatening condition, can cause profound physiological

* **Corresponding author Mina Ghaly:** Department of Anesthesiology, George Washington School of Medicine and Health Sciences, Washington, DC, USA; E-mail: Ghaly-Mina@cooperhealth.edu

Bharathi Gourkanti, Irwin Gratz, William Marion, Rajiv Lingaraju & Grace Abramian (Eds.)

instability, while obesity introduces additional concerns, including respiratory compromise and cardiovascular strain. These conditions require meticulous perioperative management to optimize patient outcomes.

Another crucial aspect of anesthetic management in cancer patients involves the effects of tumor compression, such as in the case of a mediastinal mass. Tumor-induced anatomical changes can directly affect airway, cardiovascular, and neural function, and require careful planning to mitigate risks during surgery and anesthesia.

Additionally, paraneoplastic syndromes can further complicate anesthetic management. These syndromes, often overlooked or misdiagnosed, can manifest with neurological and endocrine disruptions that must be carefully considered when choosing anesthetic agents and monitoring parameters.

Lastly, specialized anesthetic management techniques are required in certain surgical situations. Each of these conditions presents its own unique set of challenges, ranging from optimizing fluid resuscitation and hemodynamic stability to managing organ function and preventing complications.

In this chapter, we will explore these critical topics, emphasizing the need for a comprehensive, patient-tailored approach to anesthetic care. By understanding the multifactorial nature of cancer and its associated conditions, anesthesiologists can enhance the safety, comfort, and outcomes of cancer patients undergoing surgical interventions.

SYSTEMIC AND COMORBID CONSIDERATIONS IN CANCER PATIENTS

Cancer patients often present with a unique set of challenges when it comes to anesthetic management due to the presence of systemic conditions and comorbidities that can significantly impact perioperative care. Among these, sepsis and obesity are particularly critical factors that require careful consideration in the perioperative period. Both conditions can compromise the body's response to anesthesia, complicate surgical outcomes, and increase the risks of intraoperative instability and postoperative complications.

Sepsis

Sepsis is a leading cause of mortality, with a thirty-day mortality rate of 24.4% for sepsis and 34.7% for septic shock, it is an emergency that calls for early detection and rapid treatment [1]. While sepsis mortality rates are high in all cases, patients with cancer are more likely to develop sepsis, and the mortality from sepsis in such patients is significantly higher [2]. Treatment for sepsis can vary, as no pharmacologic intervention has been shown to consistently reduce mortality [2].

The first six hours of resuscitation of patients with sepsis are referred to as the golden hours due to the critical nature of the disease, to provide the patient with the highest chance of survival. Pre-operative treatment of patients with sepsis includes assessment and optimization. Prior to induction, anesthesiologists must ensure that the patient is as stable as possible to reduce the risk of complications during surgery. This includes ensuring hemodynamic stability, respiratory stability, renal function, and infection control. IV antimicrobial therapy should be administered immediately after the diagnosis of sepsis or septic shock is made. Currently, there is no benefit for delaying treatment until culture results or the start of surgery [3, 4].

Hemodynamic optimization in a timely manner is critical as treatment before organ failure can reduce mortality by 23% compared to patients treated after the onset of organ failure [1]. Hypovolemia can be corrected with a balanced crystalloid solution of up to 30 ml/kg during the first three hours. A patient is determined to be responsive if there is an increase in stroke volume of more than 10-15%. Alternative measures of determining responsiveness can be an increase in pulse pressure of >10% [1].

Respiratory function must also be monitored to avoid respiratory depression and injury during ventilation. Patients with sepsis may have comorbid conditions such as acute respiratory distress syndrome (ARDS), lung inflammation, or metabolic acidosis, which can alter the patient's respiratory function compared to baseline [1]. Therefore, physical examination as well as chest imaging are critical to identifying and treating lung injury.

For elective patients, de-nitrogenation of the lungs with patients breathing 100% O2 through a tightly fitted facemask for up to 3 minutes is recommended. However, patients with sepsis or septic shock often require emergent surgical intervention, making modified rapid sequence induction the preferred approach for initiating general anesthesia. Depending on the urgency and their laboratory values, succinylcholine or rocuronium can be used to facilitate tracheal intubation. Given the frequent presence of hemodynamic instability and compromised hepatic and renal function in septic patients, it is crucial to account for these alterations during induction, as both intravenous and inhalational agents can exacerbate myocardial depression or vasodilation [4]. Induction of anesthesia can be done with commonly used agents such as propofol or with more cardiovascular stable agents such as etomidate or ketamine. Current evidence does not clearly favor one over the other, but care should be taken to use smaller doses given the hemodynamic instability of septic patients [1]. To minimize the hemodynamic burden of induction agents, reduced doses may be employed in conjunction with short-acting opioids such as fentanyl. Continuous and vigilant hemodynamic monitoring is essential; invasive arterial lines and central venous access should be established, and vasopressors should be kept readily available, as anesthetic induction can precipitate profound hypotension in this patient population [1]. Remifentanil is especially advantageous in this context as its metabolism is unaffected by hepatic or renal dysfunction, which can be common in septic patients. While remifentanil may cause bradycardia, this side effect can actually be beneficial in septic patients, who are frequently tachycardic [4].

There is currently no evidence supporting the superiority of volatile versus intravenous anesthetic maintenance techniques, and anesthesiologists are encouraged to base their choice on individual patient risk factors and their own clinical experience [4]. Volatile anesthetics exhibit immunomodulatory effects such as the inhibition of neutrophil function and suppression of cytokine release, but most supporting data derive from *in vitro* and animal model studies [1]. Importantly, sepsis and septic shock significantly reduce the minimum alveolar concentration (MAC) of inhaled agents. In patients with compromised lung function, intravenous anesthesia may provide more reliable brain drug levels due to unpredictable alveolar gas exchange [1]. To avoid awareness or anesthetic overdose in this high-risk group, depth of anesthesia should be monitored with processed EEG tools such as the bispectral index.

Intraoperative hypotension is common and often exacerbated by anesthetic agents and mechanical ventilation. Early and continued volume resuscitation, alongside vasopressors like norepinephrine, is recommended to mitigate these effects [4]. Dynamic markers such as pulse pressure and stroke volume variation are more reliable than static pressure-based estimates such as CVP for assessing fluid responsiveness, especially in patients receiving controlled ventilation with a regular heart rhythm [4]. Intraoperative use of transesophageal echocardiography or esophageal Doppler can further guide fluid therapy. The goal is to optimize tissue oxygen delivery rather than to achieve fixed targets for cardiac output or arterial pressure, with serum lactate and mixed venous oxygen saturation serving as useful global indicators [4].

Mechanical ventilation strategies should be lung-protective, emphasizing low tidal volumes and permissive hypercapnia to prevent ventilator-induced lung injury, except in cases with contraindications such as raised intracranial pressure or late pregnancy [4]. If hypoxia persists despite elevated FiO_2, incremental PEEP may be added cautiously, provided the patient remains hemodynamically stable [4].

Recruitment maneuvers may be considered in select cases but should be approached with caution in patients at risk of barotrauma [4].

Peripheral nerve blocks may reduce sympathetic stimulation and opioid requirements, though their effectiveness may be diminished in the presence of acidosis or infection [4]. Neuraxial techniques, including epidural and spinal anesthesia, should be used with extreme caution, as they may provoke profound hypotension in the already compromised septic circulation and carry increased risks of complications in this setting [4]. Ultimately, the anesthetic strategy in septic cancer patients must be highly individualized, balancing physiological derangements with surgical demands while optimizing oxygen delivery and minimizing harm.

Following surgical source control in patients with sepsis or septic shock, postoperative care frequently requires intensive monitoring and ongoing organ support, necessitating admission to the intensive care unit [1]. These patients may remain hemodynamically unstable and hypoperfused, with ongoing requirements for mechanical ventilation, vasopressor support, and renal replacement therapy.

Given the critical and fast-acting nature of sepsis, being able to predict and act fast can be highly advantageous. Preoperative predictive factors include the Charlson comorbidity index and the American Society of Anesthesiologists (ASA) physical status. ASA physical status is commonly used to determine co-morbidity in high-risk surgical patients. However, it is a highly subjective score compared to the Charlson comorbidity index. The Charlson comorbidity index weighs co-morbid variables and demonstrated a correlation with risk of postoperative severe sepsis [3]. The Charlson comorbidity index and post-operative factors such as logistic organ dysfunction (LOD) can be used to determine the risk of developing sepsis [3]. LOD score provides a value derived from a multiple logistic regression model that incorporates dysfunction in six organ systems, thus quantifying multiple organ dysfunction that can be tracked over time [3]. An LOD score of 1 or more is predictive for developing severe sepsis with a sensitivity of 80% and a specificity of 72% [3]. ICU mortality was also associated with an LOD score in the diagnosis of catheter-related bacteremia [3].

Gender was also discovered to play a role in the risk of developing sepsis. Mice studies have shown that male gender increases the risk for developing sepsis, although the exact cause for this gender difference in the development of sepsis is unclear [3].

Overall treatment should be personalized as each patient with sepsis will have different inciting factors, demographics, environment, and co-morbidities. This can affect both treatment and prediction, as outcomes can vary from patient to patient even when treated with the same intervention.

Obesity

Obesity presents a significant challenge to anesthetic management due to a variety of physiological and metabolic changes that alter the pharmacokinetics and pharmacodynamics of anesthetic agents. Obese patients often exhibit altered airway anatomy, which can complicate intubation and increase the risk of difficult airways. Excess fat deposition around the neck and chest can reduce the size of the upper airway, making airway management more difficult and requiring careful consideration during both induction and maintenance of anesthesia.

The respiratory system is particularly affected by obesity, with many obese patients experiencing obstructive sleep apnea (OSA) or hypoventilation syndrome. These conditions increase the risk of intraoperative hypoxia, hypercapnia, and respiratory complications, making airway management even more crucial. Additionally, obesity leads to a decrease in functional residual capacity (FRC) and total lung capacity (TLC), which can result in impaired oxygenation and ventilation during anesthesia [5].

In terms of drug metabolism, obesity affects the distribution and elimination of many anesthetic agents. Fat-soluble drugs, such as propofol, may have an increased volume of distribution, leading to longer onset times and prolonged effects [5]. Conversely, water-soluble drugs, such as muscle relaxants, may have a reduced volume of distribution in obese patients, requiring careful dosing to avoid prolonged effects or inadequate paralysis [5].

Obesity also increases the risk of cardiovascular complications during anesthesia, including hypertension, increased cardiac output, and the development of heart failure in some cases [5]. The elevated work of breathing and increased oxygen demand may place additional strain on the heart, particularly in patients with underlying cardiovascular disease. Furthermore, obese patients may have a higher incidence of venous thromboembolism, which necessitates careful consideration of thromboprophylaxis during the perioperative period [5].

The renal system in obese patients is also often affected, with some patients showing signs of impaired renal function or altered pharmacokinetics of renally cleared drugs [5]. The increased adiposity can affect drug clearance, especially for those drugs that are excreted by the kidneys, leading to prolonged drug half-life and an increased risk of toxicity [5]. The presence of obesity-related comorbidities, such as diabetes, hypertension, and dyslipidemia, complicates anesthesia further by increasing the risk of intraoperative and postoperative complications [5]. These comorbidities can affect wound healing, increase the risk of infections, and contribute to poor postoperative outcomes [5].

Finally, pain control can be difficult in obese patients due to the high prevalence of OSA. General recommendations include multimodal analgesic therapy with the minimal use of sedatives, preference for regional techniques, and head of bed elevation to 30 degrees with early mobilization if possible [5].

PARANEOPLASTIC SYNDROMES AND THEIR EFFECT ON ANESTHETIC MANAGEMENT

Paraneoplastic syndromes represent a complex and often underrecognized group of disorders that arise from the indirect effects of malignancy, rather than direct tumor invasion or metastasis. Among these, conditions such as Lambert-Eaton Myasthenic Syndrome (LEMS) and Cushing's Syndrome (CS) are particularly significant due to their profound impact on perioperative management and anesthetic care. Although these syndromes are rare, their clinical consequences can be life-threatening and demand a nuanced, individualized approach to anesthetic planning. Paraneoplastic syndromes can frequently precede the diagnosis of the underlying malignancy, meaning anesthesiologists may encounter these conditions before oncologists do. Moreover, the presentation of these syndromes can mimic or mask other perioperative concerns, leading to delayed diagnosis and increased morbidity. For example, unrecognized LEMS may present only as unexplained postoperative weakness, while occult CS may manifest intraoperatively as refractory hypertension or glucose instability. Without heightened clinical awareness and dedicated research to guide decision-making, the risks for perioperative complications remain high.

Lambert-Eaton Myasthenic Syndrome

Lambert-Eaton myasthenic syndrome (LEMS) is a rare autoimmune disorder affecting the neuromuscular junction (NMJ), characterized by proximal muscle weakness, autonomic symptoms, bulbar dysfunction, and, notably, heightened sensitivity to neuromuscular blocking agents. Muscle weakness is caused by autoimmune-mediated destruction of presynaptic voltage-gated calcium channels, resulting in reduced acetylcholine release at the NMJ. Importantly, LEMS has a strong paraneoplastic association, most commonly small cell lung cancer (SCLC), with nearly half of cases linked to malignancy [6]. Neurologic symptoms often precede the diagnosis of cancer, with a median interval of six months between the onset of LEMS and cancer detection, though this can range from several years before to years after a malignancy is identified [6]. In the perioperative setting, patients with LEMS are at increased risk of complications, particularly postoperative respiratory failure, especially if the syndrome is undiagnosed or untreated at the time of surgery. LEMS patients show increased sensitivity to both non-depolarizing and depolarizing neuromuscular blocking agents (NMBs), making regional anesthesia preferred to general anesthesia. For general anesthesia, intraoperative use of NMBs must be approached with caution and best avoided, when possible, as it has been linked to delayed recovery from paralysis and difficulty weaning from mechanical ventilation [6]. Reduce your dose of NMB agents and titrate to quantitative twitch monitoring. Reversal with neostigmine may be ineffective, and it is best to use suggamadex if available. Minimize the use of medication that depresses the respiratory function, such as opioids. There is a potential aspiration risk due to bulbar dysfunction, particularly in patients with a history of oropharyngeal symptoms or recurrent aspiration, underscoring the need for careful airway assessment and planning [6]. There is also potential for autonomic dysfunction due to the relative lack of acetylcholine [7]. Postoperative considerations are centered around predicting the patient's need for ventilator support.

Cushing's Syndrome

Cushing's syndrome (CS) is a rare but clinically significant endocrine disorder resulting from excessive glucocorticoid levels, often manifesting with hallmark features such as central obesity, hyperglycemia, metabolic alkalosis, hypokalemia, hypertension, and impaired wound healing. Approximately 70% of endogenous CS cases are caused by Cushing's disease, a pituitary adenoma secreting adrenocorticotropic hormone (ACTH), while about 15% result from ectopic ACTH production and another 15% from primary adrenal tumors [8]. This link between ectopic ACTH secretion and certain cancers, particularly lung cancer in men, highlights the syndrome's relevance in oncologic contexts.

From an anesthetic perspective, CS poses substantial challenges due to potential difficult airway management, glucose intolerance, hypokalemia, volume overload, and hemodynamic instability [8]. Pre-operative evaluation should include airway (evaluate patients for possible obesity, poor mouth opening and OSA), cardiovascular function (review ECG and echo for possible left ventricular hypertrophy, pulmonary hypertension/right ventricular failure, systolic and diastolic dysfunction), metabolic derangements (review labs for possible hypokalemic metabolic alkalosis due to mineralcorticoid effect of glucocorticoids), osteoporosis (need for careful patient positioning in the operating room). There should also be a discussion between the anesthesiologist, surgical, and endocrine teams regarding perioperative steroid replacement, including stress dose and postoperative replacement, if needed. No specific anesthetic technique is universally recommended for CS. Total intravenous anesthesia with propofol and remifentanil is frequently preferred due to stable hemodynamic profiles and rapid recovery [8]. Etomidate, despite its adrenal suppression, may be used during Cushing's surgery due to its favorable profile in this population [8]. Ketamine should be avoided due to its sympathetic stimulation, which may exacerbate hypertension and tachycardia [8]. Postoperative management must prioritize respiratory function through effective analgesia (*via* systemic or epidural routes), respiratory exercises, and early mobilization to prevent atelectasis and thromboembolic events. Continued monitoring of cortisol, glucose, and electrolytes is crucial with appropriate treatment. Antihypertensive medications and insulin therapy should be titrated based on hemodynamic and metabolic status.

SPECIALIZED ANESTHETIC MANAGEMENT TECHNIQUES

Anesthetic management in complex surgical cases demands not only technical expertise but also a nuanced understanding of the underlying pathophysiology and the unique vulnerabilities of specific patient populations. As surgical procedures become increasingly sophisticated and patient demographics skew older and more comorbid, the role of the anesthesiologist has expanded well beyond the operating room to encompass perioperative optimization, critical care coordination, and hemodynamic modulation. Certain conditions, such as mesenteric ischemia, hematopoietic stem cell transplantation, and lung resection for malignancy, pose distinct physiological challenges and necessitate tailored anesthetic approaches. These scenarios require not only rapid and accurate clinical decision-making but also the thoughtful selection of anesthetic agents, monitoring modalities, and postoperative strategies to improve patient outcomes and reduce perioperative risks.

Mesenteric Ischemia

Mesenteric ischemia, particularly in elderly patients, is a life-threatening condition that demands rapid diagnosis, usually *via* angiography, followed by timely revascularization and surgical resection of necrotic bowel. In this critical scenario, the anesthesiologist plays a central role in orchestrating resuscitative measures through the careful administration of crystalloids, colloids, and vasoactive agents, along with continuous, intensive monitoring of hemodynamics and tissue oxygenation. Mesenteric venous thrombosis (MVT), though less common, accounts for 5-15% of mesenteric ischemia cases and is often associated with risk factors like abdominal malignancies, cirrhosis, abdominal trauma, hypercoagulable states, cardiovascular disease, and advanced age [9]. Elevated D-dimer levels are typically the most consistent laboratory finding in MVT, while other diagnostic tests lack sufficient specificity and sensitivity.

Given the emergent nature of bowel ischemia, there is minimal time for comprehensive preoperative optimization. Clinical signs of hypoperfusion signal critical illness and must be addressed before proceeding with anesthesia. Standard preoperative preparation includes establishing large-bore intravenous access, placement of intra-arterial lines for blood sampling and continuous pressure monitoring, and central venous access for vasoactive drug infusion and advanced hemodynamic monitoring if warranted by the patient's hemodynamic status. Blood gases and lactate levels offer insights into global tissue perfusion, and hourly urine output greater than 0.5 mL/kg/h may indicate adequate organ perfusion, although it is not definitive. Given the high aspiration risk, sufficient pre-oxygenation followed by rapid sequence induction (RSI) with cricoid pressure is recommended with care to avoid hypotension during induction [9].

While no clear guidelines exist regarding the optimal maintenance technique in patients with bowel ischemia, studies have shown no significant differences between intravenous anesthesia (TIVA) with propofol vs inhalational agents [9]. Isoflurane and desflurane have shown comparable outcomes in preserving tissue oxygenation during colorectal procedures [9]. Moderate doses of opioids, such as morphine, appear beneficial by improving splanchnic perfusion and lowering intestinal oxygen demand [9]. The choice of anesthetic agents may be severely limited by patient fragility and hemodynamic instability, often necessitating a lighter anesthetic plan. In such high-risk situations, awareness is a valid concern, and bispectral index (BIS) monitoring is recommended to prevent both under- and overdosing of anesthetics.

Elderly patients frequently suffer from impaired thermoregulation, and open abdominal procedures can result in significant heat loss [9]. Core temperature monitoring and proactive warming strategies are crucial to prevent hypothermia, which may exacerbate splanchnic vasoconstriction, impair clotting, and increase the likelihood of wound infections [9]. Patients requiring reoperation or those with persistent acidosis, hypoxemia, or instability should remain intubated postoperatively and be admitted to the intensive care unit (ICU) for continued support and stabilization.

Stem Cell Transplantation

Hematopoietic stem cell transplantation (HSCT) involves the reconstitution of blood cell lineages using donor stem cells and engages complex interactions between the host's immune cells, such as T lymphocytes and natural killer (NK) cells, and donor antigen-presenting cells and lymphocytes. In allogeneic HSCT, the beneficial graft-versus-tumor (GVT) effect, which helps prevent cance recurrence, is counterbalanced by the risk of graft-versus-host disease (GVHD), often necessitating prolonged immunosuppression.

Post-HSCT patients face increased susceptibility to opportunistic infections, particularly before engraftment, and early signs of infection may be subtle or missed during preoperative evaluation [10]. Surgical interventions during this period are further complicated by delayed wound healing, and both enhanced immune responses and excessive immunosuppression pose risks, GVHD in the former, and opportunistic infections or viral reactivation (such as cytomegalovirus) in the latter [10].

From an anesthetic standpoint, preoperative assessments must account for long-term chemotherapy effects, which can include difficult airway management due to gum hypertrophy from cyclosporine or lymphadenopathy from post-transplant lymphoproliferative disorders (PTLD) [10]. Acute GVHD may affect multiple organ systems, leading to complications such as acute lung injury, hepatic veno-occlusive disease, and thrombotic microangiopathy (TMA), all of which necessitate thorough evaluation prior to the start of anesthesia.

Surgical stress induces transient immunosuppression through mechanisms involving elevated catecholamines, angiogenic factors, matrix metalloproteinases (MMPs), and decreased NK cell and cell-mediated immunity activity [10]. Certain anesthetic agents can further modulate immune function, and volatile agents like isoflurane may promote tumor progression by suppressing NK cells and enhancing angiogenesis through upregulation of hypoxia-inducible factor (HIF-1 alpha), while nitrous oxide contributes to bone marrow suppression. In contrast, sevoflurane is a potentially safer alternative as it stabilizes tumor-suppressor genes such as P38 [10].

Similarly, intravenous agents such as ketamine and thiopentone may decrease immune surveillance by inducing T cell apoptosis and suppressing NK cell activity, while propofol helps preserve T cell function and inhibits angiogenesis, making it an advantageous choice in oncology cases. Though midazolam may impair macrophage and monocyte function, it is still considered relatively safe [10].

The action of neuromuscular blockers can be prolonged in patients on immunosuppressants such as cyclosporine which is a phenomenon also observed in renal transplant recipients. Although opioids reduce immune cell activity at high doses, they may paradoxically enhance tumor lysis *via* stabilization of tumor suppressors like P53 and activation of apoptotic pathways such as NF KB and Fas-FasL [10]. When feasible, regional anesthesia should be strongly considered, as local anesthetics can enhance NK cell activity and have been associated with reduced tumor burden, particularly in certain cancer types such as estrogen receptor-negative breast cancer [10].

Lung Resection

In patients undergoing open lung resection, the choice of anesthetic technique can influence perioperative outcomes. Compared to the sole use of general anesthesia, studies have shown that the use of neuraxial anesthesia in conjunction with general anesthesia was associated with a reduced need for blood transfusion and decreased rates of mechanical ventilation postoperatively, indicating improved hemodynamic control and respiratory function [11]. These benefits may be caused by the sympathetic blockade induced by neuraxial anesthesia, which improves blood pressure stability and reduces intraoperative blood loss. Additionally, the technique has been linked to reduced neurohumoral stress responses, enhanced intestinal perfusion, accelerated return of gastrointestinal function, and opioid-sparing effects, which could contribute to improved recovery and potentially better oncologic outcomes [11].

Main risk with neuraxial anesthesia was an increased incidence of thromboembolic complications such as deep vein thrombosis (DVT), pulmonary embolism (PE), and cerebrovascular events thought to be secondary to discontinuation of the anticoagulant medications in patients receiving neuraxial techniques [11]. Other potential side effects associated with neuraxial anesthesia include intraoperative hypotension, pruritus, urinary retention, respiratory depression, post-dural puncture headache, and the rare but serious risk of permanent neurologic injury.

In conclusion, the combined use of neuraxial and general anesthesia during open lung resection for cancer offers notable benefits in terms of reduced transfusion requirements and mechanical ventilation, but it necessitates cautious thromboembolic risk assessment and tailored anticoagulation strategies to mitigate its associated complications.

CONCLUSION

Anesthetic management in cancer patients is an intricate process that requires a deep understanding of the complexities presented by both the disease itself and its associated comorbidities. Throughout this chapter, we have explored the unique challenges posed by systemic conditions such as sepsis and obesity, the critical impact of tumor compression on organ function, the complications introduced by paraneoplastic syndromes, and the specialized techniques necessary for managing high-risk situations like mesenteric ischemia, stem cell treatments, and lung resections.

The anesthesiologist must adopt a comprehensive and individualized approach, balancing the need for effective pain management, hemodynamic stability, and minimizing the risk of perioperative complications. This often involves close collaboration with multidisciplinary teams, an awareness of underlying pathophysiology, and real-time adjustments to anesthetic techniques as the clinical situation evolves.

Ultimately, the goal of anesthesia in cancer patients is to optimize surgical outcomes while minimizing the risks inherent in their often-compromised physiological state. By considering the full spectrum of cancer-related factors, anesthesiologists can significantly improve the safety, recovery, and quality of life for cancer patients undergoing surgery. As cancer treatments and patient profiles continue to evolve, ongoing research and clinical practice refinement will remain essential to meeting the unique anesthetic needs of this complex patient population.

REFERENCES

[1] Carsetti A, Vitali E, Pesaresi L, *et al.* Anesthetic management of patients with sepsis/septic shock. Front Med (Lausanne) 2023; 10: 1150124. [http://dx.doi.org/10.3389/fmed.2023.1150124] [PMID: 37035341]

[2] Williams JC, Ford ML, Coopersmith CM. Cancer and sepsis. Clin Sci (Lond) 2023; 137(11): 881-93. [http://dx.doi.org/10.1042/CS20220713] [PMID: 37314016]

[3] Mokart D, Leone M, Sannini A, *et al.* Predictive perioperative factors for developing severe sepsis after major surgery. Br J Anaesth 2005; 95(6): 776-81. [http://dx.doi.org/10.1093/bja/aei257] [PMID: 16227337]

[4] Eissa D, Carton EG, Buggy DJ. Anaesthetic management of patients with severe sepsis. Br J Anaesth 2010; 105(6): 734-43. [http://dx.doi.org/10.1093/bja/aeq305] [PMID: 21030391]

[5] Schug SA, Raymann A. Postoperative pain management of the obese patient. Baillieres Best Pract Res Clin Anaesthesiol 2011; 25(1): 73-81. [http://dx.doi.org/10.1016/j.bpa.2010.12.001] [PMID: 21516915]

[6] Weingarten TN, Araka CN, Mogensen ME, *et al.* Lambert-Eaton myasthenic syndrome during anesthesia: a report of 37 patients. J Clin Anesth 2014; 26(8): 648-53. [http://dx.doi.org/10.1016/j.jclinane.2014.09.009] [PMID: 25468580]

[7] Kesner VG, Oh SJ, Dimachkie MM, Barohn RJ. Lambert-Eaton Myasthenic Syndrome. Neurol Clin 2018; 36(2): 379-94. [http://dx.doi.org/10.1016/j.ncl.2018.01.008] [PMID: 29655456]

[8] Domi R. Cushing's surgery: Role of the anesthesiologist. Indian J Endocrinol Metab 2011; 15(8): 322. [http://dx.doi.org/10.4103/2230-8210.86975]

[9] Vitin AA, Metzner JI. Anesthetic management of acute mesenteric ischemia in elderly patients. Anesthesiol Clin 2009; 27(3): 551-67. [http://dx.doi.org/10.1016/j.anclin.2009.07.017] [PMID: 19825492]

[10] Chowdhury SR, Roy A, Maitra S, Baidya DK. Anesthetic concerns in recipients of hematopoietic stem cell transplant. J Anaesthesiol Clin Pharmacol 2023; 39(1): 155-7. [http://dx.doi.org/10.4103/joacp.joacp_212_21] [PMID: 37250234]

[11] Özbek U, Poeran J, Mazumdar M, Memtsoudis SG. Patient Safety and Comparative Effectiveness of Anesthetic Technique in Open Lung Resections. Chest 2015; 148(3): 722-30. [http://dx.doi.org/10.1378/chest.14-3040] [PMID: 25812171]

CHAPTER 9

Post Operative Care of Cancer Patients

Flore Macenat Sulzynski[1,*] and **William Marion**[2]

[1] *Temple University at Fox Chase Cancer Center, Philadelphia, USA*

[2] *Department of Anesthesiology, Cooper Medical School of Rowan University, Cooper University Health Care, Camden, NJ, USA*

Abstract: Postoperative management of cancer patients demands a nuanced and collaborative approach, extending beyond the operating room to ensure optimal outcomes. Anesthesiologists play a pivotal role in managing pain, minimizing complications, and supporting early recovery and rehabilitation. This chapter explores evidence-based strategies, including Enhanced Recovery After Surgery (ERAS), multimodal analgesia, and regional anesthesia techniques. It also highlights the importance of psychological support, nutritional optimization, complication prevention, and long-term pain and palliative care. The chapter highlights the anesthesiologist's unique position to lead multidisciplinary teams in delivering comprehensive, patient-centered postoperative care for oncology patients.

Keywords: Cancer recovery, ERAS, Multimodal analgesia, Opioid-sparing strategies, Pain Management, Postoperative care, Palliative care, Regional anesthesia.

INTRODUCTION

The anesthesiologist's role in the care of surgical cancer patients does not end when the patient leaves the operating room. Postoperative management represents a critical extension of perioperative care—particularly for oncology patients, whose complex needs demand vigilance, precision, and a personalized approach. These patients often arrive at the operating table with a host of pre-existing challenges stemming from chemotherapy, radiation, immunosuppression, and chronic cancer pain [1]. Each of these factors increases the risk of complications and demands that require coordinated postoperative care.

* **Corresponding author Flore Macenat Sulzynski:** Temple University at Fox Chase Cancer Center, Philadelphia, USA; E-mail: Flore.Macenat@tuhs.temple.edu

POSTOPERATIVE PAIN MANAGEMENT: A CENTRAL CONCERN

Managing Pain in Cancer Patients

Postoperative pain in cancer patients is layered atop other types of pain, such as tumor-related pain, chemotherapy-induced neuropathy, post-radiation fibrosis, or chronic pain syndromes from prior cancer surgeries [2]. This pain can be intensified by both the surgery and pre-existing opioid tolerance in patients who have relied on chronic opioid therapy. These patients may benefit from a multimodal approach, which may include techniques such as regional anesthesia and the use of ketamine as an adjuvant to pain control.

Early Recovery after Surgery

Enhanced Recovery After Surgery (ERAS) is an evidence-based multidisciplinary approach to perioperative care that aims to reduce surgical stress, maintain physiologic function, and accelerate recovery [3]. In cancer patients, ERAS has added value as it addresses the increased risk of complications, chronic pain, and prolonged hospitalization. This protocol integrates multimodal analgesia, early ambulation, nutritional optimization, and psychological support.

Multimodal opioid-sparing pain management strategies are particularly emphasized in ERAS and critical in cancer patients who are already immunocompromised or at higher risk for postoperative complications [4, 5]. Non-opioid adjuncts such as acetaminophen, NSAIDs, gabapentinoids, NMDA antagonists like ketamine, and alpha-2 agonists such as dexmedetomidine are commonly used [6].

Regional techniques such as thoracic epidurals, paravertebral blocks, TAP blocks, or PECS blocks are frequently included in ERAS pathways for cancer surgeries [7]. These approaches reduce opioid consumption, enhance mobilization, andimprove postoperative outcomes.

Preoperative optimization, including nutrition and physical conditioning, is crucial, and psychosocial counseling can prepare the patient for both the physical and emotional stress of surgery [8].

Multimodal Analgesia

Multimodal analgesia is the cornerstone of postoperative pain management in cancer patients. This approach leverages the synergistic effects of combining various analgesic agents to reduce opioid requirements and improve pain control [5]. Drugs such as acetaminophen, NSAIDs, gabapentinoids, ketamine, and dexmedetomidine can be combined in carefully titrated regimens [6]. Regional anesthesia also plays a pivotal role—catheters placed for continuous peripheral nerve blocks or epidural infusions can provide sustained relief during the acute postoperative period [7].

Tailoring Opioid Use

In opioid-tolerant patients, anesthesiologists must anticipate higher analgesic needs. They may incorporate patient-controlled analgesia (PCA), long-acting opioids, and adjuncts such as ketamine and dexmedetomidine infusions to enhance analgesia and reduce side effects [4]. Coordination with the chronic pain or palliative care team is essential.

Neuropathic Pain Management

Neuropathic pain, a common feature in oncology patients, often responds poorly to opioids and instead requires agents like gabapentinoids, serotonin-norepinephrine reuptake inhibitors (SNRIs), or tricyclic antidepressants [2]. Care must be taken to balance efficacy with side effect profiles. In severe cases, interventional techniques such as epidural steroid injections, nerve blocks, or intrathecal therapies may be considered [9].

POSTOPERATIVE COMPLICATIONS IN CANCER PATIENTS

Nausea and Vomiting (N/V)

Cancer patients are predisposed to postoperative nausea and vomiting (PONV), particularly if they have had previous chemotherapy. Preventive strategies include multimodal antiemetics, minimizing opioid use, and using total intravenous anesthesia (TIVA) when appropriate [10].

Infection Control

Anesthesiologists must remain vigilant for signs of infection, given the immunosuppressed state of many patients with oncology. Strict aseptic technique, perioperative antibiotics, and glycemic control are critical [1].

Wound Healing Delays

Poor wound healing is common in patients undergoing chemotherapy or radiation therapy. Nutritional optimization, adequate pain control to allow movement, and attention to pressure points are key factors in prevention and management [1].

Thromboembolic Events

Cancer is a hypercoagulable state, and patients are at high risk for deep vein thrombosis (DVT) and pulmonary embolism. Prophylactic anticoagulation, mechanical prophylaxis, and early mobilization should be implemented [3].

Respiratory Complications

Patients undergoing thoracic or abdominal cancer surgery are at increased risk for atelectasis, pneumonia, and respiratory failure. Regional techniques that reduce opioid use can help mitigate these risks [11].

NUTRITIONAL SUPPORT FOR RECOVERY

Nutritional Challenges

Cancer patients are often nutritionally depleted prior to surgery. Poor appetite, nausea, vomiting, or cachexia contribute to increased morbidity in the postoperative period. Nutritional consultation, early enteral nutrition, and management of nausea are critical [8].

Optimizing Nutritional Status

Total parenteral nutrition (TPN) should be reserved for cases where enteral feeding is not feasible. Monitoring electrolytes, glucose, and renal function is essential in these patients [1].

ROLE OF PHYSICAL REHABILITATION AND EARLY MOBILIZATION

Anesthesiologist's Contribution to Early Mobilization

By using opioid-sparing techniques and regional anesthesia, anesthesiologists can facilitate early mobilization and reduce complications such as DVT, ileus, and muscle wasting [3].

Rehabilitation Support

Collaboration with physical therapy to initiate early ambulation and breathing exercises can hasten recovery and reduce the length of stay. Enhanced pain control allows greater participation in rehabilitation [7].

MANAGING PSYCHOLOGICAL AND EMOTIONAL STRESS

Psychological Impact of Surgery and Cancer Treatment

Anxiety, depression, and distress are common in cancer patients and may be intensified in the perioperative period. Anesthesiologists should consider using anxiolytics such as midazolam and work closely with the perioperative and palliative care teams to address these concerns [7, 12].

Psycho-Social Support in Postoperative Care

Involvement of chaplaincy services, social workers, and mental health professionals can improve the overall patient experience and assist in coping with the challenges of cancer treatment [8]. While the anesthesiologist may not be directly involved in these aspects of care, it is important to be aware of the presence of these services as their discussions can help drive the patient's decision-making and can significantly impact the course of acute resuscitation the patient is willing to undergo.

LONG-TERM POSTOPERATIVE CARE AND PAIN MANAGEMENT

Chronic Post-Surgical Pain in Cancer Patients

Certain surgeries, such as mastectomies, thoracotomies, and amputations, are associated with high rates of chronic post-surgical pain. Early use of regional anesthesia, nerve-sparing techniques, and referral to pain specialists may mitigate long-term pain [4].

Ongoing Monitoring for Cancer Recurrence and Metastasis

Persistent or new pain after surgery should prompt a thorough evaluation for tumor recurrence or metastasis, particularly in cases where the pain is localized and refractory to treatment [13].

Anesthesiologist's Role in Palliative Care

In patients with advanced cancer, anesthesiologists may work closely with palliative care teams to manage refractory pain using methods such as intrathecal pumps, neurolytic blocks, or coordinated opioid management [7, 12].

CONCLUSION

Postoperative management of the cancer patient is a dynamic, multidisciplinary endeavor that extends well beyond the operating room. Anesthesiologists are uniquely positioned to guide these patients through their recovery by employing evidence-based strategies in pain management, physiological optimization, complication prevention, and psychological support. By collaborating with surgical, oncological, palliative, and rehabilitative services, anesthesiologists make meaningful contributions to improved patient outcomes and quality of life during one of the most vulnerable periods in cancer care.

REFERENCES

[1] Extermann M, Aapro M, Bernabei R, *et al.* Use of comprehensive geriatric assessment in older cancer patients. Crit Rev Oncol Hematol 2005; 55(3): 241-52. [http://dx.doi.org/10.1016/j.critrevonc.2005.06.003] [PMID: 16084735]

[2] Fallon MT. Neuropathic pain in cancer. Br J Anaesth 2013; 111(1): 105-11. [http://dx.doi.org/10.1093/bja/aet208] [PMID: 23794652]

[3] Kehlet H, Wilmore DW. Multimodal strategies to improve surgical outcome. Am J Surg 2002; 183(6): 630-41. [http://dx.doi.org/10.1016/S0002-9610(02)00866-8] [PMID: 12095591]

[4] Schug SA, Chandrasena C. Postoperative pain management of the cancer patient. Curr Opin Support Palliat Care 2015; 9(2): 118-22.

[5] Macintyre PE, Schug SA, Scott DA, Visser EJ, Walker SM. Acute Pain Management: Scientific Evidence. 4th ed., Melbourne: Australian and New Zealand College of Anaesthetists and Faculty of Pain Medicine 2015.

[6] Practice guidelines for acute pain management in the perioperative setting: an updated report by the American Society of Anesthesiologists Task Force on Acute Pain Management. Anesthesiology 2012; 116(2): 248-73. [http://dx.doi.org/10.1097/ALN.0b013e31823c1030] [PMID: 22227789]

[7] Balaban DY, Martin E, Wysocki J, *et al.* Enhanced Recovery After Surgery (ERAS) protocols for patients undergoing major abdominal oncologic surgery: a meta-analysis and systematic review. Am J Surg 2021; 221(4): 691-701.

[8] Ferrell BR, Temel JS, Temin S, *et al.* Integration of palliative care into standard oncology care: American Society of Clinical Oncology clinical practice guideline update. J Clin Oncol 2017; 35(1): 96-112. [http://dx.doi.org/10.1200/JCO.2016.70.1474] [PMID: 28034065]

[9] Wiffen PJ, Derry S, Bell RF, *et al.* Gabapentin for chronic neuropathic pain in adults. Cochrane Libr 2017; 2020(2): CD007938. [http://dx.doi.org/10.1002/14651858.CD007938.pub4] [PMID: 28597471]

[10] Apfel CC, Korttila K, Abdalla M, *et al.* A factorial trial of six interventions for the prevention of postoperative nausea and vomiting. N Engl J Med 2004; 350(24): 2441-51. [http://dx.doi.org/10.1056/NEJMoa032196] [PMID: 15190136]

[11] Sessler DI, Meyhoff CS, Zimmerman NM, *et al.* Period-analytic risk factors for postoperative pulmonary complications. Anesthesiology 2021; 134(6): 892-903.

[12] Levy MH, Smith TJ. Pain management in palliative care. In: Hanks G, Cherny NI, Christakis NA, Eds. Oxford Textbook of Palliative Medicine. Oxford: Oxford University Press 2011; pp. 580-602.

[13] National Comprehensive Cancer Network (NCCN). Clinical Practice Guidelines in Oncology: Adult Cancer Pain. Version 1.2023.

CHAPTER 10

The Pediatric Cancer Patient

Ian Brotman[1,*], **Cathy Lee**[1], **Jason Vaz**[2] and **Nathalie Peiris**[3]

[1] *Department of Anesthesiology, Cooper Medical School of Rowan University, Cooper University Health Care, Camden, NJ, USA*

[2] *Alberta Children's Hospital, Calgary, Alberta, Canada*

[3] *Nemours Children's Hospital, Wilmington, DE, USA*

Abstract: Children with cancer have a number of pre- and perioperative risk modifiers when they undergo surgical procedures. These can be a direct result of their pathology or treatment and can persist for years after the completion of therapy. In this chapter, we explore the various sequelae of the most common pediatric malignancies and the anesthetic considerations required to deliver optimum care to this vulnerable population.

Keywords: Pediatric anesthesia, Anesthesiology, Oncology, Cancer, Chemotherapy, Hematology, Leukemia, Lymphoma, Neuroblastoma, Radiation therapy, Wilms tumor.

INTRODUCTION

Pediatric oncology patients are a subset of cancer patients who require knowledge of both children and their unique disease pathology to administer anesthesia safely. While these patients are rare, with approximately 1 in 285 children being diagnosed before the age of 20 [1], and the 5-year survival is over 80% in developed countries [2], cancer is still the second leading cause of pediatric mortality, second to trauma [3]. Childhood cancer carries a range of pathologies, and the peak incidence of various malignancies varies by age. The most common oncologic pathologies for all pediatric patients are hematologic, central nervous system tumors, and lymphoma [4, 5]. These children undergo a variety of procedures during workup, treatment, and post-therapy that require anesthesia. In the following chapter, we will explore the various sequelae that the anesthesiologist must consider in the most prevalent pediatric malignancies to deliver safe, optimal care in this vulnerable population.

* **Corresponding author Ian Brotman:** Department of Anesthesiology, Cooper Medical School of Rowan University, Cooper University Health Care, Camden, NJ, USA; E-mail: brotman-ian@cooperhealth.edu

Bharathi Gourkanti, Irwin Gratz, William Marion, Rajiv Lingaraju & Grace Abramian (Eds.)

ORGAN SYSTEM CONSIDERATIONS

Neurologic

Primary intracranial tumors are the most common pediatric solid cancers, with astrocytomas accounting for over half of these neurologic malignancies [6, 7]. These patients typically present with signs and symptoms of increased intracranial pressure (ICP), including vomiting, irritability, altered mentation, and macrocephaly [8, 9]. Older children may report nausea, headache, and vision changes [8, 9]. Focal neurologic findings such as seizures, gait disturbances, and hemiparesis may also be present, indicating significant mass effect [10, 11]. Spinal tumors are uncommon, but those patients may have signs of spinal cord compression, including gait changes, extremity weakness, and, in older children, new onset incontinence [12].

Neurologic toxicity from chemotherapy is common, and symptoms can be a multifactorial result of both malignancy and constitutional dysfunction from treatments [11]. Platinum agents, L-asparaginase, methotrexate, cyclosporin, and a host of other chemotherapeutic drugs are the most likely to cause direct central toxicity and are typically dose-limited and reversible [13]. Leukoencephalopathy, vision loss, ototoxicity, and peripheral neuropathy from cisplatin and vincristine are all possible chronic chemotherapy-induced neurotoxicities unrelated to the patient's underlying disease process [14]. Radiation therapy has been documented to cause focal necrosis, myelitis, stroke, seizures, and chronic vision changes even at relatively small doses [13, 15].

Anesthetic Considerations

Total tumor resection is the principal treatment for neurologic malignancies [16]. Increased ICP can be an immediate danger to these children. The risk of premedication and sedation must be weighed with the risk of preinduction intravenous access and patient irritation, as both plans can result in worsening ICP [17]. Careful titration of premedication allowing for quick induction, intravenous access, and intubation is required to control end-tidal carbon dioxide (CO2) and cerebral blood flow (CBF). As such, all patients with concerns for increased ICP require a definitive airway, avoiding profound hypertension during laryngoscopy, which again would further increase CBF and ICP.

Cardiac

Cardiac sequelae from malignancy in children are usually the result of noncardiac cancers, as primary cardiac tumors are uncommon [18]. When rhabdomyomas, fibromas, teratomas, or myxomas do occur, they have a high survival rate and may regress spontaneously or with medical treatment [19]. Noncardiac cancers cause cardiac dysfunction *via* several pathologies, including anterior mediastinal masses, pericardial effusions, or hypertension, and side effects of cancer therapies can cause cardiomyopathy and heart failure [20 - 22]. Cancer survivors have a 30-year increased risk of chronic cardiac disease, including coronary artery disease, cerebral vascular disease, and heart failure [22]. The anthracyclines, specifically the cytostatic antibiotics such as doxorubicin, are the most cardiotoxic, suspected to be related to free radical generation, interfering with myocyte metabolism [15, 23]. Mitoxantrone cardiac toxicity has been compared to anthracyclines [24].

Anterior Mediastinal Mass

Perhaps the most feared tumor for the anesthesiologist is the anterior mediastinal mass. Primary or metastatic disease of the chest organs, lymph nodes, or thymus can cause compression of the great vessels, tracheobronchial tree, or heart chambers, leading to dangerous hemodynamic compromise [9, 25]. Lymphomas are the most common malignancies causing anterior mediastinal masses, which are present at the time of diagnosis [26]. Patients can present with a spectrum of symptoms, including dyspnea, orthopnea, stridor, wheezing, or superior vena cava syndrome [11].

Pericardial Effusion

Pericardial effusions occur as a result of infection, obstruction, pericardial metastasis, or cancer treatment (Diamond 2018). Hematopoietic stem cell treatment and mediastinal tumors are the most common causes of pericardial effusions [27]. The presentation may be similar to an anterior mediastinal mass or intracardiac tumor and will vary depending on the degree of tamponade physiology.

Anesthetic Considerations

Anterior mediastinal masses may require tissue biopsy for definitive diagnosis before treatment can begin to try to shrink the tumor burden [28]. A CT scan is recommended for all patients with a suspected anterior mediastinal mass to assess anatomic location and involvement with surrounding structures [28]. A CT scan may also reveal pericardial or pleural effusions that may further hone the anesthetic plan, although the clinical symptoms may not match the radiographic findings [29, 30]. Transthoracic echocardiography may give important information regarding great vessel or heart compression and mass effect on ventricular function and should be considered in all patients with cardiovascular symptoms or those unable to give an accurate history [25, 30]. It is important to remember that symptomatic heart failure is rare in children, but subclinical cardiac compromise can reveal itself under general anesthesia [31].

A history and physical examination should be performed prior to induction to assess the optimal position that minimizes dyspnea and vascular compromise, as well as the position that the patient feels most comfortable in [30]. This information is incredibly useful to find the optimal induction and surgical position to help minimize cardiovascular compromise and can further help the anesthesiology provider create a repositioning strategy in the event of a hemodynamic emergency [29, 32]. Fig. (**1**) below presents a simplified algorithm for assessing a patient's safety for general anesthesia.

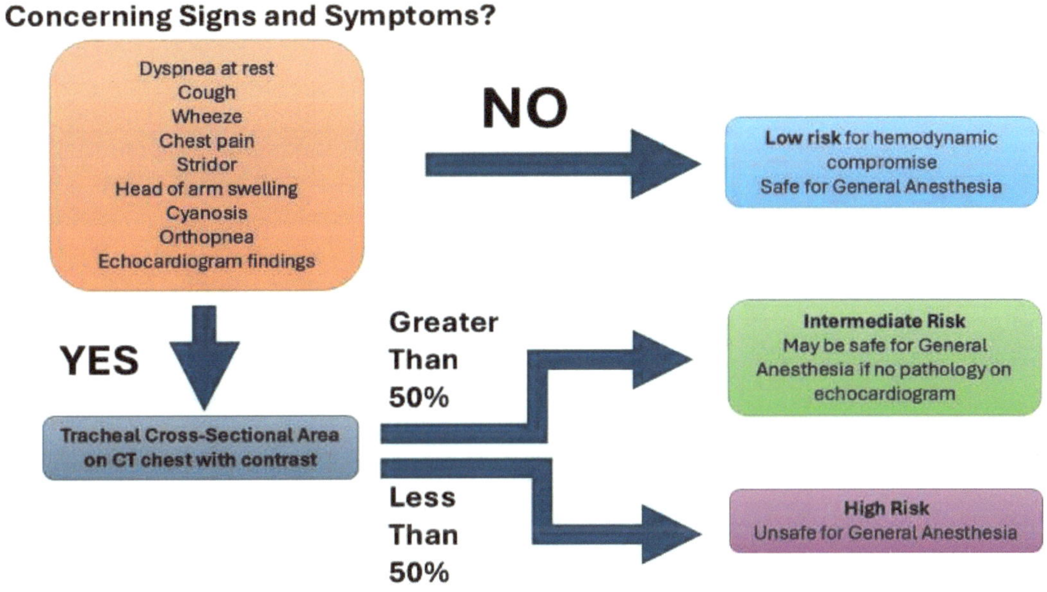

Fig. (1). Anterior mediastinal mass anesthesia decision tree [34].

If a general anesthetic is necessary, some basic principles can help avoid emergency situations. A spontaneously breathing patient is commonly advocated to maintain the transpleural pressure gradient, which may limit dangerous airway compression [33]. Neuromuscular blockade should be avoided to maintain chest wall tone and limit compression of vital chest structures [32]. In the pediatric patient, an inhalational agent is an excellent choice for the above induction goals, even in a patient with an IV in place. When cardiac compromise is unavoidable or extremely high risk, an extracorporeal membrane oxygenation (ECMO) team should be immediately available.

Pulmonary

Similar to pediatric cardiac cancer, primary lung tumors are rare in children, with the majority of lung pathology occurring from indirect effects of other cancers [35]. Pulmonary embolism, pleural effusions, chylous effusions, hyperleukocytosis-induced pulmonary leukostasis, anterior mediastinal mass effect, and opportunistic infection can be seen in a variety of pediatric patients with oncologic disease [36]. Bleomycin is a chemotherapeutic agent known to cause pneumonitis, which usually resolves with cessation of treatment but can progress to chronic pulmonary fibrosis [37]. Other chemotherapies and chest radiation treatments also have the potential to cause pneumonitis or pulmonary edema [38].

Anesthetic Considerations

Patients should have a baseline pulmonary status established for inducing anesthesia. Pulmonary function tests are controversial because both their utility and the accuracy of the results in young children are debated [39]. There is little variation outside of standard anesthetic pulmonary considerations in pediatric oncologic patients, except those with bleomycin pulmonary fibrosis. In those patients who do, unfortunately, develop bleomycin-induced lung injury, data have shown that a higher inspired oxygen concentration is associated with exacerbation of their restrictive lung disease. Thus, in that specific patient population, extra vigilance is necessary to ensure the concentration of inhaled oxygen is titrated to the minimum amount necessary [40].

Renal

Wilm's Tumor

Wilm's tumor (WT), also termed nephroblastoma, was first described by Dr. Max Wilm in 1899. It is the most common renal cancer and abdominal cancer in the pediatric population, and the fourth most common of all childhood cancers. In the century since its description, the management and available therapy for children with WT has been the subject of international attention and large-scale clinical trials [41].

WT develops from persistent embryonic cells of the renal parenchyma, also known as Wilms tumorlet cells, metanephric blastema cells, or nephrogenic rests. In the normal kidney, these cells spontaneously regress, contributing to <1% of all cell types. In the pathogenesis of WT, the loss of function of several tumor suppressor genes results in the proliferation of these cells in the periphery of the kidney, enclosed by a pseudocapsule. With aggressive palpation and surgical manipulation, this pseudocapsule may rupture. Although WT may present in the context of familial predisposition and genetic syndromes, the vast majority of presentations are sporadic. Tumors can enlarge significantly before detection, at which point compression of adjacent parenchyma and surrounding anatomic structures may occur. Histologic detection of anaplastic cells, occurring in 4% of WT and typically in older patients, correlates to a poor prognosis and worsened long term survival [42].

The typical presentation of WT is a painless abdominal mass in a well-appearing child less than 5 years of age, without racial or gender predominance. The overwhelming majority of cases present prior to age 10, with neonatal and adult presentation being rare. Table **1** below lists the congenital abnormalities associated with Wilm's tumors [43 - 45]. The tumor is unilateral and palpable in the majority of cases, and while typically painless, it can sometimes be painful. 6% of cases have bilateral renal involvement, which is associated with poorer outcomes and greater pathogenicity. Patients can also present with generalized symptoms, which include fever, anemia, malaise, loss of appetite, and weight loss. Hypertension is found in 25-50% of cases, presumed to be secondary to hyperreninemia. Renal function is typically unaffected by the presence of WT [42]. Microscopic hematuria is present in 25% of cases, and while rare, gross hematuria may be observed and suggests the involvement of collecting duct system. On examination, genitourinary abnormalities, hemihypertrophy, and aniridia are often present.

Disease staging is defined by the National Wilms' Tumor Study Group (NWTS) criteria, specifically the NWTS-5, which incorporates capsular extension, lymph node involvement, hematogenous and non-hematogenous metastases, and the presence of bilateral disease. Metastasis is most commonly found in the lungs, and metastatic spread occurs primarily *via* lymphatic and hematogenous channels. Up to 40% of cases show tumor invasion or thrombus in the adjacent vasculature, including the renal vein, and less commonly in the hepatic vein, inferior vena cava, and right atrium.

Anesthetic Considerations

Radical nephrectomy is the mainstay of surgical therapy for WT. Surgical staging, which includes radical nephrectomy and retroperitoneal lymph node sampling, as well as histologic evaluation, is recommended by the NWTSG. Two staging systems, the Children's Oncology Group (COG) and the International Society of Pediatric Oncology (SIOP), differ in the timing of surgical intervention [46]. The COG approach denotes upfront surgery followed by adjuvant chemotherapy, while the SIOP approach delays surgery after neoadjuvant chemotherapy. Both approaches advocate for upfront chemotherapy in cases of bilateral WT, unresectable tumors, or with IVC or cardiac extension. In cases where neoadjuvant chemotherapy is offered prior to surgery, the surgical date should be timed for 12 weeks, as this maximizes the tumor shrinkage effect while limiting the exposure and risk of systemic toxicity [46]. The timing of surgical intervention in relation to chemotherapy is of great relevance to the anesthesiologist; upfront surgery increases the likelihood of intraoperative tumor spillage and greater mass effect to surrounding structures, whereas upfront chemotherapy may result in preoperative cardiopulmonary toxicity, liver impairment, and chemotherapy-induced nausea and vomiting [41].

A thorough preoperative evaluation should occur in children with WT presenting for radical nephrectomy. Preoperative hypertension should be optimized prior to surgery with the initiation of angiotensin-converting enzyme (ACE) inhibitors or another agent. A review of blood work and imaging studies should be performed by the anesthesiologist. A variety of hematologic disturbances are observed in WT, including anemia, polycythemia (secondary to tumor-induced excess erythropoietin production), acquired Von Willebrand disease (8%), and polycythemia (rare). Coagulation studies should be evaluated to plan for intraoperative hemostasis, particularly if a neuraxial technique is being considered for postoperative analgesia. Cardiovascular status should be evaluated, particularly in patients with presurgical anthracycline exposure, such as doxorubicin or Adriamycin. Cardiac function may be further affected by chronic hypertension, leading to intravascular volume contraction and left ventricular hypertrophy, or if there is inferior vena cava or right atrial involvement. If intravascular extension is suspected or diagnosed, the anesthesiologist should plan for the potential for massive blood loss, major fluid shifts, and the need for transesophageal echocardiography or the use of cardiopulmonary bypass. Pulmonary function may be compromised secondary to metastatic lung disease.

Airway management may be complicated by coexisting overgrowth syndromes, such as Beckwith-Wiedemann and Simpson-Golabi-Behmel, or a higher risk of aspiration if abdominal distention is significant. Vascular access should be considered, including placement of intravenous access above the diaphragm, particularly with IVC or RA involvement. Arterial line placement should be considered as labile blood pressures may be observed due to long-standing hypertension, intravascular volume contraction, IVC compression, and during tumor handling and compression. Intraoperative tumor spillage, intestinal obstruction, major blood loss, and vascular injury may complicate the intraoperative and postoperative course.

Various techniques for effective postoperative analgesia have been described, including epidural analgesia, truncal, and quadratus lumborum blocks [47 - 50]. Moon *et al.* described their institution's experience with an enhanced recovery after surgery protocol for children undergoing unilateral radical nephrectomy for WT [51]. Analysis of their program suggests that transverse surgical incision, avoidance of epidural catheter placement or shorter epidural catheter duration, earlier return to regular diet, routine use of intravenous ketorolac, and minimizing postoperative opioid use are associated with earlier discharge [51].

Table 1. Congenital syndromes and anomalies associated with Wilms' Tumor [43 - 45].

Anomaly Class	Wilms' Tumor Risk	Clinical Features
Overgrowth		
Beckwith–Wiedemann Syndrome	7.5%	Macrosomia, macroglossia, visceromegaly, congenital hyperinsulinemia
Isolated Hemihypertrophy	<5%	Asymmetric overgrowth
Sotos Syndrome	<5%	Cerebral gigantism
Perlman Syndrome	64%	Fetal gigantism with renal dialysis
Simpson–Golabi–Behmel Syndrome (SGBS)	10%	Similar presentation to Beckwith–Wiedemann syndrome
Nonovergrowth		
WAGR Syndrome	45–57%	Wilms' tumor, aniridia, genitourinary anomalies, range of intellectual disabilities
Denys–Drash Syndrome (DDS)	74%	Triad of progressive renal disease, male pseudohermaphroditism, and Wilms' tumor
Sporadic Aniridia	33%	PAX6 gene mutation leading to absence of iris
Trisomy 18 (Edward's Syndrome)	<5%	Microcephaly, micrognathia, hypotonia, congenital heart disease, developmental delay, small stature
Horseshoe Kidney	0.5%	Congenital fusion of both kidneys

Neuroblastoma

Extrarenal tumors are rare occurrences in pediatrics. Adrenal gland tumors may present within the cortex (adrenal adenoma) or medulla and sympathetic chain (neuroblastoma, ganglioneuroma). These tumors may be hyperfunctioning or nonfunctioning. This results in a wide array of presentations and pathophysiologic alterations. Neuroblastoma, commonly presenting within the adrenal medulla, is the most common cause of adrenal malignancy in pediatrics [52].

Neuroblastoma arises from primordial neural crest cells in the sympathetic nervous system, which are primitive cells of the adrenal medulla and sympathetic neural ganglia. The malignant evolution of these cells results in a heterogeneous disease presentation and histology. These primordial cells can differentiate into a variety of cell types, including undifferentiated small round cells, found in neuroblastoma, to mature ganglion cells, found in ganglioneuroblastoma [52].

Clinical Presentation

Neuroblastoma is the second most common pediatric solid extracranial tumor, and the second most common abdominal tumor in children (secondary to Wilm's tumor). The majority of cases present between 1 and 5 years of age, with 2 years being the median age of presentation, with no sex predominance. Neonatal presentations are well described, while familial neuroblastoma is a rare phenomenon.

Due to the heterogeneous site of primary disease, neuroblastoma has a markedly varied presentation. Neuroblastoma arises most commonly from the abdominal sympathetic ganglia. Seventy-five percent of cases arise within the abdomen, with one-third of these occurring within the adrenal gland [53]. Children most commonly present with a palpable abdominal mass that can be associated with pain and fullness. About 50% of children present with metastases at the time of presentation [53]. The most common sites of metastases are the lymph nodes, bone marrow, liver, and skin (which results in a distinctive appearance termed "blueberry muffin skin"). Unlike Wilms' tumor, pulmonary metastases are rare. The primary tumor site or metastatic disease may result in compression or mass effect of adjacent structures. The remaining 25% of neuroblastoma that present outside the abdomen may arise anywhere along the sympathetic chain, including the thoracic, cervical, and pelvic sympathetic ganglia (second most common to least common) [53].

Functional neuroblastomas result in neurohumoral activation. Catecholamine-secreting neuroblastoma results in hypertension in 10-19% of cases [52]. The mechanism is thought to be not only due to the direct effects of circulating catecholamines, but also from stimulation of the renin-angiotensin-aldosterone system secondary to renal vascular compression [54]. In more than 90% of these cases, urinary catecholamines or their metabolites (dopamine, homovanillic acid and vanillylmandelic acid) can be detected [55]. Catecholamine release peaks most frequently with surgical manipulation of the tumor and with neoadjuvant chemotherapy due to tumor remodeling [52]. Chronic hyperadrenergic states can result in myocardial remodelling, including left ventricular hypertrophy and hypertrophic obstructive cardiomyopathy [52]. In the case of vasoactive intestinal peptide-secreting tumors, children may present with diarrhea, which can result in dehydration and electrolyte abnormalities. In 2% of children, paraneoplastic phenomena, including opsoclonus-myoclonus with nystagmus and ataxia, may be seen [56].

A range of associated syndromes are comorbid with neuroblastoma, including Beckwith-Wiedemann syndrome, neurofibromatosis, Hirschsprung disease, and central hypoventilation syndrome.

Two primary classification systems are commonly used for the staging of neuroblastoma: The International Neuroblastoma Staging System (INSS) and the International Neuroblastoma Risk Group (INRG) Staging System [57]. The INSS requires the information from surgical resection, and therefore cannot be used appropriately in nonsurgical patients. The INRG system incorporates clinical, imaging, and histologic information without surgical data, and therefore can be used for preoperative risk stratification. In general, age at presentation is inversely proportional to outcomes, as younger age at diagnosis and treatment is associated with improved surgical results [54]. Tumors that are localized, resectable, and have histology showing hyperploidy (higher DNA count) and no MYCN amplification have an improved prognosis [52]. With nondisseminated disease where surgical resection is favorable, chemotherapy is typically reserved for symptom relief. Advanced disease is treated with multi-agent chemotherapy, and additional therapy can include surgery, radiation, myeloablative therapy with autologous bone marrow or peripheral blood stem cell rescue, immunotherapy, and biologic agents. Tissue sampling is required prior to initiation of neoadjuvant therapy, either by surgical resection with histopathology or bone marrow aspiration and biopsy.

Anesthetic Considerations

The anesthetic requirements for neuroblastoma resection differ greatly based on the tumor location, extent, and invasiveness of the planned surgical resection, and the presence of metabolic and neuroendocrine symptoms. Anesthetic drugs used for induction, maintenance, and postoperative analgesia should minimize histamine release, which is associated with catecholamine release. Screening for systemic toxicity should take place in patients who have received preoperative chemotherapy. Patients who have received anti-GD2 immunotherapy may have ongoing pain, due to cross-reactivity with GD2 expression on peripheral nerves, which can result in and contribute to neuropathic pain [54].

Optimization of any neurohumoral symptoms should occur prior to the induction of general anesthesia. Vasoactive intestinal peptide-secreting tumors may induce diarrhea, leading to dehydration, hypovolemia, and electrolyte abnormalities, which should be corrected prior to surgery.

Patients with preoperative hypertension should have an echocardiogram to assess for any hypertension-related cardiac sequelae, including heart failure, cardiomyopathy, cardiomegaly, and cardiogenic shock [52, 58]. Intraoperative hypertension occurs in 25% of children with positive urinary catecholamines, and tumor manipulation may cause a sudden increase in serum catecholamines. Patients with catecholamine-secreting tumors should have preoperative initiation of antihypertensive therapy, which may include α-adrenergic and β-adrenergic blockades. Pio *et al.* conducted a multicenter survey to evaluate the practice patterns of preoperative antihypertensive pharmacotherapy and found that there was significant heterogeneity in the medications used, but some consistency in the use of α-1 blockade intraoperatively [58]. A variety of reports describe the successful management of preoperative and intraoperative hypertension in the abdominal neuroblastoma resection [54, 59 - 63]. Magnesium sulfate has been successfully used for blood pressure stabilization in pediatric pheochromocytoma resection due to its catecholamine receptor blockade, vasodilation, and antiarrhythmic properties, and may be considered as an adjunct in neuroblastoma resection [59, 64].

Enhanced recovery after surgery protocols have been applied to neuroblastoma resection, but with some attenuated success compared to the application of similar protocols in other surgical groups [65, 66]. He *et al.* reviewed a large series of pediatric patients undergoing retroperitoneal neuroblastoma resection and found a perioperative complication rate of 45% [67]. The most common complications are lymphatic leakage, diarrhea, and injury to major structures. Despite the low mortality rate, the findings of this study suggest that the perioperative risk for patients undergoing neuroblastoma resection is significant.

Obstructive Uropathy

Significant compression of adjacent structures may occur secondary to intra-abdominal or retroperitoneal malignancies. In the case that obstruction of the urinary tract occurs secondary to tumor mass effect, children may present with acquired obstructive uropathy. Obstruction may occur anywhere along the post-renal urinary tract. Flank pain is often a primary symptom, which can be severe and spasmodic in nature, but patients may also present without pain. Based on the nature of the obstruction, patients may be oliguric to polyuric in partial obstruction, to anuric with complete obstruction [68]. Laboratory findings include increased serum creatinine, hyperkalemia with non-anion gap metabolic acidosis, and other signs of acute renal dysfunction. Initial imaging is typically performed using ultrasound to minimize renal contrast exposure, with significant findings including hydronephrosis and a renal pelvis diameter of greater than 10 mm in the anteroposterior direction, indicating obstructive uropathy [69]. A contrast-enhanced CT provided preserved renal function, or MR urography may be considered to further delineate the obstructive picture [70].

Chemotherapy Nephrotoxicity

Renal function may be affected in pediatric malignancies from the cancer itself or secondary to antitumor therapy, including chemotherapy, radiation, or iatrogenic surgical injury. A variety of cytostatic medications are known to directly induce nephrotoxicity and acute renal impairment. Similarly, a variety of non-nephrotoxic medications may require normal renal excretion, and when renal function is impaired, they may accumulate and lead to other end-organ toxicity. While terminal renal failure is a rare outcome in pediatric oncology as a result of medication nephrotoxicity, the potential for renal injury in patients undergoing chemotherapy should be of concern to the anesthesiologist.

The platinum-based antineoplastic agents, cisplatin and carboplatin, are often implicated in nephrotoxicity, which can manifest as acute kidney injury, thrombotic microangiopathy, Fanconi's syndrome, salt-wasting hyponatremia, and hypomagnesemia. The pathophysiology of cisplatin-induced nephrotoxicity (CIN) is due to the drug's accumulation in the proximal tubules, activated caspases, cyclin-dependent kinases, and p-53 [71]. This leads to inflammation and oxidative stress, resulting in proximal tubular dysfunction and tubular cell apoptosis and necrosis. This can further manifest in renal vascular injury and a decreased GFR. CIN may cause a long-lasting decrease in GFR, accompanied by renal magnesium wasting and associated hypocalcemia. Compared to cisplatin, carboplatin is far less nephrotoxic because of decreased retention in the renal tubules. The duration of most AKIs secondary to cisplatin is typically transient. In some cases, however, this renal insult can lead to chronic kidney disease secondary to chronic tubulointerstitial fibrosis and chronic tubulopathies. The effect of NSAIDs on the risk of CIN was evaluated by Okamoto *et al*. in a meta-analysis of 7 studies [72]. They concluded that NSAIDS co-administration is a risk factor for the development of CIN with an odds ratio of 1.88 [72].

Prevention of nephrotoxicity caused by a platinum agent is reliant on appropriate hydration, which may involve high fluid loading and use of hypertonic saline. Amifostine, a glutathione analog and free radical scavenger, has shown utility in cisplatin toxicity [71]. In the perioperative setting, the anesthesiologist should be vigilant for disturbances in magnesium, potassium, and calcium, and maintenance of hydration intraoperatively. Forced diuresis using mannitol and furosemide has shown nephroprotection in high-dose cisplatin therapy, but should not be used routinely in all patients receiving standard dosing of cisplatin.

The alkylating agents cyclophosphamide and ifosfamide can induce nephrotoxicity by damage to the tubular system through toxic metabolites and increased cellular oxidative stress. This can manifest as SIADH with associated severe hyponatremia and Fanconi Syndrome (a disease characterized by the dysfunction of proximal tubule resorption). Both drugs have toxic metabolites: acrolein (generated by activation of the p-450 system by cyclophosphamide) and chloroacetaldehyde (the toxic metabolite of ifosfamide). The manifestations of nephrotoxicity differ between cyclophosphamide and ifosfamide [71, 73]. Cyclophosphamide typically results in hemorrhagic cystic (which can lead to hydronephrosis), bladder cancer, and SIADH. Comparatively, ifosfamide is known to cause Fanconi Syndrome, as a result of often permanent proximal tubulopathy, particularly when co-administered with cisplatin.

Ifosfamide-induced Fanconi Syndrome results in renal phosphate and bicarbonate losses as well as dysfunctional resorption and atrophy of the proximal tubule. Collectively, this presents as hypophosphatemia, hyponatremia, hypokalemia, glucosuria and proteinuria. In more severe cases, the drug can induce extensive glomerular and distal tubular damage, causing renal tubular acidosis and nephrogenic diabetes insipidus. Risk factors for ifosfamide-induced Fanconi Syndrome include age < 5 years, unilateral nephrectomy, high dose ifosfamide, concomitant platinum chemotherapy, and preexisting renal damage and renal malformations [74].

Hyperhydration, hypertonic saline, and electrolyte replacement may all be required for alkylating agent nephrotoxicity and SIADH. Hemorrhagic cystic secondary to cyclophosphamide is treated with the coadministration of MESNA (2-mercaptoethanesulfonate), which conjugates acrolein in the urine. Specific agents such as N-acetylcysteine, carnitine and glycine may all play a role in the management of ifosfamide-induced Fanconi Syndrome [71, 75].

Methotrexate can result in multisystem end-organ toxicity, including myelosuppression, hepatotoxicity, mucositis, pulmonary fibrosis, and nephrotoxicity. There are two mechanisms of methotrexate-induced kidney injury: (i) vasoconstriction of the afferent arteries, which reduces GFR, and (ii) crystal precipitation in distal renal tubules (crystalline nephropathy), which can result in CKD with interstitial fibrosis and tubular atrophy [71]. Renal impairment can be manifested as tubular acidosis, acute kidney injury, SIADH and hyponatremia, hemolytic uremic syndrome, and thrombotic microangiopathy. However, it should be noted that typical methotrexate dosing rarely results in nephrotoxicity, and that most cases typically result in only a mild reduction in GFR [76]. Management of methotrexate nephrotoxicity involves adequate hydration and urine alkalization. Additional agents such as leucovorin, which prevents tubule crystallization, and carboxypeptidase G2, hydrolyze methotrexate to inactive metabolites thereby lowering serum concentrations, may also be used [68, 71, 77].

Several cytostatic agents are known to cause syndrome of inadequate ADH secretion (SIADH), including vincristine (vinblastine, vindesine), cyclophosphamide, ifosfamide, cisplatin, melphalan, and etoposide phosphate [75]. This typically occurs in the first few weeks following drug initiation and presents with water intoxication and hyponatremia.

Radiation Nephropathy

Various manifestations of radiation of renal injury have been described, including acute and chronic radiation nephropathy, asymptomatic proteinuria, benign and malignant hypertension, interstitial nephritis, and glomerulonephritis. Radiation-induced DNA damage to renal cells results in inflammation, oxidative stress, and cell senescence in tubular, glomerular, and endothelial cells [77]. This results in nephron loss, interstitial fibrosis and vascular dysfunction and renin–angiotensin–aldosterone system (RAAS) activation [77]. Most cases of radiation nephrotoxicity occur with radiation doses >20 Gy or following radiosensitizing chemotherapy, and rarely occur with doses <18 Gy. The kidneys of neonates and younger children have an increased sensitivity to radiation-induced injury [78]. Patients can present with azotemia, anemia, proteinuria, fluid overload, edema, and hypertension. The degree of anemia and hypertension can be severe [68, 79]. Symptoms typically occur after a 6-12-month latent period following radiation therapy. Laboratory investigations can confirm a diagnosis of acute kidney injury, microangiopathic hemolytic anemia with schistocytes, and thrombocytopenia. Cases where severe hemolytic anemia is seen suggest an underlying thrombomicroangiopathy and can also result in hemolytic uremic syndrome (HUS) or thrombotic thrombocytopenic purpura (TTP) [79]. Radiation nephropathy typically results in chronic but typically nonprogressive disease, with reports of stabilization of kidney function following treatment with angiotensin-converting-enzyme inhibitors.

Hepatic

Primary hepatic tumors are rare in children, making up 1% of all childhood cancers [80]. The most common type of tumor in young children is hepatoblastomas, followed by sarcomas, germ cell tumors, and rhabdoid tumors [80]. In older adolescents, hepatocellular carcinoma is the most prevalent [34, 80].

Children with cancer could potentially have both acute and chronic liver disease, precipitated by chemotherapy, radiation treatments, or underlying genetic syndromes. Acute liver disease may be induced by chemotherapy agents, such as methotrexate, actinomycin D, 6-mercaptopurine, and 6-thioguanine, in as little as hours to weeks after a dose [81]. This acute toxicity is typically transient and reversible [39, 81]. Acute hepatic toxicity manifests as increased liver function tests, veno-occlusive disease, and rarely pancreatitis [81]. Chronic liver disease is usually associated with coexisting genetic syndromes [39, 81]. Children exposed to radiation therapy may have self-limited acute hepatic toxicity. Chronic hepatic fibrosis more commonly occurs after large doses of radiation, greater than 40 Gy [81, 82].

Sinusoidal Obstruction Syndrome (SOS)

The most concerning hepatic complication in a child who has received hematopoietic stem cell transplantation (HSCT) is the development of sinusoidal obstruction syndrome (SOS) or veno-occlusive disease (VOD) [81, 83]. SOS is due to endothelial damage of the hepatic sinusoids, leading to hepatic necrosis and hepatorenal syndrome [84]. Up to 60% of children develop SOS within six weeks of HSCT [84]. There is an associated mortality rate of 19% to 50% [81, 85, 86]. Diagnosis of SOS is based on transjugular liver biopsy and clinical symptoms, including portal hypertension, liver failure (*e.g.*, jaundice secondary to hyperbilirubinemia > 2 mg/dL, ascites, weight gain secondary to fluid retention), and multi-organ system failure [85, 87 - 89]. Chemotherapy drugs that are implicated in the development of SOS are oral busulfan and cyclophosphamide. Treatment includes giving ursodeoxycholic acid as prophylaxis up to 90 days post-treatment or defibrotide for severe SOS, and in severe cases, liver transplant may be necessary [85, 87 - 89].

Anesthetic Considerations

Up to 20% of primary hepatic tumors are associated with genetic syndromes like Beckwith-Wiedemann Syndrome (BWS) [81]. BWS presents unique considerations for anesthesiologists, including management of abnormal airway anatomy (*e.g.*, macroglossia, malocclusion of mandible, difficulty swallowing), hypoglycemia, cardiac anomalies, prematurity, and visceromegaly [90 - 95].

Many chemotherapy agents cause hepatotoxicity. Hepatotoxic medications should be used with caution in children with cancer. Preoperative testing of liver function tests, complete blood count, and coagulation tests should be performed to rule out issues with coagulopathies or hepatic drug metabolism [39, 81]. Communication and coordination between the oncology and perioperative teams are imperative to anticipate any hepatic-specific anesthetic concerns and comorbidities.

Gastrointestinal

Primary gastrointestinal (GI) tumors are rare in the pediatric population. Children with cancer often manifest GI symptoms secondary to side effects from chemotherapy agents or radiation treatment or from intestinal obstruction from intra-abdominal malignancies. Intra-abdominal malignancies can result in intestinal obstruction, intussusception, erosive perforation, intra-abdominal hemorrhage, biliary obstruction, venous or arterial obstruction, and massive hepatomegaly [81]. Radiation doses greater than 20 to 30 Gy result in inflammation and edema of the GI system [81, 95]. Chemotherapy agents induce mild to severe GI symptoms, including a combination of nausea, vomiting, diarrhea, mucositis, pancreatitis, stomatitis, and neutropenic enterocolitis [81, 96].

Graft Versus Host Disease (GVHD)

Children after receiving HSCT can manifest with GVHD, which occurs when donor T cells recognize and attack recipient or host alloantigens [81, 83]. Many organ systems are impacted, most notably pulmonary system involvement in 30% to 60% of cases and hematology system involvement manifesting as hemolysis [81]. Acute GVHD occurs within the first 100 days in 20% to 80% of children, presenting with inflammatory dermatitis, enteritis, and hepatitis [81]. Chronic GVHD occurs after 100 days in 6% to 50% of children, presenting with autoimmune disease features that impact nearly every organ system [81].

Most cases of GVHD are mild due to prophylaxis with calcineurin inhibitors, immunosuppression *e.g.*, methotrexate or mycophenolate, corticosteroids, and salvage therapy. There is about a 10% incidence of moderate to severe GVHD. Without prompt treatment, mortality from GVHD can be very high [81].

Anesthetic Considerations

GI symptoms should be monitored in children with cancer. Consider treating chronic nausea and vomiting, preparing for gastroparesis and increased aspiration risk, and carefully titrating opioids due to delayed gastric emptying [81]. Some children may have severe GI dysfunction, such as malnutrition, dehydration, and electrolyte imbalances, that require medical optimization prior to elective surgeries [34, 81].

Endocrine

Primary endocrine tumors account for less than 5% of all childhood cancers [81, 97, 98]. They include gonadal germ cell tumors, *e.g.*, testicular, ovarian, and extragonadal, thyroid adenomas and carcinomas, and pituitary tumors, *e.g.*, craniopharyngiomas and pituitary adenomas [81, 97, 98].

Chemotherapy agents have minimal effect on endocrine function. Some chemotherapy agents can cause electrolyte abnormalities, rash, hypomagnesemia, syndrome of inappropriate antidiuretic hormone secretion (SIADH), adrenal suppression, and glucose intolerance and imbalance. However, the use of glucocorticoids can lead to a dose-dependent adrenal suppression that is temporary in the majority of children; all adrenal function will be recovered within 2 weeks of cessation of glucocorticoids. The minority remains suppressed for two to eight months [81].

Chronic neuroendocrine dysfunction can occur from cumulative doses of focal cranial radiotherapy and from total body irradiation preconditioning for HSCT [34, 99]. Symptoms range from growth hormone and gonadotropin deficiency, panhypopituitarism, and hypothyroidism [81].

Anesthetic Considerations

Consider discussion with the oncology team about intraoperative steroids for postoperative nausea and vomiting prophylaxis or for adrenal suppression, especially within the first two months after cessation of chemotherapy. Steroids are considered active anticancer drugs that may impact the child's eligibility for treatment protocols and may cause tumor necrosis or lysis syndrome and immune suppression [34].

Hematology

Malignancy can cause derangements in the hemostatic system, which can lead to both hemorrhage and thrombosis [100]. Myelosuppression is the most common direct effect of cancer in the pediatric patient. This may present as neutropenia, anemia, or thrombocytopenia.

Neutropenia is defined as having a neutrophil count less than 1.5×10^{-9} L [101]. Neutropenia is commonly seen in patients with ALL or AML due to dysfunction of normal bone marrow function and abnormal proliferation of cells. Although neutropenia can be a presenting symptom, it is more commonly seen after chemotherapy treatment. Those with neutropenia are at higher risk of developing infections and may have increased risks of morbidity and mortality. Thus, when taking care of a neutropenic patient, protective isolation precautions should be implemented [101]. In addition, anesthesia providers should always use aseptic technique with medication administration or any invasive procedures.

Anemia is defined as a reduction in red blood cell count, and in the perioperative setting, transfusion thresholds are between 7-8 g/dL [101]. Over 90% of pediatric leukemia and lymphoma patients have anemia [101]. This is often due to bone marrow replacement with cancer cells, and anemia is often seen most at the time of cancer diagnosis [39]. Other causes of anemia may be due to chemotherapy or radiation treatment.

Thrombocytopenia in this population is typically due to malignancy infiltration or effects of chemotherapy and radiation on the bone marrow or due to platelet sequestration in the spleen. A platelet count less than 10,000 platelets per microliter has been shown to lead to a high risk of spontaneous intraventricular hemorrhage [101]. Generally, platelet counts greater than 50,000 platelets per microliter are recommended for major surgical procedures [102].

Coagulopathy in oncology patients occurs due to the increase of cytokines, procoagulants, and fibrinolytic proteins malignant cells (101). Other causes of coagulopathy in pediatric oncology patients may be due to hepatic dysfunction and vitamin K deficiency due to poor nutrition, infection, and effects of chemotherapy medications causing fibrinolysis or factor dysfunction. Medications such as asparaginase that is used to treat ALL, can cause coagulopathy by decreasing fibrinogen, plasminogen, antithrombin, and von Willebrand factor [102]. Coagulopathy usually does not have direct anesthesia implications; however, it may need to be corrected due to invasive procedures conducted by proceduralists or surgeons.

If transfusion is indicated, leukocyte-reduced and irradiated blood should be prescribed to decrease the risk of infection in patients with myelosuppression [102]. In addition, irradiation helps prevent donor blood T-cell replication and stops the development of transfusion-associated graft-versus-host disease [102].

A hypercoagulable state is typically seen in patients who have either sarcoma or other hematologic malignancies [39]. Factors that increase the risk of thromboembolism in this patient population include chronic central line catheters, chemotherapy options, infections or sepsis, or other underlying disease states and comorbidities [39].

Tumor Lysis Syndrome

Tumor Lysis Syndrome (TLS) is an oncologic emergency that typically occurs in patients with rapidly proliferating cancers, large tumor burdens, and cancers with high sensitivity to chemotherapy. High-risk malignancies for developing TLS include ALL, AML, chronic myeloid leukemia, CLL, and NHL. Although TLS is often typically described in the context of hematologic malignancies, it can also occur in non-hematologic malignancies and solid tumors.The pathophysiology of TLS is attributed to the rapid destruction of tumor cells, resulting in the release of intracellular contents, including nucleic acids, proteins, potassium, and phosphorus, as well as metabolic derangements. The release and catabolism of nucleic acids result in hyperuricemia, increasing the likelihood of uric acid precipitation in the renal tubules, leading to renal failure. Renal failure, in the context of TLS, is associated with worsened prognosis and increased morbidity [103]. In this setting, acute renal failure can further worsen the existing hyperphosphatemia and hypocalcemia.

A variety of precipitants for TLS have been described, including the onset of chemotherapy (typically at 1-3 days post-initiation), radiotherapy, cytolytic antibody therapy, fever, surgery, and anesthesia. Patients can present with laboratory findings in the absence of clinical disease, and a spectrum of disease severity exists. The Cairo-Bishop Definition can classify patients with the presence of laboratory TLS, based on electrolyte abnormalities ≥25% from baseline, and the severity of clinical TLS, based on the presence of creatinine abnormalities, cardiac arrhythmia, or seizure [103]. The hallmark laboratory findings include hyperuricemia, hyperkalemia, hyperphosphatemia, hypocalcemia, uremia, and acid-base abnormalities. Patients can present with nausea, vomiting, diarrhea, anorexia, lethargy, edema, fluid overload, muscle cramps, syncope, and hematuria. Severe clinical disease can result in acute renal failure requiring dialysis, congestive heart failure, lethal arrhythmia, cardiac arrest, seizure, tetany, multiorgan failure, and death. Risk factors that increase the risk of TLS include preexisting hyperuricemia or uremia, decreased urinary flow, dehydration, oliguria and anuria, elevated LDH, and renal insufficiency or failure [103].

Identification of high-risk patients and prevention are crucial aspects of TLS management. Adequate hydration should ensure fluid intake 1-2x maintenance, with a goal urine output of 80-100mL/m^2/hr [103]. Diuresis can be considered to meet the urine output goal but should be avoided in cases of hypovolemia and acute obstructive uropathy [103]. There is insufficient evidence to recommend urine alkalinization, and this practice may also increase the risk of urinary calcium-phosphate crystallization. Antihyperuricemic agents are indicated for the treatment of intermediate and high-risk pediatric patients [103]. Rasburicase, a recombinant urate oxidase that catabolizes uric acid, decreases uric acid levels within 4 hours of administration and shows high efficacy in normalizing uric acid levels by 3 days of treatment [103]. Allopurinol blocks the conversion of xanthine and hypoxanthine to uric acid, and can be administered orally or IV, with pediatric patients responding with decreased uric acid levels in 1 day of initiation [104]. Acute electrolyte disturbances, including hyperkalemia and hypocalcemia, require prompt attention and management. Hyperphosphatemia unresponsive to hydration may require phosphate binders, such as aluminum hydroxide, calcium carbonate, sevelamer hydroxide, and lanthanum carbonate, or the use of dialysis or hemofiltration [105].

Numerous reports have described TLS in the perioperative setting [106 - 113]. Dexamethasone, routinely administered for postoperative nausea and vomiting, has been implicated as an important potential trigger for TLS due to its rapid lymphocytic effect [108, 109]. Some authors recommend against its routine use in high-risk cases of TLS [110]. Multiple authors also comment that the use of succinylcholine, or other drugs with the potential to cause acute hyperkalemia, should also be used with caution in patients with high tumor burdens [107, 110, 111].

Retinoic Acid Syndrome

Acute promyeloid leukemia (APL) is a clinical subtype of acute myeloid leukemia. The standard treatment for APL is all-trans retinoic acid (ATRA) followed by anthracycline chemotherapy. The APL has a chromosomal dislocation injury to the retinoic acid receptor. Rapid cellular proliferation of APL, which contains a high degree of procoagulant substrate, has a high risk of disseminated intravascular coagulation and tumor lysis syndrome [114]. ATRA results in APL cells maturing and dying without cellular destruction, thereby minimizing these risks. A recognized complication of ATRA is retinoic acid syndrome, otherwise known as differentiation syndrome. The pathophysiology of retinoic acid syndrome is incompletely understood, but most likely involves the activation of inflammatory mediators resulting in hyperviscosity syndromes and leaky capillaries [115]. This results in a clinical cascade of vascular permeability, systemic inflammatory response syndrome (SIRS), and endothelial damage and multiorgan dysfunction [115].

Retinoic acid syndrome typically presents 12 days after initiation of ATRA, and presents with a constellation of fever, dyspnea, hypotension, and weight gain [116]. Patients can also present with pericardial effusion, renal failure, congestive heart failure, diffuse alveolar hemorrhage, and febrile neutrophilic dermatosis. Blood reveals leukocytosis and coagulopathy. Chest x-ray or CT scan often reveals pulmonary opacities. In addition to supportive care, the hallmark of treatment is the initiation of dexamethasone that is continued until the cessation of signs or symptoms of disease. Following this, hydroxycarbamide is administered for cytoreduction.

This syndrome has been described in the perioperative context, where a patient had ATRA initiated a day prior to time-sensitive dental surgery [117]. The patient experienced unexpected desaturations, increased difficulty with intraoperative ventilation, and increased postoperative oxygen requirements and challenges with surgical site hemostasis secondary to coagulopathy. After initiation of dexamethasone and aminocaproic acid, the patient experienced a successful recovery [117].

Common Oncology Patient Procedures

Often, an anesthesia provider will encounter pediatric oncology patients for diagnostic procedures, such as tumor, lymph node, or bone marrow biopsies, imaging, or lumbar punctures, as well as for treatment therapies, including tumor resections, line placement, and radiation therapy. Particular to this patient population, procedures often need to occur multiple times during diagnosis or treatment period, which can cause pain and distress to both the patient and the patient's family. In a retrospective study of childhood cancer survivors, invasive procedures have been reported as the most difficult part of treatment, leading to posttraumatic stress symptoms in some long-term survivors [118]. Anesthetic considerations for these patients include the fact that these procedures are done in a non-operating room environment. Thus, challenges in the non-operating room environment include a lack of familiarity with the area, variability in anesthesia supplies and monitoring equipment, and a lack of experienced anesthesia staff nearby in case of an emergency which all make anesthetizing these patients a high-risk procedure [119 - 121]. In addition, these patients typically have long-term intravenous access, such as a port with central venous access, and are at higher risk of line infections. It is important as anesthesia providers to maintain aseptic techniques when administering medications to avoid risks of infection. These procedures can typically be done with either general anesthesia or sedation, depending on the patient's other comorbidities.

Radiation beam therapy is used as a treatment for certain cancers and works by targeting specific areas and destroying cancer cells or shrinking tumors *via* a high-energy radiation beam. A mold is created of the patient's head while under anesthesia and is used to target how radiation is delivered for each session. The radiation treatments are typically split over multiple days or weeks. Often, anesthesia is required for these patients due to anxiety from the head mold and their inability to lie still for the treatment.

Anesthetic considerations for radiation beam therapy include the evaluation of airway, respiratory, and cardiac status preoperatively. Once the head mold is created and areas of radiation targeted, any manipulation of the airway may cause a need to restart the treatment plan completely due to the inability to use the mold created. One must determine whether anesthesia can be done with a natural airway or with an airway device at the beginning of the treatment sessions and commit to that plan for the multiple sessions involved. In addition, once treatment sessions have begun, cases cannot be cancelled for minor respiratory illnesses due to the risks associated with postponing therapy. Also, only the patient is allowed to be in the radiation area, and thus, the anesthesia provider must monitor the patient while under general anesthesia from another room. In addition, the proton beam centers are often in a remote place in the hospital with all the unique anesthetic challenges of a non-operating room environment described previously.

Preoperative Testing

Preoperative testing in children with cancer is not typically indicated unless there is clinical concern from their underlying condition or for their specific procedure. Specific laboratory testing should be based on history and physical examination, comorbidities, and the type of surgical procedure, such as obtaining a platelet count in a patient undergoing lumbar puncture [81]. It is crucial to have multidisciplinary communication, collaboration, and discussion for the safety of the patient [81].

Cardiac Toxicity Screening

Table **2** shows that the risk for cardiomyopathy is based on the dose of anthracycline, chest radiation, and the combination of the two [34].

Table 2. Risk factors for cardiomyopathy. Adapted from Cote 2024 [34].

High Risk for Cardiomyopathy	Moderate Risk for Cardiomyopathy	Low Risk for Cardiomyopathy
Anthracycline dose > 250 mg/m^2	Anthracycline dose 100 to 250 mg/m^2	Anthracycline dose <100 mg/m^2
Chest radiation dose > 35 Gy	Chest radiation dose 15+ to < 35 GY	Surveillance may be reasonable
Combined anthracycline and chest radiation 100 + mg/m2 and 15 + Gy		

Recommendations for chronic cardiotoxicity screening are based on the International Late Effects of Childhood Cancer Guidelines Harmonization Group. These recommendations are for childhood cancer survivors who were treated with anthracyclines, mitoxantrone, or chest radiation. The recommendations include cardiac surveillance within 2 years after treatment, then 5 years post-treatment, and then every 5 years after [34, 81]. Further chemotherapeutic agents carry other organ toxicities as outlined in Table **3** [34].

Table 3. Common Chemotherapeutic agents and organ system toxicity. Adapted from Cote 2024 [34].

Organ System Dysfunction	**Toxic Chemotheraphy Agent**
Cardiomyopathy	Anthracyclines Mitoxantrone
Pulmonary Fibrosis	Bleomycin
Clotting Dysfunction	1-Asparaginase
Renal Injury	Cisplatin Ifosfamide Methotrexate
Hepatic Failure	1-Asparaginase
Pancreatitis	1-Asparaginase

Pain Management

Acute and chronic pain is a common consequence of cancer and subsequent therapy [34, 81]. Around 70% of children with cancer suffer from acute pain [122]. Opioids are still the mainstay treatment of cancer pain, but are associated with adverse effects like constipation, tolerance, dependence, and increased respiratory events. Commonly used opioids include morphine, hydromorphone, methadone, and fentanyl. Longer-acting opioids, codeine, and tramadol are not recommended in the pediatric population. Breakthrough pain is treated as needed with an immediate-acting opioid at 10% of the total daily dose. Severe pain requiring hospitalization in age-appropriate patients with cancer can incorporate a continuous infusion with a patient-controlled analgesia bolus [61, 122, 124].

A multi-modal approach for pain management is integral to combating opioid tolerance in patients with cancer. Oftentimes, pain is associated with other symptoms like insomnia and anxiety, so those must also be addressed for effective pain management. The risks and benefits of other forms of analgesia techniques must be carefully weighed. For instance, regional anesthesia is a highly effective analgesic method but can be risky in a patient with coagulopathy or significant chemotherapy-induced neuropathy [81]. Interventional pain management also includes neurolysis and nerve blocks [81, 123]. A multi-disciplinary team discussion should include team members from anesthesia, surgery, oncology, psychiatry, and acute/chronic pain to determine an effective plan for pain management during cancer treatment and for post-survival [61, 123, 124].

CONCLUSION

Pediatric cancer patients have anesthetic implications that are numerous and constantly evolving as newer treatments emerge. All the organ system derangements mentioned above can have profound morbidity and mortality implications, and providers should be familiar with the most encountered complications before caring for a pediatric cancer patient.

REFERENCES

[1] Ward E, DeSantis C, Robbins A, Kohler B, Jemal A. Childhood and adolescent cancer statistics, 2014. CA Cancer J Clin 2014; 64(2): 83-103. [http://dx.doi.org/10.3322/caac.21219] [PMID: 24488779]

[2] MJ H. SEER cancer statistics review, 1975-2006. Available from: http://seer. cancer. gov/csr/1975_2006/

[3] Goldstick JE, Cunningham RM, Carter PM. Current causes of death in children and adolescents in the United States. N Engl J Med 2022; 386(20): 1955-6. [http://dx.doi.org/10.1056/NEJMc2201761] [PMID: 35443104]

[4] World Health Organization. CureAll framework: WHO global initiative for childhood cancer: increasing access, advancing quality, saving lives. InCureAll framework: WHO global initiative for childhood cancer: increasing access, advancing quality, saving lives 2021.

[5] Bhakta N, Force LM, Allemani C, *et al.* Childhood cancer burden: a review of global estimates. Lancet Oncol 2019; 20(1): e42-53. [http://dx.doi.org/10.1016/S1470-2045(18)30761-7] [PMID: 30614477]

[6] Legler JM, Ries LAG, Smith MA, *et al.* Cancer surveillance series [corrected]: brain and other central nervous system cancers: recent trends in incidence and mortality. J Natl Cancer Inst 1999; 91(16): 1382-90. [http://dx.doi.org/10.1093/jnci/91.16.1382] [PMID: 10451443]

[7] El-Ayadi M, Ansari M, Sturm D, *et al.* High-grade glioma in very young children: a rare and particular patient population. Oncotarget 2017; 8(38): 64564-78. [http://dx.doi.org/10.18632/oncotarget.18478] [PMID: 28969094]

[8] Pollack IF. Pediatric brain tumors. InSeminars in surgical oncology 1999 Mar (Vol. 16, No. 2, pp. 73-90). New York: John Wiley & Sons, Inc. [http://dx.doi.org/10.1002/(SICI)1098-2388(199903)16:2<73::AID-SSU2>3.0.CO;2-0]

[9] Rheingold SR. Oncologic emergency. Principles and practice of pediatric oncology. 2006:1202-30.

[10] Isaacs H Jr. I. Perinatal brain tumors: a review of 250 cases. Pediatr Neurol 2002; 27(4): 249-61. [http://dx.doi.org/10.1016/S0887-8994(02)00472-1] [PMID: 12435562]

[11] Latham GJ, Greenberg RS. Anesthetic considerations for the pediatric oncology patient – part 2: systems-based approach to anesthesia. Paediatr Anaesth 2010; 20(5): 396-420. [http://dx.doi.org/10.1111/j.1460-9592.2010.03260.x] [PMID: 20199611]

[12] Binning M, Klimo P Jr, Gluf W, Goumnerova L. Spinal tumors in children. Neurosurg Clin N Am 2007; 18(4): 631-58. [http://dx.doi.org/10.1016/j.nec.2007.07.001] [PMID: 17991588]

[13] Reddy AT, Witek K. Neurologic complications of chemotherapy for children with cancer. Curr Neurol Neurosci Rep 2003; 3(2): 137-42. [http://dx.doi.org/10.1007/s11910-003-0065-2] [PMID: 12583842]

[14] Board PP. Late effects of treatment for childhood cancer (PDQ®). PDQ Cancer Information Summaries. US: National Cancer Institute 2004. Internet

[15] Adamson PC, Balis FM, Berg S, Blaney SM. General principles of chemotherapy. Principles and practice of pediatric oncology. 2006;5:290-365.

[16] Lang SS, Beslow LA, Gabel B, *et al.* Surgical treatment of brain tumors in infants younger than six

months of age and review of the literature. World Neurosurg 2012; 78(1-2): 137-44. [http://dx.doi.org/10.1016/j.wneu.2011.09.012] [PMID: 22120270]

[17] Szabó EZ, Luginbuehl I, Bissonnette B. Impact of anesthetic agents on cerebrovascular physiology in children. Paediatr Anaesth 2009; 19(2): 108-18. [http://dx.doi.org/10.1111/j.1460-9592.2008.02826.x] [PMID: 19040505]

[18] Burke A, Virmani R. Pediatric heart tumors. Cardiovasc Pathol 2008; 17(4): 193-8. [http://dx.doi.org/10.1016/j.carpath.2007.08.008] [PMID: 18402818]

[19] Tzani A, Doulamis IP, Mylonas KS, Avgerinos DV, Nasioudis D. Cardiac tumors in pediatric patients: a systematic review. World J Pediatr Congenit Heart Surg 2017; 8(5): 624-32. [http://dx.doi.org/10.1177/2150135117723904] [PMID: 28901236]

[20] Kühn B, Peters J, Marx GR, Breitbart RE. Etiology, management, and outcome of pediatric pericardial effusions. Pediatr Cardiol 2008; 29(1): 90-4. [http://dx.doi.org/10.1007/s00246-007-9014-1] [PMID: 17674083]

[21] Armstrong GT, Liu Q, Yasui Y, *et al.* Late mortality among 5-year survivors of childhood cancer: a summary from the Childhood Cancer Survivor Study. J Clin Oncol 2009; 27(14): 2328-38. [http://dx.doi.org/10.1200/JCO.2008.21.1425] [PMID: 19332714]

[22] Armstrong GT, Kawashima T, Leisenring W, *et al.* Aging and risk of severe, disabling, life-threatening, and fatal events in the childhood cancer survivor study. J Clin Oncol 2014; 32(12): 1218-27. [http://dx.doi.org/10.1200/JCO.2013.51.1055] [PMID: 24638000]

[23] Gewirtz D. A critical evaluation of the mechanisms of action proposed for the antitumor effects of the anthracycline antibiotics adriamycin and daunorubicin. Biochem Pharmacol 1999; 57(7): 727-41. [http://dx.doi.org/10.1016/S0006-2952(98)00307-4] [PMID: 10075079]

[24] van Dalen EC, van der Pal HJH, Bakker PJM, Caron HN, Kremer LCM. Cumulative incidence and risk factors of mitoxantrone-induced cardiotoxicity in children. Eur J Cancer 2004; 40(5): 643-52. [http://dx.doi.org/10.1016/j.ejca.2003.12.006] [PMID: 15010064]

[25] Slinger P, Karsli C. Management of the patient with a large anterior mediastinal mass: recurring myths. Curr Opin Anaesthesiol 2007; 20(1): 1-3. [http://dx.doi.org/10.1097/ACO.0b013e328011390b] [PMID: 17211158]

[26] King DR, Patrick LE, Ginn-Pease ME, McCoy KS, Klopfenstein K. Pulmonary function is compromised in children with mediastinal lymphoma. J Pediatr Surg 1997; 32(2): 294-300. [http://dx.doi.org/10.1016/S0022-3468(97)90197-4] [PMID: 9044140]

[27] Diamond M, Ruiz-Mesa C, Corrales-Medina FF, Tamariz LJ, Ziga E, Swaminathan S. Incidence and outcome of pericardial effusion in pediatric patients after hematopoietic stem cell transplant: a single-institution experience. J Pediatr Hematol Oncol 2018; 40(2): 132-6. [http://dx.doi.org/10.1097/MPH.0000000000000974] [PMID: 28945662]

[28] Hack HA, Wright NB, Wynn RF. The anaesthetic management of children with anterior mediastinal masses. Anaesthesia 2008; 63(8): 837-46. [http://dx.doi.org/10.1111/j.1365-2044.2008.05515.x] [PMID: 18547295]

[29] Scrace B, McGregor K. Anterior mediastinal masses in paediatric anaesthesia. ATOTW 2015; 320: 1-7.

[30] McLeod M, Dobbie M. Anterior mediastinal masses in children. BJA Educ 2019; 19(1): 21-6. [http://dx.doi.org/10.1016/j.bjae.2018.10.001] [PMID: 33456850]

[31] Smibert E, Carlin JB, Vidmar S, Wilkinson LC, Newton M, Weintraub RG. Exercise echocardiography reflects cumulative anthracycline exposure during childhood. Pediatr Blood Cancer 2004; 42(7): 556-62. [http://dx.doi.org/10.1002/pbc.20016] [PMID: 15127409]

[32] Hammer GB. Anaesthetic management for the child with a mediastinal mass. Paediatr Anaesth 2004; 14(1): 95-7.
[http://dx.doi.org/10.1046/j.1460-9592.2003.01196.x] [PMID: 14717880]

[33] Culshaw V, Yule M, Lawson R. Considerations for anaesthesia in children with haematological malignancy undergoing short procedures. Paediatr Anaesth 2003; 13(5): 375-83.
[http://dx.doi.org/10.1046/j.1460-9592.2003.00932.x] [PMID: 12791109]

[34] Coté CJ, Lerman J, Anderson B, Eds. A Practice of Anesthesia for Infants and Children. Elsevier 2024: pp. 1416.

[35] McCahon E. Lung tumours in children. Paediatr Respir Rev 2006; 7(3): 191-6.
[http://dx.doi.org/10.1016/j.prrv.2006.05.002] [PMID: 16938641]

[36] Meyer S, Reinhard H, Graf N, Nunold H, Graf N. Pulmonary dysfunction in pediatric oncology patients. Pediatr Hematol Oncol 2004; 21(2): 175-95.
[http://dx.doi.org/10.1080/08880010490272894] [PMID: 15160517]

[37] Fauroux B, Meyer-Milsztain A, Boccon-Gibod L, *et al.* Cytotoxic drug-induced pulmonary disease in infants and children. Pediatr Pulmonol 1994; 18(6): 347-55.
[http://dx.doi.org/10.1002/ppul.1950180602] [PMID: 7892068]

[38] Limper AH. Chemotherapy-induced lung disease. Clin Chest Med 2004; 25(1): 53-64.
[http://dx.doi.org/10.1016/S0272-5231(03)00123-0] [PMID: 15062597]

[39] Latham GJ. Anesthesia for the child with cancer. Anesthesiol Clin 2014; 32(1): 185-213.
[http://dx.doi.org/10.1016/j.anclin.2013.10.002] [PMID: 24491657]

[40] Luis M, Ayuso A, Martinez G, Souto M, Ortells J. Intraoperative respiratory failure in a patient after treatment with bleomycin: previous and current intraoperative exposure to 50% oxygen. Eur J Anaesthesiol 1999; 16(1): 66-8.
[http://dx.doi.org/10.1097/00003643-199901000-00013] [PMID: 10084104]

[41] Whyte SD, Mark Ansermino J. Anesthetic considerations in the management of Wilms' tumor. Paediatr Anaesth 2006; 16(5): 504-13.
[http://dx.doi.org/10.1111/j.1460-9592.2006.01866.x] [PMID: 16677259]

[42] Vujanić GM, Mifsud W. Anaplasia in Wilms tumor: A critical review. Pediatr Blood Cancer 2024; 71(7): e31000.
[http://dx.doi.org/10.1002/pbc.31000] [PMID: 38605554]

[43] Neville H, Ritchey ML, Shamberger RC, Haase G, Perlman S, Yoshioka T. The occurrence of Wilms tumor in horseshoe kidneys: A report from the National Wilms Tumor Study Group (NWTSG). J Pediatr Surg 2002; 37(8): 1134-7.
[http://dx.doi.org/10.1053/jpsu.2002.34458] [PMID: 12149688]

[44] Meni D. Wilms tumor and associated predisposing syndromes and conditions. JAAPA 2025; 38(1): 27-33.
[http://dx.doi.org/10.1097/01.JAA.0000000000000165] [PMID: 39654521]

[45] Geller E, Kochan PS. Renal neoplasms of childhood. Radiol Clin North Am 2011; 49(4): 689-709, vi.
[http://dx.doi.org/10.1016/j.rcl.2011.05.003] [PMID: 21807169]

[46] Glick RD, Romao RLP, Pachl M, *et al.* Current surgical approaches to pediatric renal tumors. Pediatr Blood Cancer 2025; 72(S2) (Suppl. 2): e31118.
[http://dx.doi.org/10.1002/pbc.31118] [PMID: 38809413]

[47] Chen SY, Laifman E, Mack SJ, Zhou S, Stein JE, Kim ES. Epidural analgesia is associated with reduced inpatient opioid consumption and length of stay after wilms tumor resection. J Surg Res 2023; 290: 141-6.
[http://dx.doi.org/10.1016/j.jss.2023.04.018] [PMID: 37267703]

[48] Aksu C, Gürkan Y. Ultrasound guided erector spinae block for postoperative analgesia in pediatric

nephrectomy surgeries. J Clin Anesth 2018; 45: 35-6.
[http://dx.doi.org/10.1016/j.jclinane.2017.12.021] [PMID: 29274546]

[49] El Sherif F, Sayed D, Fares KM, *et al.* Magnesium Sulfate in Pediatric Abdominal Cancer Surgery: Safety and Efficacy in Ultrasound-Guided Transversus Abdominis Plane (US-TAP) Block in Conjugation with Levobupivacaine. Local Reg Anesth 2023; 16: 133-41.
[http://dx.doi.org/10.2147/LRA.S425649] [PMID: 37719936]

[50] Chakraborty A, Goswami J, Patro V. Ultrasound-guided continuous quadratus lumborum block for postoperative analgesia in a pediatric patient. A A Case Rep 2015; 4(3): 34-6.
[http://dx.doi.org/10.1213/XAA.0000000000000090] [PMID: 25642956]

[51] Moon JK, Hwang R, Balis FM, Mattei P. An enhanced recovery after surgery protocol in children who undergo nephrectomy for Wilms tumor safely shortens hospital stay. J Pediatr Surg 2022; 57(10): 259-65.
[http://dx.doi.org/10.1016/j.jpedsurg.2022.05.020] [PMID: 35768311]

[52] Tognon C, Pulvirenti R, Fati F, *et al.* Anesthesia in children with neuroblastoma, perioperative and operative management. Children (Basel) 2021; 8(5): 395.
[http://dx.doi.org/10.3390/children8050395] [PMID: 34068896]

[53] Balassy C, Navarro OM, Daneman A. Adrenal masses in children. Radiol Clin North Am 2011; 49(4): 711-727, vi.
[http://dx.doi.org/10.1016/j.rcl.2011.05.001] [PMID: 21807170]

[54] Gómez-Ríos MÁ, Nuño FC, Barreto-Calvo P. [Anesthetic management of an infant with giant abdominal neuroblastoma]. Rev Bras Anestesiol 2017; 67(2): 210-3.
[PMID: 28081907]

[55] Iwanaka T, Horie H, Hiyama E, *et al.* High diagnostic accuracy of extended catecholamine metabolite profiling in neuroblastoma. Clin Chim Acta. 2017; 471: 263-8.
[PMID: 28061374]

[56] Gupta A, Kundal R, Pandey M. Opsoclonus-myoclonus Syndrome with Neuroblastoma in Children and their Anaesthetic Management. J Coll Physicians Surg Pak 2022; 32(8): 1086-8.
[http://dx.doi.org/10.29271/jcpsp.2022.08.1086] [PMID: 35932142]

[57] Ikeda H, Iehara T, Tsuchida Y, *et al.* Experience with international neuroblastoma staging system and pathology classification. Br J Cancer 2002; 86(7): 1110-6.
[http://dx.doi.org/10.1038/sj.bjc.6600231] [PMID: 11953858]

[58] Pio L, Avanzini S, Mattioli G, *et al.* Perioperative management of hypertensive neuroblastoma: A study from the Italian Group of Pediatric Surgical Oncologists (GICOP). J Pediatr Surg 2017; 52(10): 1633-6.
[http://dx.doi.org/10.1016/j.jpedsurg.2017.06.027] [PMID: 28711167]

[59] Hernandez MR, Shamberger RC, Seefelder C. Catecholamine-secreting neuroblastoma in a 4-mont--old infant: perioperative management. J Clin Anesth 2009; 21(1): 54-6.
[http://dx.doi.org/10.1016/j.jclinane.2008.06.021] [PMID: 19232942]

[60] Selldén H, Kogner P, Sollevi A. Adenosine for per-operative blood pressure control in an infant with neuroblastoma. Acta Anaesthesiol Scand 1995; 39(5): 705-8.
[http://dx.doi.org/10.1111/j.1399-6576.1995.tb04151.x] [PMID: 7572024]

[61] Seefelder C, Sparks JW, Chirnomas D, Diller L, Shamberger RC. Perioperative management of a child with severe hypertension from a catecholamine secreting neuroblastoma. Paediatr Anaesth 2005; 15(7): 606-10.
[http://dx.doi.org/10.1111/j.1460-9592.2005.01631.x] [PMID: 15960647]

[62] Liu J, Zurakowski D, Weldon C, Umaretiya P, Holzman R, Lin YC. Perioperative hypertension and anesthetic management in patients undergoing resection of neuroblastoma. Paediatr Anaesth 2023; 33(7): 577-82.

[http://dx.doi.org/10.1111/pan.14673] [PMID: 37052325]

[63] Kako H, Taghon T, Veneziano G, Aldrink JH, Ayoob R, Tobias JD. Severe intraoperative hypertension after induction of anesthesia in a child with a neuroblastoma. J Anesth 2013; 27(3): 464-7.
[http://dx.doi.org/10.1007/s00540-012-1544-x] [PMID: 23292755]

[64] Minami T, Adachi T, Fukuda K. An effective use of magnesium sulfate for intraoperative management of laparoscopic adrenalectomy for pheochromocytoma in a pediatric patient. Anesth Analg 2002; 95(5): 1243-4.
[http://dx.doi.org/10.1097/00000539-200211000-00024] [PMID: 12401602]

[65] He J, Wang Z, Yu X, Su Y, Hong M, Zhu K. Promoting application of enhanced recovery after surgery protocols during perioperative localized abdominal and thoracic neuroblastomas. Pediatr Surg Int 2024; 40(1): 286.
[http://dx.doi.org/10.1007/s00383-024-05884-w] [PMID: 39487870]

[66] Wang L, Peng Y, Zhang H, et al. Promoting application of enhanced recovery after surgery protocols during perioperative localized abdominal and thoracic neuroblastomas. J Pediatr Surg. 2024; 59(6): 1190-1196.
[PMID: 39487870]

[67] Lee WG, Lascano D, Palmer SB, *et al.* Optimizing the postoperative management of children undergoing resection of high-risk abdominal neuroblastoma. Am Surg 2024; 90(6): 1290-7.
[http://dx.doi.org/10.1177/00031348241227199] [PMID: 38243794]

[68] Finkel KW, Foringer JR. Renal disease in patients with cancer. Nat Clin Pract Nephrol 2007; 3(12): 669-78.
[http://dx.doi.org/10.1038/ncpneph0622] [PMID: 18033226]

[69] Tsai TC, Lee HC, Huang FY. The size of the renal pelvis on ultrasonography in children. J Clin Ultrasound 1989; 17(9): 647-51.
[http://dx.doi.org/10.1002/jcu.1870170906] [PMID: 2514199]

[70] Handa A, Nozaki T, Makidono A, *et al.* Pediatric oncologic emergencies: Clinical and imaging review for pediatricians. Pediatr Int 2019; 61(2): 122-39.
[http://dx.doi.org/10.1111/ped.13755] [PMID: 30565795]

[71] Chiruvella V, Annamaraju P, Guddati AK. Management of nephrotoxicity of chemotherapy and targeted agents: 2020. Am J Cancer Res 2020; 10(12): 4151-64.
[PMID: 33414992]

[72] Okamoto K, Saito Y, Narumi K, Furugen A, Iseki K, Kobayashi M. Non-steroidal anti-inflammatory drugs are a risk factor for cisplatin-induced nephrotoxicity: A meta-analysis of retrospective studies. Anticancer Res 2020; 40(3): 1747-51.
[http://dx.doi.org/10.21873/anticanres.14128] [PMID: 32132083]

[73] Skinner R. Nephrotoxicity--what do we know and what don't we know? J Pediatr Hematol Oncol 2011; 33(2): 128-34.
[http://dx.doi.org/10.1097/MPH.0b013e3181f8cac0] [PMID: 21285904]

[74] Ruggiero A, Ferrara P, Attinà G, Rizzo D, Riccardi R. Renal toxicity and chemotherapy in children with cancer. Br J Clin Pharmacol 2017; 83(12): 2605-14.
[http://dx.doi.org/10.1111/bcp.13388] [PMID: 28758697]

[75] Rossi R, Kleta R, Ehrich JHH. Renal involvement in children with malignancies. Pediatr Nephrol 1999; 13(2): 153-62.
[http://dx.doi.org/10.1007/s004670050585] [PMID: 10229006]

[76] Sharbaf FG, Farhangi H, Assadi F. Prevention of chemotherapy-induced nephrotoxicity in children with cancer. Int J Prev Med 2017; 8(1): 76.
[http://dx.doi.org/10.4103/ijpvm.IJPVM_40_17] [PMID: 29114374]

[77] Klaus R, Niyazi M, Lange-Sperandio B. Radiation-induced kidney toxicity: molecular and cellular pathogenesis. Radiat Oncol 2021; 16(1): 43.
[http://dx.doi.org/10.1186/s13014-021-01764-y] [PMID: 33632272]

[78] Dawson LA, Kavanagh BD, Paulino AC, *et al.* Radiation-associated kidney injury. Int J Radiat Oncol Biol Phys 2010; 76(3) (Suppl.): S108-15.
[http://dx.doi.org/10.1016/j.ijrobp.2009.02.089] [PMID: 20171504]

[79] Breitz H. Clinical aspects of radiation nephropathy. Cancer Biother Radiopharm 2004; 19(3): 359-62.
[http://dx.doi.org/10.1089/1084978041425106] [PMID: 15285883]

[80] Litten JB, Tomlinson GE. Liver tumors in children. Oncologist 2008; 13(7): 812-20.
[http://dx.doi.org/10.1634/theoncologist.2008-0011] [PMID: 18644850]

[81] Ojo B, Ross FJ, and Latham GJ. Practice of Anesthesia for Infants and Children. 10th edition. 2025. 9, 261-277.

[82] Board PP. Late effects of treatment for childhood cancer (PDQ®). InPDQ Cancer Information Summaries [Internet] 2004 Apr 23. National Cancer Institute (US).

[83] Gooley TA, Chien JW, Pergam SA, *et al.* Reduced mortality after allogeneic hematopoietic-cell transplantation. N Engl J Med 2010; 363(22): 2091-101.
[http://dx.doi.org/10.1056/NEJMoa1004383] [PMID: 21105791]

[84] Fathi E, Valipour B, Jafari S, Kazemi A, Montazersaheb S, Farahzadi R. The role of the hematopoietic stem/progenitor cells-derived extracellular vesicles in hematopoiesis. Heliyon 2024; 10(15): e35051.
[http://dx.doi.org/10.1016/j.heliyon.2024.e35051] [PMID: 39157371]

[85] Cefalo MG, Maurizi P, Arlotta A, *et al.* Hepatic veno-occlusive disease: a chemotherapy-related toxicity in children with malignancies. Paediatr Drugs 2010; 12(5): 277-84.
[http://dx.doi.org/10.2165/11531840-000000000-00000] [PMID: 20799757]

[86] Hasegawa S, Horibe K, Kawabe T, *et al.* Veno-occlusive disease of the liver after allogeneic bone marrow transplantation in children with hematologic malignancies: incidence, onset time and risk factors. Bone Marrow Transplant 1998; 22(12): 1191-7.
[http://dx.doi.org/10.1038/sj.bmt.1701506] [PMID: 9894723]

[87] Bearman SI. The syndrome of hepatic veno-occlusive disease after marrow transplantation. Blood 1995; 85(11): 3005-20.
[http://dx.doi.org/10.1182/blood.V85.11.3005.bloodjournal85113005] [PMID: 7756636]

[88] Andersson BS, Madden T, Tran HT, *et al.* Acute safety and pharmacokinetics of intravenous busulfan when used with oral busulfan and cyclophosphamide as pretransplantation conditioning therapy: A phase I study. Biol Blood Marrow Transplant 2000; 6(5): 548-54.
[http://dx.doi.org/10.1016/S1083-8791(00)70064-4] [PMID: 11071260]

[89] Cheuk DKL. Hepatic veno-occlusive disease after hematopoietic stem cell transplantation: Prophylaxis and treatment controversies. World J Transplant 2012; 2(2): 27-34.
[http://dx.doi.org/10.5500/wjt.v2.i2.27] [PMID: 24175193]

[90] Lagoo J, Shah V. Anaesthetic considerations in an infant with Beckwith-Weidemann syndrome and hepatoblastoma for partial hepatectomy. Indian J Anaesth 2015; 59(2): 121-3.
[http://dx.doi.org/10.4103/0019-5049.151377] [PMID: 25788746]

[91] Whizar-Lugo V, Sigler-Moreno A, Ontiveros-Morales P, *et al.* Anesthesia for partial glossectomy in a toddler with Beckwith-Wiedemann syndrome. Anestesia en Mexico. 2006;18(3).

[92] Jacob R. Anaesthesia for biliary atresia and hepatectomy in paediatrics. Indian J Anaesth 2012; 56(5): 479-84.
[http://dx.doi.org/10.4103/0019-5049.103965] [PMID: 23293387]

[93] Bicer C, Eskitascioglu T, Aksu R, Madenoglu H. The anesthetic management of a case of Beckwith-Weidemann syndrome presenting with a large tongue. Erciyes Tip Derg 2011; 33: 251-4.

[94] Redhu S, Jalwal G, Saxena M, Shrivastava OP. A comparative study of induction, maintenance and recovery characteristics of sevoflurane and halothane anaesthesia in pediatric patients (6 months to 6 years). J Anaesthesiol Clin Pharmacol 2010; 26(4): 484-7. [http://dx.doi.org/10.4103/0970-9185.74591] [PMID: 21547175]

[95] FitzGerald TJ, Aronowitz J, Cicchetti MG, Fisher G, Kadish S, Lo YC, Mayo C, McCauley S, Meyer J, Pieters R, Sherman A. The effect of radiation therapy on normal tissue function. Hematology/Oncology Clinics. 2006 Feb 1;20(1):141-63. [http://dx.doi.org/10.1016/j.hoc.2006.01.005]

[96] Greco C, Berde C. Pain management for the hospitalized pediatric patient. Pediatr Clin North Am 2005; 52(4): 995-1027, vii-viii. [http://dx.doi.org/10.1016/j.pcl.2005.04.005] [PMID: 16009254]

[97] Singh SD, Henley SJ, Ryerson AB. Surveillance for cancer incidence and mortality—United States, 2012. MMWR Morb Mortal Wkly Rep 2016; 63(55): 17-58. [http://dx.doi.org/10.15585/mmwr.mm6355a4] [PMID: 27736826]

[98] Pizzo PA, Poplack DG. Principles and practice of pediatric oncology. Lippincott Williams & Wilkins; 2015 Jun 24.

[99] Blijdorp K, van Waas M, van der Lely AJ, Pieters R, van den Heuvel-Eibrink M, Neggers S. Endocrine sequelae and metabolic syndrome in adult long-term survivors of childhood acute myeloid leukemia. Leuk Res 2013; 37(4): 367-71. [http://dx.doi.org/10.1016/j.leukres.2012.12.008] [PMID: 23312900]

[100] Falanga A, Marchetti M, Vignoli A. Coagulation and cancer: biological and clinical aspects. J Thromb Haemost 2013; 11(2): 223-33. [http://dx.doi.org/10.1111/jth.12075] [PMID: 23279708]

[101] Kostense Z, de Ruiter J. Anaesthesia for children with cancer. BJA Educ 2024; 24(7): 231-7. [http://dx.doi.org/10.1016/j.bjae.2024.03.007] [PMID: 38899313]

[102] Practice guidelines for perioperative blood management: an updated report by the American Society of Anesthesiologists Task Force on Perioperative Blood Management*. Anesthesiology 2015; 122(2): 241-75. [http://dx.doi.org/10.1097/ALN.0000000000000463] [PMID: 25545654]

[103] Coiffier B, Altman A, Pui CH, Younes A, Cairo MS. Guidelines for the management of pediatric and adult tumor lysis syndrome: an evidence-based review. J Clin Oncol 2008; 26(16): 2767-78. [http://dx.doi.org/10.1200/JCO.2007.15.0177] [PMID: 18509186]

[104] Smalley RV, Guaspari A, Haase-Statz S, Anderson SA, Cederberg D, Hohneker JA. Allopurinol: intravenous use for prevention and treatment of hyperuricemia. J Clin Oncol 2000; 18(8): 1758-63. [http://dx.doi.org/10.1200/JCO.2000.18.8.1758] [PMID: 10764437]

[105] Friedman EA. An introduction to phosphate binders for the treatment of hyperphosphatemia in patients with chronic kidney disease. Kidney Int 2005; 68(96): S2-6. [http://dx.doi.org/10.1016/S0085-2538(15)51226-X] [PMID: 15954946]

[106] Chubb EA, Maloney D, Farley-Hills E. Tumour lysis syndrome: an unusual presentation. Anaesthesia 2010; 65(10): 1031-3. [http://dx.doi.org/10.1111/j.1365-2044.2010.06414.x] [PMID: 20645952]

[107] Lee MH, Cheng KI, Jang RC, Hsu JH, Dai ZK, Wu JR. Tumour lysis syndrome developing during an operation. Anaesthesia 2007; 62(1): 85-7. [http://dx.doi.org/10.1111/j.1365-2044.2006.04873.x] [PMID: 17156233]

[108] McDonnell C, Barlow R, Campisi P, Grant R, Malkin D. Fatal peri-operative acute tumour lysis syndrome precipitated by dexamethasone. Anaesthesia 2008; 63(6): 652-5. [http://dx.doi.org/10.1111/j.1365-2044.2007.05436.x] [PMID: 18477278]

[109] Lerza R, Botta M, Barsotti B, *et al.* Dexamethazone-induced acute tumor lysis syndrome in a T-cell malignant lymphoma. Leuk Lymphoma 2002; 43(5): 1129-32. [http://dx.doi.org/10.1080/10428190290021452] [PMID: 12148896]

[110] Dhar M, Prakash S, Pandey V, Pai V. Intraoperative tumor lysis syndrome in a child with Wilms' tumor. Anesth Essays Res 2016; 10(1): 145-7. [http://dx.doi.org/10.4103/0259-1162.171446] [PMID: 26957712]

[111] Verma A, Mathur R, Chauhan M, Ranjan P. Tumor lysis syndrome developing intraoperatively. J Anaesthesiol Clin Pharmacol 2011; 27(4): 561-3. [http://dx.doi.org/10.4103/0970-9185.86611] [PMID: 22096300]

[112] Farley-Hills E, Byrne AJ, Brennan L, Sartori P. Tumour lysis syndrome during anaesthesia. Paediatr Anaesth 2001; 11(2): 233-6. [http://dx.doi.org/10.1046/j.1460-9592.2001.00625.x] [PMID: 11240885]

[113] Zhang G, Duan M, Zhou Z, Yang J, Peng YG. Intraoperative tumor lysis-induced fatal hyperkalemia. J Anesth 2012; 26(6): 945-6. [http://dx.doi.org/10.1007/s00540-012-1428-0] [PMID: 22684215]

[114] Usoltsev NA, Dhamee MS. Perioperative retinoic acid syndrome in a patient with acute promyelocytic leukemia. J Clin Anesth 2012; 24(4): 315-7. [http://dx.doi.org/10.1016/j.jclinane.2011.10.009] [PMID: 22608587]

[115] Stahl M, Tallman MS. Differentiation syndrome in acute promyelocytic leukaemia. Br J Haematol 2019; 187(2): 157-62. [http://dx.doi.org/10.1111/bjh.16151] [PMID: 31410848]

[116] Montesinos P, Bergua JM, Vellenga E, *et al.* Differentiation syndrome in patients with acute promyelocytic leukemia treated with all-trans retinoic acid and anthracycline chemotherapy: characteristics, outcome, and prognostic factors. Blood 2009; 113(4): 775-83. [http://dx.doi.org/10.1182/blood-2008-07-168617] [PMID: 18945964]

[117] Beebe DS, Belani KG. Hematopoietic Stem Cell Transplantation: History and Perioperative Care of Patients Undergoing HSCT. Curr Anesthesiol Rep 2018; 8(2): 197-201. [http://dx.doi.org/10.1007/s40140-018-0279-0]

[118] Afessa B, Abdulai RM, Kremers WK, Hogan WJ, Litzow MR, Peters SG. Risk factors and outcome of pulmonary complications after autologous hematopoietic stem cell transplant. Chest 2012; 141(2): 442-50. [http://dx.doi.org/10.1378/chest.10-2889] [PMID: 21778261]

[119] Fitch T, Myers KC, Dewan M, Towe C, Dandoy C. Pulmonary complications after pediatric stem cell transplant. Front Oncol 2021; 11: 755878. [http://dx.doi.org/10.3389/fonc.2021.755878] [PMID: 34722309]

[120] Chowdhury SR, Roy A, Maitra S, Baidya DK. Anesthetic concerns in recipients of hematopoietic stem cell transplant. J Anaesthesiol Clin Pharmacol 2023; 39(1): 155-7. [http://dx.doi.org/10.4103/joacp.joacp_212_21] [PMID: 37250234]

[121] Khurmi N, Patel P, Koushik S, Daniels T, Kraus M. Anesthesia practice in pediatric radiation oncology: Mayo Clinic Arizona's Experience 2014–2016. Paediatr Drugs 2018; 20(1): 89-95. [http://dx.doi.org/10.1007/s40272-017-0259-8] [PMID: 28786083]

[122] Simon JDHP, Van Loon FRAA, Van Amstel J, Elmont GS, Zwaan CM, Fiocco M, Schepers SA, Tissing WJE, Michiels EMC. Pain at home during childhood cancer treatment: Severity, prevalence, analgesic use, and interference with daily life. Pediatr Blood Cancer. 2020 Dec; 67(12) :e28699. [http://dx.doi.org/10.1002/pbc.28699] [PMID: 32926551]

[123] Oeffinger KC, Hudson MM. Long-term complications following childhood and adolescent cancer: foundations for providing risk-based health care for survivors. CA Cancer J Clin 2004; 54(4): 208-36. [http://dx.doi.org/10.3322/canjclin.54.4.208] [PMID: 15253918]

[124] Yoshimoto-Suzuki Y, Hasegawa D, Hosoya Y, *et al.* Significance of active screening for detection of health problems in childhood cancer survivors. Front Pediatr 2022; 10: 947646. [http://dx.doi.org/10.3389/fped.2022.947646] [PMID: 36275067]

CHAPTER 11

Cancer Patients and Critical Care

Crystal Adams[1] and **Akhil Patel**[1,*]

[1] *Department of Anesthesiology, George Washington School of Medicine and Health Sciences, Washington, DC, USA*

Abstract: Advances in both detection and management strategies have improved survival rates among cancer patients. As a result, more patients may benefit from ICU admission over the course of their disease. Considerations for admission to ICU should include both the short- and long-term prognoses as well as the reversibility of the acute illness. Cancer patients may be admitted to the ICU for a host of reasons, which may be due to the underlying malignancy, treatment related effects, or non-oncologic acute illnesses. Regardless of the indication for admission, these patients require complex coordination of care and a thoughtful and methodical approach to their ICU management.

Keywords: Acute respiratory failure, Cardiac tamponade, Cytokine release syndrome, Hypercalcemia, Hyperleukocytosis, Immune effect cell-associated neurotoxicity syndrome, Leukostasis, Neutropenic fever, Superior vena cava syndrome, Tumor lysis syndrome.

INTRODUCTION

Historically, the admission of cancer patients to the intensive care unit (ICU) has been widely debated. Reasons cited include the depletion of already limited resources and anticipated poor outcomes [1, 2]. However, advances in cancer therapies and early detection methods have improved overall survival rates [3, 4]. Not only that but studies have shown that the survival rate of cancer patients requiring ICU admission has also increased. Proposed reasons include advances in both oncologic therapies and management of organ dysfunction [5]. As a result, the number of cancer patients who may benefit from ICU admission has substantially increased [1, 4].

* **Corresponding author Akhil Patel:** Department of Anesthesiology, George Washington School of Medicine and Health Sciences, Washington, DC, USA; E-mail: ap1189@gmail.com

Bharathi Gourkanti, Irwin Gratz, William Marion, Rajiv Lingaraju & Grace Abramian (Eds.)

TRIAGE AND PROGNOSTICATION

Triage of the critically ill cancer patient is quite complex. Predicting which patients will benefit from ICU admission can be challenging. The decision of whether a cancer patient should be admitted to the ICU should take into account the short-term intensive care prognosis as well as the patient's long-term prognosis and anticipated quality of life [6]. In general, ICU admission should be considered if the patient has a reversible condition and his or her oncologic prognosis justifies aggressive therapies [6]. Of course, this is assuming that ICU admission is within the patient's goals of care.

Prognostic scores are often used to predict outcomes and aid in clinical decision making within the general ICU population. However, studies assessing the utility of these scores in cancer patients are limited and the results have been mixed [7 - 10]. Soares *et al* conducted a prospective study assessing the performance of 5 general severity of illness scores (Acute Physiology and Chronic Health Evaluation II and IIIJ (APACHE II/IIIJ), Simplified Acute Physiology Score II (SAPS II), Mortality Probability Models at admission and 24 hours (MPM0/24)) and one cancer-specific predictive model (ICU Cancer Mortality Model (ICMM)). They found that none of the scoring models accurately predicted mortality in the critically ill cancer patients [7]. Similarly, Schellongowski *et al* found that while the APACHE II, SAPS II, and ICCM scores could accurately describe the severity of illness and predict outcomes within a group of cancer patients, they failed to reliably predict individual prognosis [8]. Interestingly, both groups also found that the ICCM, which is a cancer-specific predictive model that takes into account hospital days prior to ICU admission, did not perform better than general predictive models [7, 8].

Studies looking at predictors of short-term prognosis among cancer patients admitted to the ICU have identified several risk factors associated with increased mortality. These include severity and number of organ failures, acute respiratory failure, need for mechanical ventilation, late ICU admission, the need for vasopressor support, and performance status prior to admission [6, 11, 12]. The development of acute respiratory failure has been identified as the most important risk factor for mortality in critically ill cancer patients [6, 13]. In contrast, the stage of malignancy has little to no effect on short-term survival [12, 14]. However, the primary determinants of long-term outcomes in this patient population relate to the characteristics of the underlying malignancy [6, 14].

Studies have demonstrated the inadequacy of ICU admission triage criteria, particularly in cancer patients' population. In a prospective study by Thiery *et al.*, 20% of patients denied ICU admission because they were deemed "too well" and died before discharge. Similarly, 25% of the patients, not admitted to the ICU because they were "too sick", survived [5, 15]. As a result, some have called for broader ICU admission criteria among the cancer patient population. In response to this, an international expert consensus released evidence-based ICU admission criteria recommendations for critically ill cancer patients. While these recommendations are evidence-based, they are founded mostly on observational studies. The recommendations place patients into one of three categories: full code management, ICU trial, or no ICU admission. Patients recommended for full code management include patients with a newly diagnosed cancer with expected survival of longer than 1 year, patients whose cancer is in remission, and patients with malignancies that have either curative therapies or therapies, which can extend survival beyond one year [5, 6]. The guidelines recommend not pursuing ICU admission whenexpected survival is less than one year despite ongoing treatments, when there are no further life-extending treatments available, and when the patient has a poor functional status [6]. Outside of these specific circumstances, an ICU trial is suggested. An ICU trial consists of initial unlimited ICU support followed by re-evaluation after a period of 3-5 days. The recommendation of 3-5 days is based on data that suggests that only after 3 days could the degree of organ dysfunction differentiate between survivors and non-survivors [5, 6, 16].

INDICATIONS FOR ICU ADMISSION

Cancer patients comprise 15% of all ICU admissions [17, 18]). Solid organ malignancies are more commonly encountered than hematologic malignancies. Lung cancer is the most common solid organ malignancy seen in cancer patients admitted to the ICU while leukemia and lymphoma are the most common hematologic malignancies identified [12, 19]. Reasons for admission to the ICU can be divided into malignancy related, cancer therapy related, and acute illness unrelated to malignancy [12]. The most common indications for ICU admission in cancer patients are post-operative recovery, respiratory failure, and sepsis [4, 20]. In a prospective study by Soares *et al* looking at characteristics of cancer patients requiring ICU admission, post-operative care represented 57%, acute respiratory failure represented 10%, and sepsis represented 15% of ICU admissions [20].

Malignancy Related Indications

Acute cancer-related complications often necessitate ICU admission in both solid organ and hematologic cancer patients. Some complications are common to all types of malignancy whereas others may be attributed to a specific subtype.

Superior Vena Cava Syndrome

Superior vena cava syndrome (SVC syndrome) results when obstruction of the SVC causes decreased venous return to the heart from the head, neck, thorax, and upper extremities. Approximately 70% of SVC syndrome cases are associated with malignancy, though non-malignant causes have been cited [21, 22]. Tumoral related causes include tumor invasion into the vessel, external compression from either a mass or lymph nodes, and intravascular thrombosis. SVC syndrome is most commonly seen with non-small cell lung cancer, small cell lung cancer, and non-Hodgkin lymphoma [21 - 23]. Metastases make up the remaining percentage, with breast cancer being the most common primary cancer. SVC syndrome may be the initial presenting symptom of an undiagnosed malignancy in up to 60% of cases [22]. The estimated life expectancy in patients with malignant SVC syndrome is approximately 6 months [22].

The clinical presentation of SVC syndrome varies depending on the degree of obstruction, anatomic location of obstruction, speed of onset, and degree of venous collaterals [22]. SVC obstruction can lead to upper airway obstruction, pericardial tamponade, cerebral edema, and pleural effusions. Symptoms can include face and upper extremity swelling, flushing, shortness of breath, coughing, chest pain, venous dilation, hoarseness, stridor, and neurologic symptoms [21].

Diagnosis of SVC syndrome combines clinical evaluation with confirmatory radiographic imaging. Several imaging modalities can be used to confirm SVC obstruction including chest radiography (CXR), computed tomography (CT) scan with contrast, duplex ultrasound, and magnetic resonance venogram (MRV). However, contrasted CT scan has the most utility as it can identify the degree of obstruction, venous collaterals, as well as the underlying cause of obstruction [22]. In the case of malignant SVC syndrome, tissue sampling for histologic confirmation is sometimes necessary [22].

Specific guidelines regarding the management of SVC syndrome are lacking. While many patients recover without active management, some patients require urgent intervention. Which patients require active management has historically not been well defined. However, Yu *et al.*, developed a scoring system to help define the severity of illness and identify which patients require urgent intervention. This classification system is based on the degree of laryngeal and/or cerebral edema as well as hemodynamic status. The patient's SVC syndrome is then classified as life-threatening (grade 4), severe (grade 3), or non-lif--threatening (grade 0-2). This can then be used to guide clinical decision making [22, 24]. The goals of treatment for SVC syndrome are two-fold: symptomatic improvement and treatment of the underlying cause. Head elevation, which decreases hydrostatic pressure, improving head and neck swelling, is the hallmark of initial supportive management [22, 25]. Glucocorticoids may be prescribed to decrease tumor burden in certain steroid-sensitive malignancies. Loop diuretics may also be prescribed to reduce venous return and relieve pressure. However, studies supporting the utility of these two classes of medication are limited [22, 25]. Treatment modalities aimed at relieving the obstruction include radiation therapy, systemic chemotherapy, open surgery, and endovascular recanalization. Historically, radiation therapy was the gold standard treatment for malignant SVC syndrome. However, endovascular therapy is now the standard of care for symptomatic malignancy-related SVC syndrome requiring urgent intervention. Endovascular therapy is faster and has higher efficacy rates than radiation therapy. It can also be combined with radiation and systemic chemotherapy treatments [22, 25].

Hyperleukocytosis and Leukostasis

Hyperleukocytosis is classically defined as a white blood cell (WBC) count greater than 100,000 μL [26]. It is typically associated with hematologic malignancies, most often acute lymphoblastic leukemia and acute myeloblastic leukemia. The incidence of hyperleukocytosis is 5-13% in adult AML patients and 10-30% in ALL [26, 27]. However, the incidence of symptomatic hyperleukocytosis is greater in AML. There have been very few reports of hyperleukocytosis associated with chronic myelogenous leukemia (CML) in the literature(28). Hyperleukocytosis is more commonly associated with certain subtypes of leukemia, including myelomonocytic leukemia, monocytic leukemia, and the microgranular variant of acute promyelocytic leukemia [26]. The particular WBC count at which a patient becomes symptomatic varies depending on the type of leukemia. As a result, patients with WBC counts below the arbitrary threshold of 100,000 μL may present with symptoms and complications of hyperleukocytosis [28].

Studies have shown that hyperleukocytosis is a poor prognostic indicator in patients with AML. However, the literature is mixed as to which factors are specifically affected. Dutcher *et al.*, found that AML patients with hyperleukocytosis had lower complete remission, disease-free survival, and overall survival rates [27, 29]. In contrast, Greenwood *et al.*, showed that only high early mortality could be attributed to hyperleukocytosis among AML patients [27, 30]. Similarly, the literature shows that the presence of hyperleukocytosis is a poor prognostic indicator in ALL [27]. Some have proposed that it is the high tumor burden associated with hyperleukocytosis that contributes to the worsened prognosis. However, others suggest that those leukemias that have a high WBC count may represent a distinct clinical entity with different underlying pathophysiology [27]. In addition, hyperleukocytosis can induce conditions such as disseminated intravascular coagulation (DIC), leukostasis, and tumor lysis syndrome, which subsequently lead to increased morbidity and mortality [27].

Leukostasis occurs when a high leukocyte level leads to vascular obstruction and subsequent tissue hypoxia [27]. It is characterized by multi-organ failure, coagulopathy, tumor lysis syndrome, and metabolic abnormalities [28]. Pathologically, it is the presence of intravascular accumulation of leukemic blasts obstructing the vascular lumen with or without the presence of fibrin [28]. There are two proposed underlying pathophysiological mechanisms. The first, rheological theory, is based on the idea that blood viscosity is based on both the deformability of cells and the volume of the cell fraction in the blood. Blasts are less deformable than mature WBCs. In addition, the high fractional percentage of leukocytes in these patients results in increased blood viscosity. The combination of these two factors results in microvascular occlusion and decreased flow. Myeloblasts are larger than lymphoblasts and lymphocytes, and, as a result, leukostasis is more often seen in AML than in ALL. The second proposed mechanism relates to the interaction between blast cells and the endothelium. Endothelial cells activated by blasts secrete cytokines TNF-α and IL1β, and specific adhesion receptors, including VCAM-1 and selectins, mediate the blast-endothelium interaction. The combination of these factors promotes blast cell recruitment [27, 28].

The central nervous system (CNS), lung, and renal vasculature are the most common sites for symptomatic leukostasis to occur. CNS symptoms are variable and range from headaches and dizziness to delirium and coma. Cranial imaging may reveal an intracranial hemorrhage. Respiratory symptoms include shortness of breath, tachypnea, and hypoxia. Patients may have rales on physical exam. Chest imaging often reveals bilateral interstitial or alveolar infiltrates. Patients may also develop renal tubular dysfunction and subsequent renal failure [26 - 28].

The symptoms associated with leukostasis are relatively non-specific. As a result, it is difficult to prove with a high degree of confidence, and there are no agreed-upon diagnostic criteria [27, 28]. In reality, leukostasis can only be proven at autopsy. However, Novotny *et al.*, developed a grading system to predict the likelihood of the presence of leukostasis. In this study, patients were assigned a grade of 0-3 (0-no leukostasis, 1-possible leukostasis, 2-probable leukostasis, 3-highly probably leukostasis) based on the severity of symptoms in several organ systems [27, 28, 31]. Subsequently, Piccirillo *et al.*, found that patients in the very high probability group had higher rates of early mortality [27, 32].

Leukostasis is considered a medical emergency and should be treated quickly and aggressively [27]. Given the severity of potential downstream complications of leukostasis, including the development of DIC and tumor lysis syndrome, physicians often begin aggressive treatment at the first sign of respiratory or CNS symptoms even in the absence of a definitive diagnosis [27].

Management of both hyperleukocytosis and leukostasis involves supportive care combined with leukoreduction. Supportive care includes hyper-hydration with the goal of hemodilution, decreasing viscosity and waste product concentration, and maintaining adequate renal blood flow and glomerular filtration rate(GFR). The rate of fluid administration is determined by the degree of leukocytosis, tumor burden, hemoglobin, and the presence of any respiratory or cardiac comorbidities [26 - 28]. In addition, other goals of supportive care are to prevent tumor lysis syndrome and the development of DIC. The prevention of tumor lysis syndrome is accomplished in part by correction of electrolyte abnormalities. In addition, the administration of allopurinol or rasburicase is recommended to decrease uric acid levels [26, 27]. The prevention of DIC primarily involves the treatment of the underlying cause with the infusion of platelets and plasma as necessary. Transfusions increase whole blood viscosity, which may worsen leukostasis. As a result, it is recommended that transfusions be avoided unless the patient has symptomatic anemia [28]. Induction chemotherapy is the other mainstay of treatment for hyperleukocytosis. Induction chemotherapy consists of cytarabine plus anthracycline, hydroxyurea, and steroids [26]. It is recommended that standard or high-dose chemotherapy be used, as low-dose chemotherapy has not been shown to be effective. In contrast, high-dose chemotherapy has been shown to produce rapid and sustained bone marrow remission [26, 33, 34]. Historically, cranial radiation was also considered in patients with neurological symptoms associated with hyperleukocytosis. However, there have been no randomized controlled trials proving the efficacy of this practice. In addition, Pui *et al* showed that with intensive and effective chemotherapy, cranial radiation can be omitted without negatively affecting overall survival in ALL patients [26, 35]. Leukapheresis is considered for patients who are not able to immediately undergo induction chemotherapy. Leukapheresis involves the removal of circulating blast cells and reinfusion of leukocyte-poor plasma using blood cell separators. One session of leukapheresis lowers the peripheral WBC count by 20-50%. However, routine use of leukapheresis is limited by potential complications, including symptomatic hypocalcemia, paresthesias, muscle cramps, loss of blood/platelets, and general risks associated with central venous catheter use [26, 28].

Hypercalcemia

Hypercalcemia is a well-known malignancy-related complication. It is seen in roughly 30% of cancer patients at some point during their disease course [36]. While it can be associated with any malignancy, it is most commonly seen in patients with non–small-cell lung cancer, breast cancer, multiple myeloma, squamous-cell cancers of the head and neck, urothelial carcinoma, or ovarian cancer [37, 38]. Malignancy-related hypercalcemia is typically associated with advanced stage cancers and portends a poor prognosis. Studies have shown a median survival ranging from 25 to 52 days after the onset of hypercalcemia [37, 39].

The clinical presentation of hypercalcemia is variable depending upon severity. Both the degree of hypercalcemia and the rapidity of onset determine the severity of symptoms. The primary organ systems where symptoms manifest include neurological, gastrointestinal (GI), cardiovascular (CV), and renal [38]. Neurologic symptoms range from fatigue to altered mental status and coma. GI symptoms include nausea and vomiting, constipation, peptic ulcer disease, and pancreatitis. CV symptoms include hypertension, malignant ventricular arrhythmias, shortened QT, and ST segment changes. Renal manifestations include acute kidney injury and nephrogenic diabetes insipidus [38].

Malignancy related hypercalcemia is classically divided into four subtypes based on the underlying pathophysiology [37, 38]. Humoral hypercalcemia occurs when tumor cells secrete parathyroid hormone-related protein (PTHrP) resulting in increased osteoclastic bone resorption and reabsorption of calcium at the renal tubules. This type of hypercalcemia is most frequently associated with breast cancer, urothelial cancer, and squamous cancers of the lungs and head/neck [37, 38]. Local osteolytic hypercalcemia is most often seen in patients with breast cancer or multiple myeloma. In this subtype, tumor cells within bony metastases release cytokines, which increase osteoclastic activity while also inhibiting osteoblastic activity. Osteolytic hypercalcemia results when the amount of calcium released from bone exceeds renal clearance [37, 38]. 1,25-dihydroxyvitamin D–mediated hypercalcemia results from tumor upregulation of Cyp27B1, which encodes 1-alpha-hydroxylase. Subsequently, this causes increased conversion of 25-hydroxyvitamin D to 1,25-dihydroxyvitamin D. Excess 1,25-dihydroxyvitamin D then results in increased intestinal calcium absorption and bone resorption leading to hypercalcemia [36, 37]. The final subcategory of hypercalcemia results from ectopic hyperparathyroidism. This subtype is extremely rare and results from tumor cells which produce parathyroid hormone (PTH). Malignancies that have been implicated include small cell lung cancer, squamous cell carcinoma, ovarian cancer, thymoma, papillary thyroid cancer, bladder cancer, rhabdomyosarcoma, pancreatic cancer, and lymphoma [40]. While malignancy associated hypercalcemia has historically been subdivided into these four classes, newer data suggests that the underlying pathophysiology is likely more complex [36, 37].

Diagnosis of hypercalcemia of malignancy involves both confirming hypercalcemia and identifying the underlying pathophysiology. Serum calcium values represent the total of both protein bound and ionized calcium. Alterations in serum protein affect total calcium levels but may not affect physiologically active ionized calcium levels. Corrected calcium levels can be calculated or ionized calcium levels can be obtained to further guide management strategies. Once hypercalcemia has been confirmed, the next step is to check PTH and PTHrP levels. If PTHrP levels are low, the next step is to send 1,25-dihydroxyvitamin D levels [37, 38].

Management of hypercalcemia of malignancy is guided by the degree of hypercalcemia, the rate of increase in calcium levels, and the presence or absence of neurologic manifestations. Situations where urgent intervention is indicated include a corrected calcium greater than 13 mg/dL, a rate of rise more than 1mg/dL in 24 hours, or the presence of altered mental status. The three goals of treatment include correction of volume depletion, inhibition of bone resorption, and treatment of the underlying malignancy [37].

The initial step in management of hypercalcemia is aggressive rehydration. The rate and duration of fluid administration is guided by the severity of dehydration, degree of hypercalcemia, and the patient's comorbidities. The fluid of choice is a normal saline bolus of 1-2 liters followed by a continuous infusion of 200-500mL/hr. Loop diuretics, such as furosemide, may be used in conjunction with normal saline to further promote calciuresis. However, they should only be used after rehydration has been achieved [37, 38, 41].

Since excess bone resorption is the most common underlying etiology of hypercalcemia of malignancy, antiresorptive agents are a mainstay of treatment. The most used classes are bisphosphonates, denosumab, and calcitonin. Bisphosphonates, namely pamidronate, zoledronate, and ibandronate inhibit osteoclast activity by inducing cell death [37]. Studies have shown that that administration of bisphosphonates results in temporary normalization of calcium levels in 60-90% of patients after 4-7 days [37, 42]. Zoledronate is the bisphosphonate of choice as studies have shown that it is superior to pamidronate in successfully treating hypercalcemia(37). Denosumab is a monoclonal antibody that binds to the receptor activator of nuclear factor-κB ligand (RANKL) blocking it. This leads to decreased bone resorption by inhibiting osteoclast formation and activity [37, 43]. Henry *et al* conducted a randomized controlled trial comparing the efficacy of denosumab to zoledronic acid in delaying or preventing skeletal related events in patients with bone metastases or multiple myeloma. They found that denosumab was non inferior with a trend toward superior to zoledronic acid [43]. An additional study by Hu *et al.* showed that use of denosumab reduced calcium levels below 11.5mg/dL 80% of the time in patients with bisphosphonate resistant hypercalcemia [44]. Calcitonin, which is secreted by the parafollicular cells of the thyroid gland works by inhibiting both osteoclast activity and renal calcium reabsorption. While calcitonin is rapid-acting, its longevity is limited by the development of tachyphylaxis within 48 hours of administration [37, 45].

Additional therapeutic adjuncts include glucocorticoids and hemodialysis. Glucocorticoids are the preferred treatment for 1,25-dihydroxyvitamin D–mediated hypercalcemia. They work to lower calcium by both decreasing vitamin D 1α-hydroxylase activity and inhibiting osteoclast activity by decreasing tumor production of local cytokines [45]. Glucocorticoids can also be used in conjunction with other therapies. For example, patients who have elevated levels of both PTHrP and 1,25-dihydroxyvitamin D are often somewhat resistant to bisphosphonate therapy and may benefit from co-administration of glucocorticoids. Finally, hemodialysis with a low-calcium dialysate has been shown to effectively reduce calcium levels. However, its use is limited to those patients who need a rapid reduction in calcium levels [37, 45].

Coagulopathy

There is a well-known link between malignancy and coagulopathies. In fact, laboratory evidence of coagulation abnormalities can be seen in up to 95% of patients with metastatic cancer [46]. Thrombosis may even be the initial presentation of a previously undiagnosed malignancy [47]. However, the exact underlying pathophysiologic mechanisms are incompletely understood. The phenotype of malignancy-associated coagulopathy is a hypercoagulable and hypofibrinolytic state [48]. Nand *et al.*, classified coagulopathies seen in cancer patients into 4 categories based upon underlying pathophysiology: 1) increased platelet aggregation and activation, 2) abnormal coagulation cascade activation, 3) release of plasminogen activator, and 4) decreased hepatic synthesis of anticoagulant proteins [46]. Tissue factor (TF) and other procoagulant molecules may be expressed by cancer cells, leading to activation of the coagulation cascade. Some cancers, such as mucinous adenocarcinoma, work to induce platelet aggregation and development of platelet microthrombi *via* interaction with P and L selectins [49]. In addition, many tumor cells express fibrinolytic proteins, such as urokinase-type plasminogen activator (uPA) and tissue plasminogen activator (tPA). Finally, the vascular endothelium plays a large role in the development of coagulation abnormalities in cancer patients *via* several mechanisms. Endothelial cells synthesize, store, and release Von Willebrand Factor, tPA, and uPA, and may also express TF and thrombomodulin on their surface. Therefore, endothelial cell damage can result in dysregulation of the coagulation process in multiple ways. This is of particular interest for cancer patients undergoing chemotherapy, which may lead to vascular endothelial damage [49].

The clinical presentation of malignancy-induced coagulopathy is highly variable, ranging from subclinical laboratory abnormalities to venous thromboembolism (VTE) and disseminated intravascular coagulation (DIC). Coagulation derangements can be divided into thrombotic and hemorrhagic types. Thrombotic complications are more common and have higher morbidity and mortality [50].

Thrombotic complications can include deep vein thrombosis (DVT)/pulmonary embolism (PE), arterial thrombosis, thrombotic endocarditis, veno-occlusive disease, and thrombotic microangiopathy (TMA). The risk of development of VTE is 4-7 times higher in cancer patients than in the general population [51]. Arterial thromboembolism (ATE) is more commonly seen in patients with gastric, lung, pancreatic, and myeloproliferative malignancies. Clinically, patients present most commonly with signs of stroke, myocardial infarction, or peripheral arterial occlusion. Veno-occlusive disease is characterized by microvascular occlusion within the intrahepatic venules. Mortality is high in patients with severe disease. Thrombotic endocarditis is seen in 0.9-1.3% of cancer patients and is most common in patients with myeloproliferative malignancies. These patients develop valve vegetations from fibrin and platelet deposits, which are then at risk for embolization. Finally, TMA is characterized by hemolytic anemia, thrombocytopenia, and evidence of schistocytes on peripheral blood smear. Patients develop microvascular occlusion leading to organ dysfunction. Chemotherapy drugs are the most common cause of TMA. Implicated agents include: mitomycin-C, gemcitabine, bortezomib, carfilzomib, sunitinib, and vascular endothelial growth factor inhibitors. However, TMA may also be caused by certain malignancies, including gastric, breast, pancreatic, prostate, and lung cancer, in the absence of chemotherapy. Treatment of TMA is mainly supportive therapy, and the prognosis is generally poor [50, 52].

Cancer patients are also at increased risk of hemorrhagic complications. Patients may develop thrombocytopenia, DIC, or acquired Von Willebrand's disease, among other complications. Thrombocytopenia is most often caused by chemotherapy drugs. In one study by Wu *et al*, the reported overall prevalence of chemotherapy-associated thrombocytopenia was 21% [50, 53]. Carboplatin therapies are the most frequently implicated [54]. DIC is characterized by both hemorrhage and thrombosis secondary to abnormal activation of the clotting cascade, resulting in clot formation and consumptive coagulopathy. The reported incidence of DIC in cancer patients is 7-10% in patients with solid tumors and 15-20% in patients with hematologic malignancies. In contrast to DIC seen with sepsis and trauma, malignancy-associated DIC has a more insidious onset and protracted course. Some patients may even develop subclinical DIC. DIC-associated bleeding complications are more commonly seen in hematological malignancies and particularly promyelocytic leukemia. These patients can develop life-threatening intracerebral or pulmonary hemorrhage. In contrast, thrombotic complications are more commonly seen with solid tumors [49, 50]. Treatment of DIC consists primarily of treating the underlying etiology and supportive care. Data has shown that DIC will resolve if the underlying malignancy is adequately treated. Patients with clinically apparent thrombosis are treated with anticoagulation. Heparin has been shown to partially negate the abnormal clotting activation seen in DIC [50]. Acquired Von Willebrand's disease is most commonly seen in patients with hematologic malignancies. Plasma cell dyscrasias and lymphoproliferative disorders are most often implicated. Malignant cells may express autoantibodies or adsorb von Willebrand factor (vWF) to their surface, resulting in lower circulating plasma levels. Management involves treatment of the underlying malignancy as well as other adjuvant therapies. Desmopressin can increase plasma levels of vWF and Plasma-derived vWF replacements can also be given. Antifibrinolytics may also be given to control bleeding [50, 55].

Pericardial Disease and Tamponade

Malignant pericardial disease can manifest as pericarditis, pericardial effusion, cardiac tamponade, or pericardial constriction. The reported prevalence of malignancy-associated pericardial effusion ranges from 5-20% in the literature. Patients with lung cancer, breast cancer, lymphoma, and leukemia are the most likely to develop malignant pericardial effusions. Much less commonly, patients may have primary cardiac malignancies. Effusions may be related to the malignancy itself or to an underlying inflammatory process [56 - 58]. Neoplastic invasion of the pericardium can occur from either direct invasion of localized tumor cells or *via* lymphatic or hematogenous spread. Patients may also develop pericardial effusions secondary to radiation toxicity, chemotherapeutic toxicity, or opportunistic infections. Patients receiving mediastinal radiation can go on to develop constrictive pericarditis. In addition, the chemotherapeutic drugs anthracycline and cyclophosphamide are associated with a dose-dependent risk of both pericarditis and myocarditis. In both cases, the underlying pathophysiology involves the generation of reactive oxygen species, which activate neutrophils and predispose the patient to pericardial inflammation. Finally, in the setting of immunosuppression, cancer [59] patients are at increased risk for opportunistic infections, including cytomegalovirus, candida, and aspergillus, which can cause infectious pericarditis [56, 57]. Transthoracic echocardiography is the best imaging modality for the identification of a pericardial effusion and assessment of hemodynamic effects [56, 57]. Other imaging modalities such as chest radiography (CXR), computed tomography (CT), and magnetic resonance imaging (MRI) may also be used to evaluate pericardial effusions. Cytologic evaluation is the gold standard for the diagnosis of malignant pericardial effusion [57].

Presenting symptoms vary depending on the size of the effusion, the rapidity of accumulation, and the presence or absence of tamponade physiology. Cardiac tamponade and pericardial constriction are considered oncologic emergencies and must be addressed expeditiously due to the risk of hemodynamic collapse.

Cardiac tamponade occurs when pressure from a pericardial effusion impedes ventricular filling, resulting in diastolic collapse and decreased cardiac output. Symptoms associated with tamponade can include chest pain, shortness of breath, and syncope. The classic presentation is described by Beck's triad, which involves hypotension, tachycardia, and muffled heart tones. Patients may have pulsus paradoxus, which is a decrease of systolic blood pressure of at least 10 mm Hg with inspiration, as well as jugular venous distension. While echocardiography can provide evidence of tamponade, right heart catheterization is the gold standard for definitive diagnosis. Treatment of cardiac tamponade involves immediate pericardial drainage with pericardiocentesis. Even in the absence of tamponade, urgent drainage is recommended for large malignant pericardial effusions. However, definitive therapy requires treatment of the underlying malignancy. Management of these patients is often complicated by effusion recurrence. As such, management guidelines recommend the treatment of malignant pericardial disease with systemic cancer therapies, pericardiocentesis, and extended pericardial drainage. To address the risk of recurrence, adjunct therapies including the installation of pericardial sclerosing agents, balloon pericardiotomy, and pericardial window have been proposed [57]. In a systematic review by Virk *et al.*, rates of recurrence were lower with pericardiocentesis plus adjunctive therapies compared to pericardiocentesis alone. The pericardial window had the lowest recurrence rate at 7% [57, 60].

Pericardial constriction occurs when pericardial scarring due to inflammation restricts the elasticity of the pericardial sac, leading to impaired ventricular filling. Three pericardial constriction syndromes have been described. Patients may have transient constriction, effusive-constrictive pericarditis with concomitant effusion, and chronic constrictive pericarditis. Patients may present with symptoms such as fatigue or shortness of breath. Similar to tamponade, patients may present with hypotension, tachycardia, and jugular venous distension. They may also have a pericardial friction rub on exam. An electrocardiogram may show diffuse ST-segment elevations. Echocardiography reveals a thickened pericardium, and an early diastolic mitral annular velocity value ≥8 cm/second is both sensitive and specific for constrictive pericarditis. The treatment of constrictive pericarditis is pericardiectomy. However, perioperative mortality is cited as 11%. Non-steroidal anti-inflammatory drugs can be considered in patients with transient constrictive disease. Anakinra is also considered in patients with recurrent or refractory disease [56, 59].

Treatment Related Indications

Tumor Lysis Syndrome

Tumor lysis syndrome (TLS) is a life-threatening oncologic condition characterized by massive cellular lysis resulting in the release of cellular contents and cytokines into the blood. Intracellular products released include nucleic acids, phosphates, and potassium. Nucleic acids are subsequently metabolized to xanthine and then to uric acid. The massive release of these cellular components can overwhelm the body's normal homeostatic mechanisms, leading to severe metabolic derangements. TLS is considered an oncological emergency. The classic metabolic derangements seen are hyperuricemia, hyperphosphatemia, hyperkalemia, and hypocalcemia. Such metabolic disturbances contribute to the development of acute kidney injury (AKI), thus further impairing metabolite clearance. Proposed mechanisms of AKI include calcium phosphate deposition, uric acid crystal deposition in the renal tubules, and a systemic inflammatory response [61, 62]. Tumor lysis syndrome is most often seen in patients with hematologic malignancies after the initiation of cytotoxic therapy. However, it can also occur spontaneously prior to initiation of therapy. It may also be seen in other types of malignancies with a high proliferative rate, large tumor burden, or high sensitivity to cytotoxic chemotherapy [63 - 65]. The prognosis of TLS greatly depends on the severity of the illness. The development of acute renal failure is an independent risk factor for worsening morbidity and mortality [66].

TLS can be subdivided into laboratory TLS, where patients are clinically asymptomatic, and clinical TLS. The Cairo-Bishop diagnostic criteria for laboratory TLS requires the presence of a 25% change in at least two biochemical variables (uric acid, calcium, phosphorus, potassium) within 3 days prior to 7 days after the start of chemotherapy, despite adequate hydration and use of uric acid-lowering agents. Clinical TLS requires the presence of at least one clinical feature defined as kidney injury, arrhythmia, or seizure, which is not attributable to a chemotherapy drug. Clinical TLS can then be graded 0-5 based on severity [63, 65].

Much of the management of TLS centers around preventive strategies. A delay in diagnosis and treatment initiation can be life-threatening. As such, it is important to identify patients who are at high risk and maintain a high index of clinical suspicion. Risk factors can be subdivided into those related to the tumor type, disease-specific characteristics, and patient-related factors [67]. Cairo *et al.*, proposed a risk stratification system that stratifies malignancies into high, intermediate, and low risk groups for the development of TLS. High-risk malignancies include Burkitt lymphomas, acute B cell lymphoblastic leukemia, ALL with leukocyte count greater than 100,000, and ALL with leukocyte count greater than 50,000. Intermediate risk malignancies include diffuse large B-cell lymphoma, ALL with leukocyte count 50,000-100,000, AML with leukocyte count 10,000-50,000, CLL with leukocyte count 10,000-100,000, and any other malignancies with rapid cellular proliferation. Low-risk malignancies include Non-Hodgkin's lymphoma and other malignancies with a low proliferation rate [62, 65, 67, 68]. Guidelines for management of low-risk patients recommend intravenous hydration to ensure maintenance of adequate urine output from 48 hours prior to 72 hours after the start of chemotherapy. Goal urine output should be at least 100cc/hr. Patients considered intermediate or high risk are recommended for ICU admission prior to chemotherapy initiation for close laboratory and clinical monitoring. Some papers recommend laboratory monitoring as frequently as every 4-6 hours [65, 69]. It is recommended that these patients receive hyperhydration as well as anti-hyperuricemia prophylaxis. Allopurinol is the recommended initial anti-hyperuricemic medication for intermediate risk patients without hyperuricemia and should be started at least 12 hours prior to the start of chemotherapy. In addition, rasburicase is recommended for all patients who develop TLS-associated hyperuricemia as well as for prophylaxis in high-risk patients, and is continued for at least 72 hours. Clinical trials have shown that rasburicase is superior to allopurinol at controlling uric acid levels in high risk patients. Loop diuretics may also be used to maintain adequate urine output but only in patients with adequate volume repletion [65, 67]. In some cases, renal replacement therapy may also be required. Additional tenets of TLS management focus on the prevention and treatment of acute kidney injury (AKI) and treatment of other metabolic derangements, including hyperphosphatemia, hypocalcemia, and hyperkalemia. Early renal replacement therapy is favored for the treatment of oliguric AKI. Hyperphosphatemia may be treated with phosphate binders, adequate volume resuscitation, and maintenance of adequate urine output. Hyperkalemia may be treated with shifting agents or with removal agents such as lokelma. However, in the setting of oliguric AKI, renal replacement therapy may be necessary for treatment of both hyperkalemia and hyperphosphatemia. Symptomatic hypocalcemia should also be treated [67].

Cytokine Release Syndrome/ Immune Effector Cell-Associated Neurotoxicity Syndrome

Advances in cancer research have led to the development of more targeted therapies such as tyrosine kinase inhibitors, monoclonal antibodies, immune checkpoint inhibitors, and immune effector cell therapy. Each novel therapy has associated toxicities that clinicians must be aware of. Of particular interest for intensivists are those associated with immune effector cell therapies, as many of those patients end up requiring ICU admission [70].

Immune effector cell therapies include chimeric antigen receptors (CARs) and T-cell receptors (TCRs). CAR T-cells are autologous T-cells that are genetically modified to express an antibody that recognizes a specific tumor antigen, resulting in tumor lysis. CAR T-cell therapy has been shown to induce remission in up to 50% of patients with refractory ALL, large B-cell lymphoma, mantle cell lymphoma, and multiple myeloma [71]. However, toxicities associated with CAR T-cell therapy, which are due to an exaggerated inflammatory response, can be associated with significant morbidity [70, 71]. Cytokine release syndrome (CRS) and Immune effector cell-associated neurotoxicity syndrome (ICANS) are two well-known CAR T-cell associated toxicities that are reversible but may have high associated morbidity. Up to 47% of these patients require ICU admission [71].

CRS is the most common CAR T-cell-associated toxicity with reported incidences ranging from 60-94%. The incidence increases with a higher tumor burden as well as higher dosing. Symptoms of CRS usually appear within 7-14 days of the initiation of CAR T-cell therapy. Classic symptoms of CRS include fever, hypotension, and hypoxemia. Symptoms may progress to shock and multi-organ failure. Patients may develop symptoms of cardiac toxicity, including arrhythmia, hypotension, shock, and decreased ejection fraction. Patients may also develop hypoxic respiratory failure, which can progress to acute respiratory distress syndrome. This occurs secondary to capillary leak leading to non-cardiogenic pulmonary edema [70, 71]. Renal failure, hepatic toxicity, DIC, and skin lesions have also been reported [70].

Consensus grading for CRS has been developed based on the severity of illness. Patients with grade 1 CRS have a fever but no evidence of hypotension or hypoxia. These patients can typically be safely managed on the floor with supportive therapy. Grade 2 CRS is characterized by fever, mild hypotension without the need for pressors, and the need for low-level oxygen support. Grade 3 patients require pressors and increasing oxygen support. Finally, grade 4 patients require multiple pressors and positive pressure ventilation. Patients with grade 2 CRS may not immediately need ICU support, but should be monitored closely for deterioration. Patients with grade 3 or 4 CRS should be admitted to the ICU. The mainstay of treatment for patients with grade 2 CRS is anti-IL6 monoclonal antibody therapy with tocilizumab or siltuximab for a maximum of 3 doses. Patients with grade 3 or 4 CRS receive steroids in addition to either tocilizumab or siltuximab. Once these patients have improvement in symptoms to grade 2 or less for 24-48 hours, the steroids can be tapered off [70]. Supportive care for specific organ failure is also employed. A survey by Gutierrez *et al.*, found that interventions for hemodynamic support were similar among institutions surveyed, with some differences noted. While norepinephrine was always the first pressor used, there was variability in the second pressor preference. In addition, the choice of fluid used for resuscitation and the mechanisms for assessment of volume responsiveness varied between institutions. Ventilatory support practices also varied between institutions. While most institutions reported offering a trial of BIPAP for hypoxic respiratory failure, trial duration varied greatly [71].

ICANS refers to neurologic toxicity associated with CAR T-cell therapy. ICANS can be seen in 70-80% of patients receiving CAR T-cell therapy, with 30-40% of cases being severe [70]. The appearance of ICANS is often biphasic in association with CRS. It first appears concurrently with the CRS and then recurs after CRS resolution. However, it may also occur independently of CRS [72]. Risk factors for the development of ICANS include high tumor burden, high CAR T-cell dose, severe CRS, and pre-existing neurologic disease [72]. The presentation is variable and can range from tremors, headaches, and confusion to status epilepticus, global aphasia, paresis, cerebral edema, and coma [70, 72]. The underlying pathophysiology is thought to be multifactorial, with contributions from immune activation, blood-brain barrier disruption, and endothelial dysfunction leading to central nervous system inflammation. The grading of ICANS is divided into 4 grades by the ASTCT consensus criteria based on the severity of illness as determined by the Associated Encephalopathy (ICE) assessment tool score, level of consciousness, motor symptoms, seizures, and signs of elevated intracranial pressure (ICP) [70, 73]. ICANS grade 3 or 4 occurs in 12-30% of cases. It typically occurs 3-5 days after CAR T-cell infusion, but a small percentage of patients develop delayed ICANS. Recommendations for the work-up of ICANS include CT or MRI, electroencephalogram (EEG), and lumbar puncture (LP) to rule out other potential underlying causes. MRI findings may include flair abnormalities in the pons, thalamus, and white matter tracts. LP findings are often non-specific and may include pleocytosis with lymphocytic predominance and elevated protein [72]. Given the severity of symptoms and potential for rapid progression, patients with grade 3 or 4 ICANS are typically admitted to the ICU.

Treatment strategies focus on symptom management. Anti-epileptic drugs are often prescribed prophylactically. However, the ideal dose and duration of therapy are not well defined. Hypertonic saline and mannitol are utilized for the treatment of increased intracranial pressure. Steroids have been shown to improve symptoms of neurotoxicity. Dexamethasone is preferentially utilized for ICANS grades 1-3. High-dose methylprednisolone is typically reserved for grade 4 ICANS. However, steroids can potentially decrease the efficacy of CAR T-cells. Therefore, short steroid courses are preferred [74].

Non-oncologic Acute Illness Indications

The most common reasons for non-oncologic admission to the ICU include acute respiratory failure and hypotension. Additional reasons include sepsis, acute kidney injury, and post-operative care [12].

Acute Respiratory Failure

Acute respiratory failure is the most common reason for unplanned ICU admission in cancer patients and may be infectious or non-infectious in nature. These patients may have in-hospital mortality rates as high as 65% [18]. Patients who require mechanical ventilation have a reported ICU mortality higher than 40% [12].

Acute respiratory failure is more often seen in patients with ALL, AML, patients undergoing hematopoietic stem cell transplants, neutropenic patients, and patients with lung cancer. Acute respiratory failure in cancer patients is most often due to ventilation-perfusion mismatch from either infiltrates, pneumonia, pulmonary embolism, or atelectasis. Other underlying causes include: pulmonary shunting secondary to acute respiratory distress syndrome (ARDS), drug-induced interstitial lung disease, hypoventilation, or diffusion abnormalities secondary to lung metastases [18]. In 15-20% of cases, there may be more than one underlying cause.

Cancer patients are at risk for both community-acquired and opportunistic pathogens, with bacterial infections being the most common [75]. Among patients with bacterial pneumonia, Schnell *et al.*, found that community-acquired pathogens accounted for 25% of cases, with Streptococcus pneumonia being the most frequently isolated [76]. Seasonal respiratory viruses are also commonly found in cancer patients with acute respiratory failure [77]. In terms of opportunistic infections, the type of immune defect determines which pathogens the immunocompromised patient is most at risk for. For example, neutropenic patients are at higher risk for infection with staphylococcus, gram-negative, or fungal pathogens. Aspergillus is the most common fungal pathogen identified. In contrast, patients with defective cellular immunity are at increased risk for intracellular bacteria, such as Nocardia, as well as mycobacterium infections. These patients are also at risk for fungal pneumocystis infections and viral infections, such as cytomegalovirus [75, 77].

The differential diagnosis of non-infectious causes of acute respiratory failure is broad and includes aspiration pneumonia or pneumonitis, pulmonary embolism, cardiogenic pulmonary edema, noncardiogenic pulmonary edema, progression of malignancy, and chemotherapy-related complications [18, 77]. Cancer patients are at risk for both ARDS and lung diseases, which mimic the clinical and radiographic features of ARDS. The hallmarks of ARDS are acute onset, bilateral fluffy infiltrates, hypoxemia, and non-cardiogenic pulmonary edema. Examples of lung diseases that can mimic ARDS include diffuse alveolar hemorrhage, acute interstitial pneumonia, organizing pneumonia, and acute hypersensitivity pneumonitis. Malignancy, chemotherapy, and bone marrow transplantation all can predispose patients to both ARDS and ARDS-mimics. Patients undergoing radiation therapy are at risk for acute or subacute radiation pneumonitis. The risk of developing radiation pneumonitis is mediated by factors such as co-existing lung disease, type of chemotherapy, and both location and dose of radiation received. Radiation pneumonitis may develop into fibrosis over time. In addition, certain chemotherapeutic agents have well-known pulmonary toxicities. Clinical features vary depending on the offending agent but can range from organizing pneumonia to diffuse alveolar hemorrhage. Pulmonary drug toxicity is a diagnosis of exclusion, but should be considered in patients on cytotoxic chemotherapy who develop signs of respiratory failure and have new opacities on imaging [78]. Finally, cancer patients are at risk for the development of both transfusion-associated lung injury (TRALI) and transfusion-associated circulatory overload (TACO). The risk of TRALI in cancer patients arises from the need for frequent blood transfusions. In contrast, the risk of TACO is typically associated with underlying cardiac dysfunction, rapid volume administration, and positive fluid balance [75, 77].

Some causes of acute respiratory failure are specific to the hematopoietic stem cell transplant recipient population. Idiopathic pneumonia syndrome is characterized by diffuse infiltrates, hypoxia, and symptoms of pneumonia appearing weeks to months after stem cell transplant. To prove the diagnosis, infection must be ruled out by a bronchoalveolar lavage sample or biopsy. Peri-engraftment respiratory distress syndrome is characterized by the presence of fever, rash, hypoxia, and non-cardiogenic pulmonary edema during the neutrophil recovery phase. These patients often require mechanical ventilation. Finally, patients undergoing stem cell transplants are at risk for the development of diffuse alveolar hemorrhage (DAH). DAH is diagnosed by either BAL with increasingly bloody return or the presence of greater than 20% hemosiderin-filled macrophages [77].

The approach to diagnosis of the underlying etiology of acute respiratory failure in the cancer population should be methodical and streamlined. Some sources recommend following the DIRECT method outlined by Azoulay *et al* [79]. This strategy considers the duration and type of symptoms, immunosuppression characteristics, radiographic appearance on X-ray, clinical picture, and findings on high-resolution CT scan. Various invasive and non-invasive diagnostic tools may be employed, including serum and/or sputum studies and cultures, as well as possibly bronchoscopy with bronchoalveolar lavage to narrow the differential further. However, risks and benefits discussions are key prior to pursuing more invasive testing.

The management approach to acute respiratory failure in the oncology patient involves rapid diagnosis and initiation of appropriate therapies directed towards the underlying etiology. Given their complexity and unique issues, these patients should be cared for by a multidisciplinary team. Such multi-disciplinary approaches have been shown to improve outcomes in cancer patients [77, 80]. Overall, the goal of ICU admission is supportive care targeted towards the underlying etiology to prevent worsening respiratory failure. Studies have been mixed regarding the effectiveness of early introduction of non-invasive ventilation (NIV) strategies in immunocompromised patients. Early studies suggested a benefit but were limited in their generalizability [81, 82]. A newer trial by Lemiale *et al.*, showed no difference between NIV and regular oxygen therapy [83]. In addition, it has been shown that failure of NIV is associated with increased mortality. Historically, oncology patients requiring mechanical ventilation have worse outcomes. While overall outcomes in these patients have improved, there is still a subset of patients requiring mechanical ventilation who have a high associated mortality. As a result, these patients require special considerations of the severity of illness and risks of establishing an airway, including the potential for a difficult airway. Lung protective ventilation strategies should be employed, including tidal volumes of 4-8mL/kg based on ideal body weight and maintaining plateau pressures less than 30 cm H_20 [75, 77].

Neutropenic Fever and Neutropenic Sepsis

Neutropenia is a common finding among cancer patients. Neutropenia can further be stratified by severity, with absolute neutrophil count (ANC) less than 1500/mm3 being mild, less than 1000/mm3 being moderate, and less than 500/mm3 being severe [84]. Neutropenia may be secondary to the malignancy itself or a treatment-related effect. Risk factors for the development of neutropenia in cancer patients include advanced age, significant medical comorbidities, and a history of use of multiple cytotoxic chemotherapy agents [84]. Bone marrow infiltration by solid tumor cancers can result in neutropenia. Lymphoproliferative malignancies such as hairy cell leukemia, CLL, and natural killer cell lymphomas can also cause neutropenia [84]. In addition, some patients with hematologic malignancies may have normal absolute neutrophil counts but have neutrophilic dysfunction producing a qualitative neutropenia [85]. Patients receiving radiation therapy to areas with active bone marrow proliferation can also develop neutropenia. However, most cancer-related neutropenia is secondary to cytotoxic chemotherapy. The severity and duration of neutropenia vary depending on the type of chemotherapy. Chemotherapy for hematologic malignancies has been associated with longer durations of neutropenia compared to chemotherapy agents for solid tumor malignancies. Not surprisingly, the longer the duration of neutropenia, the higher the risk of infection. As a result, patients with hematologic malignancies and those who undergo hematopoietic stem cell transplants develop neutropenia-related infections more frequently [85].

Patients with isolated neutropenia may not have any associated symptoms. In some cases, fever may be the first sign. Neutropenic fever is defined as a single temperature greater than 38.3 °C or sustained temperature greater than 38.0 °C for more than an hour in the setting of an ANC less than 1500/mm3. Febrile neutropenia is considered an oncologic emergency as these patients are at high risk for increased mortality. In-hospital mortality for patients with neutropenic fever is approximately 10%. As a result, prompt recognition and initiation of broad-spectrum antibiotics is imperative [85, 86]. Antibiotics should be initiated within 1 hour of the onset of symptoms to decrease the risk of mortality. However, there is some data to suggest that even a delay of antibiotics beyond 30 minutes from presentation can result in increased mortality [86, 87]. While neutropenic patients may have non-infectious causes of fever, fevers are presumed to be infectious until proven otherwise. Risk stratification of patients is necessary to help predict which patients may benefit from a higher level of care and/or prophylactic antibiotic therapy. The Multinational Association of Supportive Care of Cancer (MASCC) risk score assesses 8 factors to help determine patients' risk of developing complications from neutropenic fever. The lower the score, the higher the risk of developing complications. A score of greater than 21 indicates a low risk. Negative prognostic indicators include age>60, hypotension, dehydration, prior fungal infection, moderate symptoms, and hospital admission [84].

Neutropenic patients are at risk for infections from bacterial, viral, and fungal pathogens. Common viral pathogens include respiratory viruses and herpes viruses. Bacterial infections can arise from many different sources, including gut translocation, pneumonias, skin and soft tissue infections, oral mucosal translocation, and urinary tract infections. Up to 25% of patients may have bacteremia with gram-positive organisms, including Staphylococci, Enterococci, and Streptococci being the most frequently isolated [84, 86]. Historically, Gram-negative infections with pathogens such as *E. coli*, klebsiella, and Pseudomonas were more common. Gram-negative infections confer an increased risk of mortality. Fungal infections are more commonly seen in patients with prolonged duration of neutropenia or profound neutropenia. Common sources for fungal infections include gut translocation, pneumonia, and central line catheters. Fungal pathogens most frequently implicated include Candida and Aspergillus [84, 86].

The true incidence of neutropenic sepsis is unknown, but it is estimated that approximately 50% of patients with neutropenic fever will develop neutropenic sepsis. While there is no consensus definition of neutropenic sepsis, it is recommended that any evidence of organ dysfunction in the presence of neutropenia should be considered sepsis until proven otherwise. Of the patients who develop neutropenic sepsis, it is estimated that 10% go on to develop severe septic shock. This is particularly common among hematopoietic stem cell patients during the engraftment period [86].

Preventive and prophylactic measures have been established to try to prevent complications in neutropenic patients. The approach to the prevention of infections in neutropenic patients involves decreasing the risk of acquisition of exogenous pathogens and suppression of potential pathogens already present. Neutropenic precautions employed may depend on the degree of neutropenia. Evidence-based practices, including strict adherence to good hand hygiene for health care providers and visitors and avoiding exposure to visitors and staff who are ill, are applicable to all neutropenic patients. For patients with prolonged or profound neutropenia, avoidance of exposure to live plants and animals is also recommended [88]. Historically, the use of flow reversal rooms, isolation, and adherence to a low microbial diet have also been recommended; however, newer data suggest that these interventions may not change infection rates [88 - 90]. The American Society of Clinical Oncology, in conjunction with the Infectious Diseases Society of America, has provided guidelines for the use of antimicrobial prophylaxis in immunosuppressed cancer patients. They recommend that the risk of febrile neutropenia be assessed systematically, considering patient, malignancy, and treatment-related factors. Those patients deemed to be high risk, including patients with profound or prolonged neutropenia, should be treated with prophylactic antibacterial and antifungal therapy. The recommended antibacterial prophylaxis is a fluoroquinolone. The addition of trimethoprim-sulfamethoxazole is recommended for patients undergoing chemotherapy regimens associated with greater than a 3.5% risk for Pneumocystis jirovecci (PCP) pneumonia. The recommended antifungal prophylaxis is either an oral triazole or an IV echinocandin. Herpes simplex virus-positive patients undergoing hematopoietic stem cell transplantation or leukemia patients undergoing induction therapy are recommended for antiviral prophylaxis with a nucleoside analog such as acyclovir. Finally, for patients at high risk for hepatitis B virus reactivation, prophylaxis with a nucleoside reverse transcriptase inhibitor, such as entecavir, is recommended [91]. An additional preventative measure is prophylactic administration of a granulocyte colony-stimulating factor (G-CSF), such as filgrastim. Studies have demonstrated that prophylactic administration in high-risk patients may reduce the risk of febrile neutropenia and early death [92].

CONCLUSION

With improving survival rates among cancer patients, more oncology patients are being admitted to the ICU at some point during their disease course. Both malignancy and patient-related factors should be considered when determining the appropriateness of an ICU admission. Patients may be admitted to the ICU for a host of reasons, ranging from malignancy-related issues, treatment-related issues, and acute non-oncologic illnesses. Regardless of the reason for ICU admission, these complex patients require a thoughtful and methodical management approach involving a multidisciplinary team to maximize patient outcomes.

REFERENCES

[1] Koutsoukou A. Admission of critically ill patients with cancer to the ICU: many uncertainties remain. ESMO Open 2017; 2(4): e000105.
[http://dx.doi.org/10.1136/esmoopen-2016-000105] [PMID: 29259818]

[2] Schapira DV, Studnicki J, Bradham DD, Wolff P, Jarrett A. Intensive care, survival, and expense of treating critically ill cancer patients. JAMA 1993; 269(6): 783-6.
[http://dx.doi.org/10.1001/jama.1993.03500060083036] [PMID: 8423662]

[3] Azoulay É, Afessa B. The intensive care support of patients with malignancy: do everything that can be done. Intensive Care Med 2006; 32(1): 3-5.
[http://dx.doi.org/10.1007/s00134-005-2835-6] [PMID: 16308682]

[4] Kostakou E, Rovina N, Kyriakopoulou M, Koulouris NG, Koutsoukou A. Critically ill cancer patient in intensive care unit: Issues that arise. J Crit Care 2014; 29(5): 817-22.
[http://dx.doi.org/10.1016/j.jcrc.2014.04.007] [PMID: 24857640]

[5] Azoulay E, Soares M, Darmon M, Benoit D, Pastores S, Afessa B. Intensive care of the cancer patient: recent achievements and remaining challenges. Ann Intensive Care 2011; 1(1): 5.
[http://dx.doi.org/10.1186/2110-5820-1-5] [PMID: 21906331]

[6] Schellongowski P, Sperr WR, Wohlfarth P, *et al.* Critically ill patients with cancer: chances and limitations of intensive care medicine—a narrative review. ESMO Open 2016; 1(5): e000018.
[http://dx.doi.org/10.1136/esmoopen-2015-000018] [PMID: 27843637]

[7] Soares M, Fontes F, Dantas J, *et al.* Performance of six severity-of-illness scores in cancer patients requiring admission to the intensive care unit: a prospective observational study. Crit Care 2004; 8(4): R194-203.
[http://dx.doi.org/10.1186/cc2870] [PMID: 15312218]

[8] Schellongowski P, Benesch M, Lang T, *et al.* Comparison of three severity scores for critically ill cancer patients. Intensive Care Med 2004; 30(3): 430-6. [http://dx.doi.org/10.1007/s00134-003-2043-1] [PMID: 14598029]

[9] Sculier JP, Paesmans M, Markiewicz E, Berghmans T. Scoring systems in cancer patients admitted for an acute complication in a medical intensive care unit. Crit Care Med 2000; 28(8): 2786-92. [http://dx.doi.org/10.1097/00003246-200008000-00018] [PMID: 10966251]

[10] Staudinger T, Stoiser B, Müllner M, *et al.* Outcome and prognostic factors in critically ill cancer patients admitted to the intensive care unit. Crit Care Med 2000; 28(5): 1322-8. [http://dx.doi.org/10.1097/00003246-200005000-00011] [PMID: 10834673]

[11] Kress JP, Christenson J, Pohlman AS, Linkin DR, Hall JB. Outcomes of critically ill cancer patients in a university hospital setting. Am J Respir Crit Care Med 1999; 160(6): 1957-61. [http://dx.doi.org/10.1164/ajrccm.160.6.9812055] [PMID: 10588613]

[12] Biskup E, Cai F, Vetter M, Marsch S. Oncological patients in the intensive care unit: prognosis, decision-making, therapies and end-of-life care. Swiss medical weekly. 2017; 147(3132): w14481-w. [http://dx.doi.org/10.4414/smw.2017.14481]

[13] Pastores SM, Voigt LP. Acute respiratory failure in the patient with cancer: diagnostic and management strategies. Crit Care Clin 2010; 26(1): 21-40. [http://dx.doi.org/10.1016/j.ccc.2009.10.001] [PMID: 19944274]

[14] Massion PB, Dive AM, Doyen C, *et al.* Prognosis of hematologic malignancies does not predict intensive care unit mortality. Crit Care Med 2002; 30(10): 2260-70. [http://dx.doi.org/10.1097/00003246-200210000-00014] [PMID: 12394954]

[15] Thiéry G, Azoulay É, Darmon M, *et al.* Outcome of cancer patients considered for intensive care unit admission: a hospital-wide prospective study. J Clin Oncol 2005; 23(19): 4406-13. [http://dx.doi.org/10.1200/JCO.2005.01.487] [PMID: 15994150]

[16] Lecuyer L, Chevret S, Thiery G, Darmon M, Schlemmer B, Azoulay É. The ICU Trial: A new admission policy for cancer patients requiring mechanical ventilation. Crit Care Med 2007; 35(3): 808-14. [http://dx.doi.org/10.1097/01.CCM.0000256846.27192.7A] [PMID: 17235261]

[17] Azoulay E, Schellongowski P, Darmon M, *et al.* The Intensive Care Medicine research agenda on critically ill oncology and hematology patients. Intensive Care Med 2017; 43(9): 1366-82. [http://dx.doi.org/10.1007/s00134-017-4884-z] [PMID: 28725926]

[18] Martos-Benítez FD, Soler-Morejón CD, Lara-Ponce KX, *et al.* Critically ill patients with cancer: A clinical perspective. World J Clin Oncol 2020; 11(10): 809-35. [http://dx.doi.org/10.5306/wjco.v11.i10.809] [PMID: 33200075]

[19] Assi HI, Halim NA, Alameh I, *et al.* Outcomes of patients with malignancy admitted to the intensive care units: a prospective study. Crit Care Res Pract 2021; 2021(1): 4792309. [PMID: 34513091]

[20] Soares M, Caruso P, Silva E, *et al.* Characteristics and outcomes of patients with cancer requiring admission to intensive care units: A prospective multicenter study. Crit Care Med 2010; 38(1): 9-15. [http://dx.doi.org/10.1097/CCM.0b013e3181c0349e] [PMID: 19829101]

[21] Morin S, Grateau A, Reuter D, *et al.* Management of superior vena cava syndrome in critically ill cancer patients. Support Care Cancer 2018; 26(2): 521-8. [http://dx.doi.org/10.1007/s00520-017-3860-z] [PMID: 28836006]

[22] Patriarcheas V, Grammoustianou M, Ptohis N, *et al.* Malignant superior vena cava syndrome: state of the art. Cureus 2022; 14(1): e20924. [http://dx.doi.org/10.7759/cureus.20924] [PMID: 35004083]

[23] Sandill S, Krishna B, Kohli S, Jaiswal B. SVC Syndrome in ICU: The Need of a Multidisciplinary

Approach. Archives of Anesthesia and Critical Care 2022; 8(3): 260-2.
[http://dx.doi.org/10.18502/aacc.v8i3.9622]

[24] Yu JB, Wilson LD, Detterbeck FC. Superior vena cava syndrome--a proposed classification system and algorithm for management. J Thorac Oncol 2008; 3(8): 811-4.
[http://dx.doi.org/10.1097/JTO.0b013e3181804791] [PMID: 18670297]

[25] Wilson LD, Detterbeck FC, Yahalom J. Clinical practice. Superior vena cava syndrome with malignant causes. N Engl J Med 2007; 356(18): 1862-9.
[http://dx.doi.org/10.1056/NEJMcp067190] [PMID: 17476012]

[26] Ruggiero A, Rizzo D, Amato M, Riccardi R. Management of Hyperleukocytosis. Curr Treat Options Oncol 2016; 17(2): 7.
[http://dx.doi.org/10.1007/s11864-015-0387-8] [PMID: 26820286]

[27] Ganzel C, Becker J, Mintz PD, Lazarus HM, Rowe JM. Hyperleukocytosis, leukostasis and leukapheresis: Practice management. Blood Rev 2012; 26(3): 117-22.
[http://dx.doi.org/10.1016/j.blre.2012.01.003] [PMID: 22364832]

[28] Giammarco S, Chiusolo P, Piccirillo N, *et al.* Hyperleukocytosis and leukostasis: management of a medical emergency. Expert Rev Hematol 2017; 10(2): 147-54.
[http://dx.doi.org/10.1080/17474086.2017.1270754] [PMID: 27967252]

[29] Dutcher JP, Schiffer CA, Wiernik PH. Hyperleukocytosis in adult acute nonlymphocytic leukemia: impact on remission rate and duration, and survival. J Clin Oncol 1987; 5(9): 1364-72.
[http://dx.doi.org/10.1200/JCO.1987.5.9.1364] [PMID: 3625254]

[30] Greenwood MJ, Seftel MD, Richardson C, *et al.* Leukocyte count as a predictor of death during remission induction in acute myeloid leukemia. Leuk Lymphoma 2006; 47(7): 1245-52.
[http://dx.doi.org/10.1080/10428190600572673] [PMID: 16923553]

[31] Novotny JR, Müller-Beißenhirtz H, Herget-Rosenthal S, Kribben A, Dührsen U. Grading of symptoms in hyperleukocytic leukaemia: a clinical model for the role of different blast types and promyelocytes in the development of leukostasis syndrome. Eur J Haematol 2005; 74(6): 501-10.
[http://dx.doi.org/10.1111/j.1600-0609.2005.00421.x] [PMID: 15876254]

[32] Piccirillo N, Laurenti L, Chiusolo P, *et al.* Reliability of leukostasis grading score to identify patients with high□risk hyperleukocytosis. Am J Hematol 2009; 84(6): 381-2.
[http://dx.doi.org/10.1002/ajh.21418] [PMID: 19391131]

[33] Cuvelier GDE, Vitali AM, Ford JC, Dix DB. Multiple intracranial tumors in Philadelphia chromosome positive acute lymphoblastic leukemia: Successful treatment following aggressive supportive care, early cranial radiation, high dose chemotherapy and imatinib. Pediatr Blood Cancer 2008; 51(1): 135-7.
[http://dx.doi.org/10.1002/pbc.21562] [PMID: 18383153]

[34] Oberoi S, Lehrnbecher T, Phillips B, *et al.* Leukapheresis and low-dose chemotherapy do not reduce early mortality in acute myeloid leukemia hyperleukocytosis: A systematic review and meta-analysis. Leuk Res 2014; 38(4): 460-8.
[http://dx.doi.org/10.1016/j.leukres.2014.01.004] [PMID: 24472688]

[35] Pui CH, Campana D, Pei D, *et al.* Treating childhood acute lymphoblastic leukemia without cranial irradiation. N Engl J Med 2009; 360(26): 2730-41.
[http://dx.doi.org/10.1056/NEJMoa0900386] [PMID: 19553647]

[36] Chukir T, Liu Y, Hoffman K, Bilezikian JP, Farooki A. Calcitriol elevation is associated with a higher risk of refractory hypercalcemia of malignancy in solid tumors. J Clin Endocrinol Metab 2020; 105(4): e1115-23.
[http://dx.doi.org/10.1210/clinem/dgz278] [PMID: 31841590]

[37] Guise TA, Wysolmerski JJ. Cancer-Associated Hypercalcemia. N Engl J Med 2022; 386(15): 1443-51.
[http://dx.doi.org/10.1056/NEJMcp2113128] [PMID: 35417639]

[38] Mirrakhimov A. Hypercalcemia of malignancy: An update on pathogenesis and management. N Am J Med Sci 2015; 7(11): 483-93.
[http://dx.doi.org/10.4103/1947-2714.170600] [PMID: 26713296]

[39] Donovan PJ, Achong N, Griffin K, Galligan J, Pretorius CJ, McLeod DSA. PTHrP-mediated hypercalcemia: causes and survival in 138 patients. J Clin Endocrinol Metab 2015; 100(5): 2024-9.
[http://dx.doi.org/10.1210/jc.2014-4250] [PMID: 25719931]

[40] Neves A, Mendonça I, Cunha Marques JA, Costa J, Almeida JS. Malignant Hypercalcemia Induced by the Ectopic Production of Intact Parathyroid Hormone (PTH). Cureus 2023; 15(2): e34770.
[http://dx.doi.org/10.7759/cureus.34770] [PMID: 36909108]

[41] Khoury N, Carmichael KA. Evaluation and therapy of hypercalcemia. Mo Med 2011; 108(2): 99-103.
[PMID: 21568230]

[42] Thomas S, Chung S-H. Management of hypercalcemia of malignancy. Integr Cancer Sci Ther 2016; 3(1): 358.

[43] Henry DH, Costa L, Goldwasser F, *et al.* Randomized, double-blind study of denosumab versus zoledronic acid in the treatment of bone metastases in patients with advanced cancer (excluding breast and prostate cancer) or multiple myeloma. J Clin Oncol 2011; 29(9): 1125-32.
[http://dx.doi.org/10.1200/JCO.2010.31.3304] [PMID: 21343556]

[44] Hu MI, Glezerman IG, Leboulleux S, *et al.* Denosumab for treatment of hypercalcemia of malignancy. J Clin Endocrinol Metab 2014; 99(9): 3144-52.
[http://dx.doi.org/10.1210/jc.2014-1001] [PMID: 24915117]

[45] Clines GA. Mechanisms and treatment of hypercalcemia of malignancy. Curr Opin Endocrinol Diabetes Obes 2011; 18(6): 339-46.
[http://dx.doi.org/10.1097/MED.0b013e32834b4401] [PMID: 21897221]

[46] Nand S, Messmore H. Hemostasis in malignancy. Am J Hematol 1990; 35(1): 45-55.
[http://dx.doi.org/10.1002/ajh.2830350111] [PMID: 2202206]

[47] Miller SP, Sanchez-Avalos J, Stefanski T, Zuckerman L. Coagulation disorders in cancer.I. Clinical and laboratory studies. Cancer 1967; 20(9): 1452-65.
[http://dx.doi.org/10.1002/1097-0142(196709)20:9<1452::AID-CNCR2820200912>3.0.CO;2-T] [PMID: 6038391]

[48] Walsh M, Moore EE, Moore H, Thomas S, Vande Lune S, Zimmer D, Eds. Use of viscoelastography in malignancy-associated coagulopathy and thrombosis: a review Seminars in thrombosis and hemostasis. Thieme Medical Publishers 2019.
[http://dx.doi.org/10.1055/s-0039-1688497]

[49] Levi M. Cancer-related coagulopathies. Thromb Res 2014; 133 (Suppl. 2): S70-5.
[http://dx.doi.org/10.1016/S0049-3848(14)50012-6] [PMID: 24862149]

[50] Deshpande SP, Henderson RA Jr, Ajith AU, Zimrin AB, Williams B. Cancer-Related Coagulopathy and Perioperative Considerations. Anesth Analg 2025; 140(4): 860-72.
[http://dx.doi.org/10.1213/ANE.0000000000007286] [PMID: 39630596]

[51] Halsema K, Mcmahon B. Cancer-Associated Thrombosis: Risk Assessment, Prevention, and Treatment. J Adv Pract Oncol 2023; 14(3): 213-7.
[http://dx.doi.org/10.6004/jadpro.2023.14.3.6] [PMID: 37197728]

[52] Falanga A, Marchetti M. Cancer-associated thrombosis: enhanced awareness and pathophysiologic complexity. J Thromb Haemost 2023; 21(6): 1397-408.
[http://dx.doi.org/10.1016/j.jtha.2023.02.029] [PMID: 36931602]

[53] Wu Y, Aravind S, Ranganathan G, Martin A, Nalysnyk L. Anemia and thrombocytopenia in patients undergoing chemotherapy for solid tumors: A descriptive study of a large outpatient oncology practice database, 2000–2007. Clin Ther 2009; 31(Pt 2): 2416-32.

[http://dx.doi.org/10.1016/j.clinthera.2009.11.020] [PMID: 20110050]

[54] ten Berg MJ, van den Bemt PMLA, Shantakumar S, *et al.* Thrombocytopenia in adult cancer patients receiving cytotoxic chemotherapy: results from a retrospective hospital-based cohort study. Drug Saf 2011; 34(12): 1151-60.
[http://dx.doi.org/10.2165/11594310-000000000-00000] [PMID: 22077503]

[55] Franchini M, Mannucci PM. Acquired von Willebrand syndrome: focused for hematologists. Haematologica 2020; 105(8): 2032-7.
[http://dx.doi.org/10.3324/haematol.2020.255117] [PMID: 32554559]

[56] Refaat MM, Katz WE. Neoplastic pericardial effusion. Clin Cardiol 2011; 34(10): 593-8.
[http://dx.doi.org/10.1002/clc.20936] [PMID: 21928406]

[57] Mudra SE, Rayes D, Kumar AK, *et al.* Malignant Pericardial Effusion: A Systematic Review "Malignant Pericardial Effusion: A Review". CJC open. 2024.

[58] Çelik S, Lestuzzi C, Cervesato E, *et al.* Systemic chemotherapy in combination with pericardial window has better outcomes in malignant pericardial effusions. J Thorac Cardiovasc Surg 2014; 148(5): 2288-93.
[http://dx.doi.org/10.1016/j.jtcvs.2014.04.031] [PMID: 24836991]

[59] Lorenzo-Esteller L, Ramos-Polo R, Pons Riverola A, *et al.* Pericardial Disease in Patients with Cancer: Clinical Insights on Diagnosis and Treatment. Cancers (Basel) 2024; 16(20): 3466.
[http://dx.doi.org/10.3390/cancers16203466] [PMID: 39456560]

[60] Virk SA, Chandrakumar D, Villanueva C, Wolfenden H, Liou K, Cao C. Systematic review of percutaneous interventions for malignant pericardial effusion. Heart 2015; 101(20): 1619-26.
[http://dx.doi.org/10.1136/heartjnl-2015-307907] [PMID: 26180077]

[61] Zafrani L, Canet E, Darmon M. Understanding tumor lysis syndrome. Intensive Care Med 2019; 45(11): 1608-11.
[http://dx.doi.org/10.1007/s00134-019-05768-x] [PMID: 31520104]

[62] Russell TB, Kram DE. Tumor lysis syndrome. Pediatr Rev 2020; 41(1): 20-6.
[http://dx.doi.org/10.1542/pir.2018-0243] [PMID: 31894070]

[63] Mirrakhimov AE, Voore P, Khan M, Ali AM. Tumor lysis syndrome: A clinical review. World J Crit Care Med 2015; 4(2): 130-8.
[http://dx.doi.org/10.5492/wjccm.v4.i2.130] [PMID: 25938028]

[64] Abdel-Nabey M, Chaba A, Serre J, *et al.* Tumor lysis syndrome, acute kidney injury and disease-free survival in critically ill patients requiring urgent chemotherapy. Ann Intensive Care 2022; 12(1): 15.
[http://dx.doi.org/10.1186/s13613-022-00990-1] [PMID: 35166948]

[65] Burghi G, Berrutti D, Manzanares W. [Tumor lysis syndrome in intensive therapy: diagnostic and therapeutic encare]. Med Intensiva 2011; 35(3): 170-8.
[http://dx.doi.org/10.1016/j.medin.2010.07.014] [PMID: 21112673]

[66] Howard SC, Pui C-H, Ribeiro RC. Tumor lysis syndrome. Renal Disease in Cancer Patients 2014; pp. 39-64.

[67] Mughal TI, Ejaz AA, Foringer JR, Coiffier B. An integrated clinical approach for the identification, prevention, and treatment of tumor lysis syndrome. Cancer Treat Rev 2010; 36(2): 164-76.
[http://dx.doi.org/10.1016/j.ctrv.2009.11.001] [PMID: 20031331]

[68] Cairo MS, Coiffier B, Reiter A, Younes A, Panel TE. Recommendations for the evaluation of risk and prophylaxis of tumour lysis syndrome (TLS) in adults and children with malignant diseases: an expert TLS panel consensus. Br J Haematol 2010; 149(4): 578-86.
[http://dx.doi.org/10.1111/j.1365-2141.2010.08143.x] [PMID: 20331465]

[69] Hochberg J, Cairo MS. Tumor lysis syndrome: current perspective. Haematologica 2008; 93(1): 9-13.
[http://dx.doi.org/10.3324/haematol.12327] [PMID: 18166779]

[70] Gutierrez C, McEvoy C, Munshi L, *et al.* Critical care management of toxicities associated with targeted agents and immunotherapies for cancer. Crit Care Med 2020; 48(1): 10-21. [http://dx.doi.org/10.1097/CCM.0000000000004087] [PMID: 31725440]

[71] Gutierrez C, Brown ART, Herr MM, *et al.* The chimeric antigen receptor-intensive care unit (CAR-ICU) initiative: Surveying intensive care unit practices in the management of CAR T-cell associated toxicities. J Crit Care 2020; 58: 58-64. [http://dx.doi.org/10.1016/j.jcrc.2020.04.008] [PMID: 32361219]

[72] Ong SY, Baird JH. A Primer on Chimeric Antigen Receptor T-cell Therapy-related Toxicities for the Intensivist. J Intensive Care Med 2024; 39(10): 929-38. [http://dx.doi.org/10.1177/08850666231205264] [PMID: 37899577]

[73] Bellal M, Malherbe J, Damaj G, Du Cheyron D. Toxicities, intensive care management, and outcome of chimeric antigen receptor T cells in adults: an update. Crit Care 2024; 28(1): 69. [http://dx.doi.org/10.1186/s13054-024-04851-0] [PMID: 38444031]

[74] Rice J, Nagle S, Randall J, Hinson HE. Chimeric antigen receptor T cell-related neurotoxicity: mechanisms, clinical presentation, and approach to treatment. Curr Treat Options Neurol 2019; 21: 1-14.

[75] Ferreyro BL, Munshi L. Acute respiratory failure in the oncologic patient: New Era, new issues. Annual Update in Intensive Care and Emergency Medicine 2019; 2019: 31-45. [http://dx.doi.org/10.1007/978-3-030-06067-1_3]

[76] Schnell D, Mayaux J, Lambert J, *et al.* Clinical assessment for identifying causes of acute respiratory failure in cancer patients. Eur Respir J 2013; 42(2): 435-43. [http://dx.doi.org/10.1183/09031936.00122512] [PMID: 23143549]

[77] Sears SP, Carr G, Bime C. Acute and chronic respiratory failure in cancer patients. Oncologic Critical Care 2020; pp. 445-75. [http://dx.doi.org/10.1007/978-3-319-74588-6_43]

[78] Roig J, Domingo C, Gea E. Pulmonary toxicity caused by cytotoxic drugs. Clin Pulm Med 2006; 13(1): 53-62. [http://dx.doi.org/10.1097/01.cpm.0000197361.07900.51]

[79] Azoulay É, Schlemmer B. Diagnostic strategy in cancer patients with acute respiratory failure. Intensive Care Med 2006; 32(6): 808-22. [http://dx.doi.org/10.1007/s00134-006-0129-2] [PMID: 16715324]

[80] Prin M, Wunsch H. International comparisons of intensive care. Curr Opin Crit Care 2012; 18(6): 700-6. [http://dx.doi.org/10.1097/MCC.0b013e32835914d5] [PMID: 22954664]

[81] Hilbert G, Gruson D, Vargas F, *et al.* Noninvasive ventilation in immunosuppressed patients with pulmonary infiltrates, fever, and acute respiratory failure. N Engl J Med 2001; 344(7): 481-7. [http://dx.doi.org/10.1056/NEJM200102153440703] [PMID: 11172189]

[82] Antonelli M, Conti G, Bufi M, *et al.* Noninvasive ventilation for treatment of acute respiratory failure in patients undergoing solid organ transplantation: a randomized trial. JAMA 2000; 283(2): 235-41. [http://dx.doi.org/10.1001/jama.283.2.235] [PMID: 10634340]

[83] Lemiale V, Mokart D, Resche-Rigon M, *et al.* Effect of noninvasive ventilation vs oxygen therapy on mortality among immunocompromised patients with acute respiratory failure: a randomized clinical trial. JAMA 2015; 314(16): 1711-9. [http://dx.doi.org/10.1001/jama.2015.12402] [PMID: 26444879]

[84] Lustberg MB. Management of neutropenia in cancer patients. Clin Adv Hematol Oncol 2012; 10(12): 825-6. [PMID: 23271355]

[85] Nesher L, Rolston KVI. The current spectrum of infection in cancer patients with chemotherapy related neutropenia. Infection 2014; 42(1): 5-13.
[http://dx.doi.org/10.1007/s15010-013-0525-9] [PMID: 23975584]

[86] Stephens RS. Neutropenic fever in the intensive care unit. Oncologic Critical Care 2020; pp. 1297-311.
[http://dx.doi.org/10.1007/978-3-319-74588-6_118]

[87] Rosa RG, Goldani LZ. Cohort study of the impact of time to antibiotic administration on mortality in patients with febrile neutropenia. Antimicrob Agents Chemother 2014; 58(7): 3799-803.
[http://dx.doi.org/10.1128/AAC.02561-14] [PMID: 24752269]

[88] Vioral AN, Wentley D. Managing oncology neutropenia and sepsis in the intensive care unit. Crit Care Nurs Q 2015; 38(2): 165-74.
[http://dx.doi.org/10.1097/CNQ.0000000000000058] [PMID: 25741957]

[89] Van Dalen EC, Leclercq E, Mulder RL, Davies M, Kersten MJ, van de Wetering MD. Low bacterial diet versus control diet to prevent infection in cancer patients treated with chemotherapy causing episodes of neutropenia. Cochrane Database of Systematic Reviews. 2016(4).
[http://dx.doi.org/10.1002/14651858.CD006247.pub3]

[90] Zitella LJ, Friese CR, Hauser J, *et al.* Putting evidence into practice: prevention of infection. Clin J Oncol Nurs 2006; 10(6): 739-50.
[http://dx.doi.org/10.1188/06.CJON.739-750] [PMID: 17193941]

[91] Taplitz RA, Kennedy EB, Bow EJ, *et al.* Antimicrobial prophylaxis for adult patients with cancer-related immunosuppression: ASCO and IDSA clinical practice guideline update. J Clin Oncol 2018; 36(30): 3043-54.
[http://dx.doi.org/10.1200/JCO.18.00374] [PMID: 30179565]

[92] Kuderer NM, Dale DC, Crawford J, Lyman GH. Impact of primary prophylaxis with granulocyte colony-stimulating factor on febrile neutropenia and mortality in adult cancer patients receiving chemotherapy: a systematic review. J Clin Oncol 2007; 25(21): 3158-67.
[http://dx.doi.org/10.1200/JCO.2006.08.8823] [PMID: 17634496]

CHAPTER 12

Anesthetic Management of Major Cancer Related Surgical Procedures, Part 1: Thoracic and Neurological Procedures

William Marion[1,*], **Amber Williams**[1] and **Colleen Naglee**[1]

[1] *Department of Anesthesiology, Cooper Medical School of Rowan University, Cooper University Health Care, Camden, NJ, USA*

Abstract: In this chapter, we will look at the anesthetic considerations and techniques that facilitate the safe and successful operative care of thoracic and neurologic tumors. Modality and drug choice will be discussed in both the context of hemodynamic stability and tumor effects. Additionally, airway management, vascular access, and invasive monitoring may change based on tumor type and location, along with patient presentation. The goal of this chapter is to provide the non-fellowship-trained anesthesiologist with a basic understanding of how to safely care for patients undergoing care that they may not commonly provide.

Keywords: Activated clotting time, Bronchial blocker, Double lumen endotracheal tube, One lung ventilation, Pulse pressure variation, Retrograde autologous priming, Sarcoma, Transesophageal echocardiography.

INTRODUCTION

Providing care for patients with thoracic tumors is a complex and challenging aspect of anesthesia practice. The tumors can broadly be categorized by anatomical location as follows:

1. Lung Tumors
2. Mediastinal Tumors
3. Pleural Tumors
4. Chest Wall Tumors
5. Tracheobronchial Tumors
6. Esophageal Tumors
7. Cardiac Tumors

* **Corresponding author William Marion:** Department of Anesthesiology, Cooper Medical School of Rowan University, Cooper University Health Care, Camden, NJ, USA; ;lE-mail: marion-william@cooperhealth.edu

Bharathi Gourkanti, Irwin Gratz, William Marion, Rajiv Lingaraju & Grace Abramian (Eds.)

Anesthetic approaches and specialized techniques depend on the variety and location of the tumor, along with its impacts on respiratory and cardiovascular function, to ensure patient safety and optimize surgical outcomes. This section will provide an overview of the principles, practices, and considerations involved in the anesthetic management of patients undergoing surgical treatment of thoracic tumors.

PREOPERATIVE ASSESSMENT

Medical History

Having a firm understanding of the patient's medical history is essential for formulating an effective and safe anesthetic plan. Patients with thoracic tumors often have significant comorbidities such as chronic obstructive pulmonary disease (COPD), cardiovascular diseases, a history of smoking, significant alcohol use, antiplatelet therapy, *etc*. All of which can significantly affect anesthetic management.

Physical Examination

A comprehensive physical examination should focus on the respiratory and cardiovascular systems. Evaluation of airway patency, lung function tests, and assessment of exercise tolerance are essential components. Additionally, uncontrolled hypertension (specifically a diastolic blood pressure of 110 mmHg or higher) on the day of surgery may merit postponing the procedure as this can lead to poor outcomes, including but not limited to uncontrollable intra- or postoperative bleeding, increased thirty-day mortality, cerebrovascular accidents (CVA), and myocardial infarction (MI).

Diagnostic Tests

Preoperative diagnostic tests such as chest X-rays, CT scans, MRI, and PET scans provide information on tumor location, size, and potential metastasis. Pulmonary function tests, arterial blood gases, and echocardiograms offer insights into the patient's baseline respiratory and cardiac status. However, basic blood work such as complete blood counts (CBC) and comprehensive metabolic panels may be even more valuable for intraoperative anesthetic management as they may reveal electrolyte and metabolic disturbances related to various cancer syndromes. These disturbances can lead to hemodynamic instability that is refractory to treatment other than correcting the disturbance itself.

ANESTHETIC PLAN

Choice of Anesthetic Technique

The choice between general anesthesia, regional anesthesia, or a combination of both depends on the tumor's location, the surgical procedure, and the patient's overall health status. General anesthesia is typically required for thoracic surgeries, while regional techniques, such as epidural or paravertebral blocks can provide effective analgesia. Although regional techniques may be contraindicated if the patient is unable to hold antiplatelet therapy or if heparinization is necessary for the procedure.

Airway Management

Airway management poses significant challenges in thoracic surgery due to potential airway obstruction by the tumor. Techniques such as double-lumen endotracheal tubes (DL ETT) or bronchial blockers are often employed to achieve lung isolation, which is crucial for surgical exposure and patient safety. However, standard endotracheal intubation is utilized when lung isolation is not required. Placement of a DL ETT starts with selecting an appropriate size based on the height and gender of the patient [1]. The choice of a right or left DL ETT must also be made, but the vast majority of cases can be managed with a left-sided DL ETT if there is no surgical involvement of the left main bronchus.

Patient Factors	DLT Size Recommendations
Height 54-65" 65-70" 71-76"	35-37 Fr 37-39 Fr 39-41 Fr
Age 8-10 yo 10-12 yo 12-13 yo 13-14 yo	~26 Fr ~28 Fr ~32 Fr ~35 Fr

n.b. 26 an 28 Fr DLT are only generally available as left-sided.

To place the DL ETT, direct laryngoscopy is best, and once the vocal cords are visualized, the DL ETT is initially advanced with the curvature to the patient's right side. As the tip passes the cords, the DL ETT is rotated 90 degrees counterclockwise as it is advanced, and the stylet is removed. It is also important to ensure the stylet is placed in the bronchial side, as it is generally longer than the tracheal side and can cause perforation. Once the DL ETT is in place, the tracheal cuff should be inflated, the Y-connector attached, the patient ventilated, and placement confirmed with the presence of EtCO2.

Next, precise placement is achieved *via* bronchoscopy [2]. First, the bronchoscope is passed through the tracheal side to identify the carina and tracheal rings to orient yourself to the patient's anterior and ensure the bronchial side is seated appropriately in the left main bronchus. A small ring of the bronchial cuff should be seen just to the left of the carina, and 2-3 ml of air should be added to the cuff while watching to prevent herniation. Once the DL ETT has been confirmed as deep enough to ensure lung isolation, the bronchoscope should be passed through the bronchial lumen and the left superior lobar bronchus visualized to ensure either ventilation or deflation of the entire left lung as needed.

n.b. A sudden drop in volume with a sharp, concurrent rise in peak pressure during ventilation of the tracheal lumen and isolation of the bronchial lumen indicates herniation of the bronchial balloon and occlusion of the distal trachea.

In patients who require video laryngoscopy or fiberoptic intubation, it may not be possible to place a DL ETT due to its shape and stiffness. In this case, endotracheal intubation with a standard ET tube and use of a bronchial blocker for the isolation of the operative lung may provide an acceptable alternative. Once the patient is intubated, the bronchial blocker is passed through the ET tube, and the curved tip is positioned in the main bronchus of the operative lung under bronchoscopy. The cuff is then inflated under visualization, ensuring that the operative bronchus is isolated without herniation above the carina or migration distally, which may occlude a lobar bronchus and prevent adequate deflation of the lung.

Ventilation Strategies

One-lung ventilation (OLV) is frequently required during thoracic surgery to provide a clear operative field. Anesthetic teams must be adept at managing OLV, adjusting ventilatory parameters to maintain oxygenation and prevent complications such as barotrauma or hypoxemia. Prior to incision, the patient should be placed on OLV to assess their tolerance of the strategy. However, some patients may initially tolerate OLV but have difficulty maintaining adequate oxygenation once surgical stress is introduced. In this case, the first step in management is to ask the surgeon to stop if possible. Next, ensure the FiO_2 is set to 1.0 and verify proper positioning of all airway devices to maximize the oxygen content of ventilated alveoli. If there is no improvement, the next steps should focus on optimizing ventilation of the nonoperative lung. This includes increasing Vt without causing excessive peak pressures, performing a gentle Valsalva maneuver to recruit alveoli, and adding PEEP to prevent atelectasis.

If hypoxia persists after these interventions, there are several techniques for managing the operative lung that may be attempted [3]. These include CPAP and passive oxygenation without ventilation by the anesthesiologist, followed by clamping the PA of the non-ventilated lung. However, caution is warranted in patients with right ventricular dysfunction, as increased afterload could precipitate ventricular failure. Finally, the operative lung can be ventilated if necessary after pausing the procedure. In this case, it may be necessary to continue two-lung ventilation with intermittent apneic pauses and stabilization of the operative lung by the surgeon.

Monitoring and Maintenance

Intraoperative monitoring should include standard measures such as ECG, pulse oximetry, capnography, and invasive arterial pressure monitoring. Advanced monitoring techniques, including esophageal Doppler and transesophageal echocardiography, can be valuable in complex cases to monitor cardiac output and fluid status. Additionally, the choice to place an arterial line depends on a confluence of patient, pathological, and procedural factors. First, all procedures that require cardiopulmonary bypass, such as intracardiac or aortic tumors, require arterial line placement. Next, tumors that do not fall into those categories but may result in significant blood loss, such as those in proximity to large vessels, necessitate placement. Additionally, patients with tumors that cause metabolic or hemodynamic derangements, thus requiring serial lab draws, should also have an arterial line placed. Finally, patients with significant cardiovascular disease, such as reduced ejection fraction, propensity for unstable arrhythmias, and coronary artery disease, should have an arterial line placed in order to rapidly detect and treat hemodynamic instability.

If there is concern for right ventricular failure or significant pulmonary hypertension, a pulmonary artery catheter (PAC) should be placed *via* central venous catheter (CVC). A CVC should also be placed if there is the possibility of cardiopulmonary bypass or if large volume resuscitation is expected. In patients who require a CVC but not a PAC, central venous pressure can still be monitored using a CVC lumen or *via* a single-lumen infusion catheter (SLIC) placed through the PAC introducer port.

INTRAOPERATIVE CONSIDERATIONS

Fluid Management

Precise fluid management is critical in thoracic surgery to avoid fluid overload and pulmonary edema. Balanced crystalloid solutions and colloids should be carefully titrated based on the patient's hemodynamic status and intraoperative blood loss. In patients with an arterial line, fluid resuscitation can be guided by the use of pulse pressure variation (PPV) monitoring. A PPV of 14 or higher suggests a fluid-responsive hemodynamic state. Attention should also be given to hemoglobin and blood loss. Significant drops or loss may necessitate the use of packed red cells (PRBC) or thawed fresh frozen plasma (FFP) rather than simple crystalloids or colloids.

Drug Administration

Selection and administration of anesthetic drugs must consider the potential impact on respiratory and cardiovascular functions. Agents such as volatile anesthetics, intravenous anesthetics, and neuromuscular blockers should be chosen based on their profile and suitability for the specific case. For example, patients who have difficulty tolerating one lung ventilation and become hypoxic may benefit from switching to total intravenous anesthesia (TIVA) as volatile gas blocks the phenomenon of hypoxic pulmonary vasoconstriction. This is a physiologic response that serves to maintain V:Q matching. In other words, the pulmonary vasculature will shunt circulation from non-ventilated to ventilated alveolar beds in response to falling oxygen concentration. Transitioning to maintenance with intravenous agents such as propofol and remifentanil may allow the non-ventilated lung to vasoconstrict, thereby increasing the amount of hemoglobin exposed to the fresh gas flow.

Induction drugs should be selected based on patient factors such as age, ejection fraction (EF), infection status, hemodynamics, and coronary artery disease (CAD). Generally, lidocaine and fentanyl are used in most cases, and midazolam may be added if appropriate, given the patient's age and mental status. In a hemodynamically stable patient without pulmonary hypertension, significant CAD, or ventricular failure, propofol is an acceptable hypnotic agent. If those conditions are present or if the patient is unstable, ketamine and etomidate are preferable options. However, those medications are not without their own considerations, as ketamine may not be appropriate for tachycardic or hypertensive patients, while etomidate should be avoided in patients with active infection or pre-existing adrenal insufficiency.

Pain Management

Effective pain management is vital to facilitate postoperative recovery and improve patient outcomes. Multimodal analgesia, including opioids, non-steroidal anti-inflammatory drugs (NSAIDs), and regional anesthesia techniques, is commonly employed. However, many of the patients undergoing thoracic procedures will bypass the PACU and go directly to the ICU, and post-op analgesia will be directed by the intensivist rather than the anesthesiologist.

ANATOMIC AND TUMOR-SPECIFIC CONSIDERATIONS

Tumors Requiring Lung Isolation

Certain tumors of the lung, pleura, mediastinum, airway, esophagus, or aorta may OLV to facilitate surgical exposure, provide the surgeon with a non-moving target or surgical field, protect the opposite lung, or provide selective ventilation if there is airway compromise. Generally, the procedures that require isolation are those addressing tumors within the lungs themselves or those where the normal ventilatory motions of the lungs would create an impedance to surgical resection. Following this guideline, tumors of the anterior mediastinum and small pleural or chest wall tumors often do not require special airway techniques. As previously stated, isolation is generally achieved through the use of a DL ETT, an endobronchial blocker or direct endobronchial intubation. This also tends to be the order of surgeon preference, as the DL ETT provides the best isolation, while endobronchial intubation is least effective and may not provide adequate decompression of the target lung.

Tumors Requiring Cardiopulmonary Bypass

Generally, any intracardiac tumor, tumors in the proximal aorta, and tumors within the pulmonary artery require cardiopulmonary bypass in order to prevent excessive blood loss, give the surgeon a clear field of view, and prevent ischemic events in both the myocardium and brain. Additionally, patients requiring bypass should also have transesophageal echocardiography by the anesthesiologist during the procedure, and are usually managed by trained cardiothoracic anesthesiologists. Although greater than 75% of intracardiac lesions are benign, they still generally require surgical resection. This is because they can cause inflow and outflow obstructions, impact valve function, and potentially cause embolic events, which can lead to stroke and MI in the case of left-sided lesions. Common benign lesions include the following [4 - 11]:

- <u>Myxoma</u>→ generally in the left atrium, often attached to the septum, high risk of embolic events
- <u>Fibroma</u>→ which tends to be ventricular and occurs in childhood; may be attached to the septum or free wall. If large enough and invades the myocardium, it may rarely require transplantation
- <u>Lipoma</u>→ rare fatty tumors, usually epicardial or endocardial, but infrequently transmural
- <u>Papillary Fibroelastoma</u>→ small tumors attached to valves, may be amenable to valve-sparing repairs if not excessively invasive

- Rhabdomyoma→ most common cardiac tumor in young children, may regress spontaneously, so surgery is reserved for symptomatic cases
- Hemangioma→ vascular tumor appearing in any chamber, resection should be pre-planned using imaging such as MRI or CTA
- Teratoma→ rare germ cell tumor containing multiple tissue types, may be within the heart, invading great vessels or attached to the pericardium

More concerning and less amenable to resection are malignant primary cardiac tumors. This minority of cardiac tumors (~10-25%) is often aggressive and invasive, leading to surgical interventions that are much more frequently palliative and not curative. These tumors are as follows:

- Angiosarcoma→ rapidly metastasizing and aggressive from endothelial cells, frequent local recurrence, most commonly in the RA attached to the atrial wall
- Undifferentiated Pleomorphic Sarcoma (UPS)→ rare and aggressive with frequent metastasis, from soft tissue progenitor cells but lacks any differentiation or morphological consistency, making classification difficult
- Rhabdomyosarcoma→ from embryonic mesenchymal cells, rare and aggressive, but the most common cardiac malignancy in infants, and can occur in any chamber
- Leiomyosarcoma→ rapidly growing and highly metastatic with poor prognosis; originates from smooth muscle cells and most commonly occurs in the left atrium.
- Fibrosarcoma→ high-grade malignancy from fibroblasts, often has non-specific symptoms that often delay diagnosis, and the median survival is only several months
- Osteosarcoma→ <10% of primary cardiac tumors, from osteoblasts, with irregular margins and density with spots of ossification, most commonly in LA, with rapid growth and poor prognosis
- Synovial Sarcoma→ rare and aggressive with poor prognosis, can originate in any chamber or pericardium, requires complete resection with chemotherapy and radiation
- Liposarcoma→ from adipose cells within the heart or pericardium, can be well-differentiated, dedifferentiated, myxoid, and pleomorphic, with a poor prognosis
- Primary cardiac lymphoma→ usually non-Hodgkin B-cell and in immunocompromised patients, rare but increasing
- Mesothelioma of the pericardium→ from mesothelial cells of the pericardium, aggressive and usually involves asbestos exposure

Although the discussion of specific surgical techniques is beyond the scope of this chapter, it is important to address anesthetic management during the initiation of and separation from bypass. Prior to arterial cannulation, the patient should be fully heparinized at a dose of 300-400 u/kg with a target activated clotting time (ACT) of at least 400 seconds [12]. Additionally, systolic blood pressure should be maintained at 90-100 mmHg during arterial cannulation. Once this is achieved and the cannula is secured, the perfusionist will initiate retrograde autologous priming (RAPping) of the bypass machine, requiring a preemptive increase in blood pressure to avoid instability loss associated with the decrease in volume. This will be repeated after venous cannulation, without the need to lower systolic blood pressure.

Once the resection is complete and separation from bypass approaches, TEE should be resumed to assess biventricular function, the presence of air in the left ventricle and integrity of the surgical site if possible. If biventricular function is decreased or poor at baseline, inotrope infusions with agents such as epinephrine or milrinone should be initiated. If the patient is hypertensive or has pulmonary hypertension, milrinone is the superior choice, while the hypotensive patient with poor ventricular function will likely derive more benefit from epinephrine. Once the venous cannula has been removed, the surgeon will ask to reverse heparinization with protamine at a 100:1 ratio. For example, a patient who received 30,000 units of heparin should be reversed with 300 mg of protamine over 5-10 minutes to an ACT within 10% of baseline [13].

Once this is achieved, the remaining blood volume should be transfused under TEE guidance to avoid ventricular dysfunction and distension. If the total volume can't be transfused, the remainder can be spun down as a cell saver and transfused through a fluid warmer. The surgeon will also remove the aortic cannula and repair the insertion site, which once again requires a systolic blood pressure of 90-100 mmHg to avoid aneurysm or dissection. Finally, the TEE should be checked once more after the chest is closed to ensure adequate function and identify any effusion that may be problematic. The patient can now be transported to the ICU with sedation, ventilatory support, and whatever pharmacological support is necessary to maintain hemodynamic stability.

POSTOPERATIVE CARE

Recovery and Extubation

Postoperative recovery involves careful monitoring of respiratory function and pain levels. Extubation criteria should include adequate oxygenation, stable hemodynamics, and sufficient pain control. Patients may require supplemental oxygen and respiratory support such as BiPAP to aid recovery. However, the settings must be carefully titrated in patients with surgical insults to the airways and lung parenchyma, as they are significantly more susceptible to barotrauma. It is also important to note that most facilities do not extubate patients in the OR after cardiopulmonary bypass but instead take them directly to the ICU to allow a more gradual recovery and thus a more hemodynamically stable recovery.

Postoperative Monitoring

Continuous postoperative monitoring in an intensive care unit (ICU) or high-dependency unit (HDU) is often necessary for complex thoracic surgery patients. Monitoring parameters should include respiratory rate, oxygen saturation, pain levels, and fluid balance.

Complications Management

Awareness and prompt management of potential complications such as respiratory distress, bleeding, infection, and cardiac events are essential. Early intervention can prevent severe outcomes and improve recovery rates. Additionally, early re-exploration may help prevent refractory decompensation. However, prompt intervention such as blood product administration or blood pressure control may obviate the need for a secondary surgical intervention.

Conclusion

Anesthetic care for thoracic tumors requires a comprehensive understanding of the unique challenges associated with thoracic surgery and the physiologic changes that a tumor may cause. Thorough preoperative assessment, meticulous intraoperative management, and vigilant postoperative care are fundamental to ensuring patient safety and achieving optimal surgical outcomes. Continued research and advancements in anesthetic techniques promise further to enhance the care of patients with thoracic tumors.

NEUROLOGICAL TUMOR SURGERY

General Overview

Spinal and brain tumor surgeries present unique challenges that require close collaboration between neurosurgeons and anesthesiologists to ensure optimal outcomes. These procedures, performed to address primary, metastatic, or locally invasive tumors, often involve extensive surgical resection aimed at alleviating pain, restoring spinal stability, and preserving or improving neurological function. However, these surgeries are inherently complex, often characterized by significant blood loss, prolonged operative times, and the challenges associated with prone positioning, which complicates anesthetic management [14].

Anesthetic management is pivotal in mitigating these risks, with primary goals including maintaining hemodynamic stability, optimizing neurophysiological monitoring conditions, ensuring effective pain control, and minimizing complications. Maintaining hemodynamic stability is crucial to preserving adequate perfusion while minimizing blood loss. Equally important is optimizing intraoperative neuromonitoring conditions to protect the functional integrity of the spinal cord and nerve roots. Effective pain management both intraoperatively and postoperatively enhances recovery, while addressing specific risks—such as intraoperative blindness, embolism, and neurological injury—is critical to reducing morbidity.

Tumors of the spine

In this section, we explore the key anesthetic considerations in spinal tumor surgeries, focusing on multimodal anesthesia, intraoperative blindness, blood loss management, monitoring considerations, and kyphoplasty.

Multimodal Anesthesia

Multimodal anesthesia (MMA) refers to the use of multiple medications and techniques that act on different pathways in the nervous system to achieve optimal pain control while minimizing side effects. It is essential in spine surgeries, such as tumor resections, which tend to be associated with significant pain and perioperative challenges. MMA for pain control has become favored as patients are less likely to have opioid consumption compared to using primarily IV opioid patient-controlled analgesia [15]. MMA generally involves optimizing non-opioid pharmacologic and non-pharmacologic interventions and reserving opioid use to treat breakthrough pain. Some of the components of multimodal analgesics include non-opioid analgesics, NMDA antagonists, regional anesthesia, and adjuncts.

Dexmedetomidine's unique sedative and analgesic properties make it valuable for enhancing patient comfort during procedures, particularly when combined with other analgesics for a more comprehensive multimodal approach. It can also aid in managing autonomic stability, thus supporting a smoother perioperative course [16]. Dexmedetomidine has opioid-sparing effects and is effective in reducing postoperative pain and nausea. It exerts its effects by reducing central sympathetic outflow, achieved through the blockade of alpha receptors in the brainstem, which in turn inhibits norepinephrine release. This stress-relieving effect contributes to enhanced recovery and better postoperative outcomes [17].

Gabapentin is an anticonvulsant medication that has gained widespread use for managing neuropathic pain. It works by binding to calcium channels in the central nervous system, modulating excitatory neurotransmitter release, and reducing neuronal excitability. Preoperative administration of gabapentinoids effectively reduces postoperative pain, lowers total morphine consumption, and minimizes morphine-related complications following spine surgery [18]. They also help reduce the incidence of nausea, vomiting, and pruritus without increasing sedation or dizziness. This opioid-sparing benefit underscores its utility in multimodal analgesia strategies [19]. Its opioid-sparing effects make it a valuable component in multimodal analgesia strategies, particularly in perioperative care.

Preoperative use of gabapentin in spinal surgery has been shown to significantly reduce postoperative opioid consumption and pain scores while also decreasing side effects such as vomiting and urinary retention, making it a valuable component in multimodal analgesia [20]. By contributing to a multimodal analgesic approach, gabapentin helps reduce reliance on opioids, promoting better pain management and overall postoperative outcomes. However, some concerns have been raised regarding oversedation and delirium, especially in the elderly [21].

NSAIDs (nonsteroidal anti-inflammatory drugs) are widely used to manage pain, inflammation, and fever. They work by inhibiting cyclooxygenase (COX) enzymes, particularly COX-1 and COX-2, and are involved in producing prostaglandins that mediate inflammation and pain. Although effective, its use can be associated with bleeding risks due to the antiplatelet effects of COX-1 inhibition. NSAIDs, particularly COX-2 selective inhibitors like celecoxib, offer significant opioid-sparing benefits in postoperative pain management. Despite concerns about bleeding risks, these drugs are generally safe at recommended doses and help reduce the reliance on opioids, promoting better recovery outcomes.

Acetaminophen, when combined with anti-inflammatory and neuropathic agents such as NSAIDs and gabapentinoids, offers the most significant opioid-sparing benefits, making it a cornerstone of effective multimodal analgesia strategies. Lidocaine is a local anesthetic used to provide perioperative analgesia. It is shown to reduce opioid consumption, lower postoperative pain scores, and potentially reduce hospital stays. Its opioid sparing effects and minimal adverse effects make it an effective adjunct in multimodal analgesia, especially for improving patient outcomes.

Intraoperative Blindness

Intraoperative blindness (IO) is a rare but severe complication that can result in partial or complete vision loss during or after surgery. It is most associated with procedures that involve significant blood loss, prolonged prone positioning, hypotension, or complex spine, cardiac, or cranial surgeries. Specifically, when related to anesthesia, intraoperative blindness is primarily associated with factors affecting ocular perfusion, oxygenation, and pressure dynamics. The primary mechanisms contributing to this condition include ischemic optic neuropathy (ION), central retinal artery occlusion (CRAO), and cortical blindness.

Management of Blood Loss

Spinal tumors are associated with significant blood loss due to their vascularity and the extensive nature of the surgeries required for their resection. The management of blood loss is crucial for maintaining hemodynamic stability, reducing the need for allogenic blood transfusion, and improving overall patient outcomes. Significant blood loss during spine surgery can result in increased morbidity and mortality. Tranexamic acid (TXA) is commonly used to reduce bleeding during surgeries. TXA works by inhibiting fibrin breakdown, a protein essential for blood clotting, stabilizing clots, and reducing excessive blood loss. Intravenous administration of TXA has demonstrated effective systemic absorption, with doses of 10 mg/kg capable of inhibiting up to 80% of fibrinolysis in tissues [22]. Common side effects of TXA include nausea, vomiting, diarrhea, and headaches. Although rare, thrombogenesis is a side effect still being researched.

Systemic (intravenous) use of TXA has been shown to significantly reduce blood loss, particularly in high-risk procedures. Multiple RCTs have demonstrated the benefit of TXA in reducing blood loss across different surgical groups [23]. Epsilon-aminocaproic acid (EACA), another antifibrinolytic agent like tranexamic acid, also helps reduce clotting by inhibiting the conversion of plasminogen to plasmin. A study using EACA in spinal fusion surgery found that patients receiving EACA experienced significantly lower total perioperative blood loss, postoperative blood loss, and reduced requirements for blood transfusions, including hemoglobin levels and red blood cell transfusions [24]. Both drugs inhibit fibrinolysis, reduce bleeding, and improve patient outcomes.

In addition to pharmacologic agents, blood conservation techniques are essential in managing blood loss. The use of cell-saver devices for autologous blood transfusion allows the collection and reinfusion of a patient's own blood during surgery, reducing the need for allogenic blood products and minimizing transfusion-related risks. Moreover, hemostatic agents, such as Floseal or

Surgicel, are used in surgical settings to control localized bleeding, further reducing overall blood loss.

Preoperative management of anemia includes erythropoietin administration, iron loading, or transfusions to minimize blood loss during surgery. Risk stratification is crucial, and patients who are at high risk for significant blood loss—such as those with highly vascular tumors or those undergoing extensive resection—should be identified early. Intraoperatively, the use of antifibrinolytics like tranexamic acid and aminocaproic acid, along with techniques such as fibrinogen concentrates, thromboelastometry, and controlled hypotension, help reduce blood loss and transfusion needs. Thromboelastometry is particularly valuable in guiding blood product use, ensuring that only the necessary products are transfused.

Monitoring Considerations

Surgery for spinal and brain tumors presents anesthetic challenges that require attentive intraoperative monitoring to ensure patient safety, optimize surgical conditions, and prevent complications.

Intraoperative neuromonitoring serves as an alternative to wake-up testing by detecting impending neurological injury and allowing adjustments in surgical technique, positioning, physiological parameters, or medication management to prevent permanent deficits [25]. Neuromonitoring techniques such as somatosensory evoked potentials (SSEPs), motor evoked potentials (MEPs), and direct spinal cord stimulation play a crucial role in preserving neurological function during spinal tumor resections, as they provide real-time feedback on spinal cord integrity and help prevent postoperative deficits.[i]

Intraoperative neurophysiological mapping and monitoring have become indispensable tools in spinal and brain tumor surgery, allowing for real-time assessment of neural structures and aiding in the prevention of iatrogenic injury [26]. Anesthetic agents can significantly impact the reliability of intraoperative neurophysiologic monitoring signals, necessitating careful selection and adjustment of anesthetic protocols to optimize signal quality and ensure accurate interpretation during spinal tumor surgery [27].

Spinal and brain surgeries carry the risk of severe neurological complications, including paraparesis, paraplegia, and quadriplegia, making intraoperative neurophysiologic monitoring a critical tool for early detection of spinal cord distress and prevention of permanent deficits. Monitoring of motor-evoked potentials (mMEPs) has proven to be a reliable method for detecting early signs of spinal cord injury, enabling timely surgical interventions to prevent permanent neurological deficits [28, 29]. Additionally, the use of D-wave monitoring during spinal tumor surgery has been shown to provide valuable prognostic information on postoperative motor function, aiding in surgical decision-making and improving patient outcomes.

Kyphoplasty

Kyphoplasty is a minimally invasive surgical procedure primarily designed to treat vertebral compression fractures (VCFs), which are mostly caused by osteoporosis, trauma, or metastatic tumors. In the context of spinal tumors, kyphoplasty plays a crucial role in pain management, spinal stability, and preserving the quality of life for patients with vertebral body involvement.

Kyphoplasty involves the percutaneous insertion of a balloon catheter into the collapsed vertebra. The balloon is inflated to restore vertebral height, followed by injection of bone cement to reinforce the vertebra's structural integrity. When integrated into a multidisciplinary treatment plan—which may include radiation therapy, chemotherapy, or surgical interventions—kyphoplasty significantly enhances patient outcomes and quality of life for those with tumor-related vertebral fractures.

ANESTHETIC CONSIDERATIONS FOR BRAIN TUMORS

An understanding of the unique physiology of the brain is critical to appropriate anesthesia management. The skull is a fixed-sized cavity that accommodates brain matter, blood, and cerebrospinal fluid (CSF). The Monro-Kellie doctrine dictates that these volumes remain constant. Thus, an intracranial mass will cause pressure effects unless compensated for by either the removal of a portion of the skull or decreases in blood or CSF. As a tumor increases in size, a small difference in volume can drastically increase intracranial pressure. Cerebral perfusion pressure is the difference between mean arterial pressure and intracranial pressure (or central venous pressure if that is higher). Autoregulation in the brain means that a range of cerebral perfusion pressures can be accommodated.

Various medications and maneuvers can be utilized to reduce the mass effect of lesions in the brain [30]. Osmotic diuretics such as mannitol and hypertonic saline remain the first line therapy for removing fluid from the brain. Furosemide is occasionally used as well, but the efficacy is less than that of other agents. Reduction of $PaCO_2$ is one of the most effective ways to lower intracranial pressure by decreasing cerebral blood flow. It can also create cerebral vasoconstriction, so hyperventilation must be done carefully. Severe reductions in $PaCO_2$, especially for a prolonged period, may correlate with cerebral ischemia [31].

There are anesthetics that are associated with favorable conditions for surgery on the brain. Volatile agents create mild increases in intracranial pressure (ICP) by increased cerebral blood flow, cerebral blood volume, and sometimes CSF production. The clinical effects of the increased ICP are very mild. Some studies suggest that total intravenous anesthesia improves operative and recovery times, but other studies demonstrate no difference [32 - 34]. Adding dexmedetomidine as an adjunct medication improved hemodynamics, anesthesia recovery, and operative conditions for transsphenoidal pituitary tumors in one study [35]. This is an active area of research.

Monitoring is frequently done for intracranial tumors. As discussed in the previous section, there are several modalities utilized. These include somatosensory evoked potentials, motor evoked potentials, and brainstem auditory evoked potentials. In addition, most cranial nerves can be monitored. There is growing interest in awake craniotomy, as it allows the surgeon to monitor more intricate functions, including speech, complex motor functions, and the identification of seizure foci.

Anesthesia for awake brain surgery can take several forms. The most common option is asleep-awake-asleep. This entails general anesthesia followed by a period of being awake, and then general anesthesia at the end. It can be modified to MAC, then awake, and MAC during closing. Finally, some centers keep the patient awake throughout surgery [36, 37]. Scalp blocks or local to Mayfield pin sites are helpful to reduce pain. Transitions from asleep to awake portions of the surgery are carefully done to reduce coughing, nausea, vomiting, agitation, and hemodynamic instability.

Blood loss can be attenuated by preoperative embolization. This is an increasingly used technique to reduce blood flow to the tumor. Various particles are injected intra-arterially using a minimally invasive radiologic approach. Studies have demonstrated that not only does embolization reduce blood loss, but it also improves surgical conditions.

CONCLUSION

Tumors of the brain, spine, and peripheral nerves have unique anesthetic considerations. Effects on the body can be due to both the size of the tumor and also surrounding edema. Some tumors are metabolically active, but this is less common. The goals of providing anesthesia to patients with neurological cancers are multifold. First, anesthesia should be designed to prevent further neurologic decline. Next, these patients often undergo specialized intraoperative monitoring, and the anesthetic has to be tailored appropriately. The neurologic exam is often critical upon awakening. And finally, attention must be paid to analgesia, which is often a significant concern for the patient.

REFERENCES

[1] Shah SB, Hariharan U, Chawla R. Choosing the correct-sized adult double-lumen tube: Quest for the holy grail. Ann Card Anaesth 2023; 26(2): 124-32. [http://dx.doi.org/10.4103/aca.aca_140_22] [PMID: 37706375]

[2] Webb WR, Gamsu G, Speckman JM. Computed tomography of the pulmonary hilum in patients with bronchogenic carcinoma. J Comput Assist Tomogr 1983; 7(2): 219-25. [http://dx.doi.org/10.1097/00004728-198304000-00002] [PMID: 6833551]

[3] Jung DM, Ahn HJ, Jung SH, *et al.* Apneic oxygen insufflation decreases the incidence of hypoxemia during one-lung ventilation in open and thoracoscopic pulmonary lobectomy: A randomized controlled trial. J Thorac Cardiovasc Surg 2017; 154(1): 360-6. [http://dx.doi.org/10.1016/j.jtcvs.2017.02.054] [PMID: 28412111]

[4] Young RJ, Brown NJ, Reed MW, Hughes D, Woll PJ. Angiosarcoma. Lancet Oncol 2010; 11(10): 983-91. [http://dx.doi.org/10.1016/S1470-2045(10)70023-1] [PMID: 20537949]

[5] Matushansky I, Charytonowicz E, Mills J, Siddiqi S, Hricik T, Cordon-Cardo C. MFH classification: differentiating undifferentiated pleomorphic sarcoma in the 21st Century. Expert Rev Anticancer Ther 2009; 9(8): 1135-44. [http://dx.doi.org/10.1586/era.09.76] [PMID: 19671033]

[6] Antunes MJ, Vanderdonck KM, Andrade CM, Rebelo LS. Primary cardiac leiomyosarcomas. Ann Thorac Surg 1991; 51(6): 999-1001. [http://dx.doi.org/10.1016/0003-4975(91)91031-P] [PMID: 2039335]

[7] Kabashi S, Hoxha N, Gashi S, *et al.* Primary fibro sarcoma of the heart. Acta Inform Med 2013; 21(3): 213-5. [http://dx.doi.org/10.5455/aim.2013.21.213-215] [PMID: 24167396]

[8] Aguilar CA, Donet JA, Galarreta CI, Yabar A. A primary cardiac osteosarcoma: Case report and review of the literature. J Cardiol Cases 2013; 7(2): e29-33. [http://dx.doi.org/10.1016/j.jccase.2012.09.010] [PMID: 30533114]

[9] Sharma M, Sharma A, Dixit S, Sharma N, Sharma O. Primary synovial cell sarcoma of the heart: A rare case. Heart Views 2015; 16(2): 62-4. [http://dx.doi.org/10.4103/1995-705X.159223] [PMID: 26240736]

[10] Uemura S, Watanabe M, Iwama H, Saito Y. Extensive primary cardiac liposarcoma with multiple functional complications. Heart 2004; 90(8): e48.

[11] Godar M, Liu J, Zhang P, Xia Y, Yuan Q. Primary pericardial mesothelioma: a rare entity. Case Rep Oncol Med 2013; 2013: 1-4. [http://dx.doi.org/10.1155/2013/283601] [PMID: 23840993]

[12] Bolliger D, Maurer M, Tanaka KA. Toward Optimal Anticoagulation Monitoring During Cardiopulmonary Bypass: It Is Still A Tough “ACT”. J Cardiothorac Vasc Anesth 2020; 34(11): 2928-30. [http://dx.doi.org/10.1053/j.jvca.2020.07.024] [PMID: 32741612]

[13] Lee MH, Beck M, Shann K. Protamine dose to neutralize heparin at the completion of cardiopulmonary bypass can be reduced significantly without affecting post-operative bleeding. J Extra Corpor Technol 2023; 55(3): 105-11. [http://dx.doi.org/10.1051/ject/2023026] [PMID: 37682208]

[14] Khanna P, Sarkar S, Garg B. Anesthetic considerations in spine surgery: What orthopaedic surgeon

should know! J Clin Orthop Trauma 2020; 11(5): 742-8.
[http://dx.doi.org/10.1016/j.jcot.2020.05.005] [PMID: 32879562]

[15] Bhatia A, Buvanendran A. Anesthesia and postoperative pain control—multimodal anesthesia protocol. J Spine Surg 2019; 5(S2) (Suppl. 2): S160-5.
[http://dx.doi.org/10.21037/jss.2019.09.33] [PMID: 31656870]

[16] Reel B, Maani CV. Dexmedetomidine. StatPearls. Published online January 2023.

[17] Blaudszun G, Lysakowski C, Elia N, Tramèr MR. Effect of perioperative systemic α2 agonists on postoperative morphine consumption and pain intensity: systematic review and meta-analysis of randomized controlled trials. Anesthesiology 2012; 116(6): 1312-22.
[http://dx.doi.org/10.1097/ALN.0b013e31825681cb] [PMID: 22546966]

[18] Liu B, Liu R, Wang L. A meta-analysis of the preoperative use of gabapentinoids for the treatment of acute postoperative pain following spinal surgery. Medicine (Baltimore) 2017; 96(37): e8031.
[http://dx.doi.org/10.1097/MD.0000000000008031] [PMID: 28906391]

[19] Hyland SJ, Brockhaus KK, Vincent WR, *et al.* Perioperative Pain Management and Opioid Stewardship: A Practical Guide. Healthcare (Basel) 2021; 9(3): 333.
[http://dx.doi.org/10.3390/healthcare9030333] [PMID: 33809571]

[20] Han C, Kuang MJ, Ma JX, Ma XL. The Efficacy of Preoperative Gabapentin in Spinal Surgery: A Meta-Analysis of Randomized Controlled Trials. Pain Physician 2017; 20(7): 649-61.
[PMID: 29149144]

[21] Park CM, Inouye SK, Marcantonio ER, *et al.* Perioperative Gabapentin Use and In-Hospital Adverse Clinical Events Among Older Adults After Major Surgery. JAMA Intern Med 2022; 182(11): 1117-27.
[http://dx.doi.org/10.1001/jamainternmed.2022.3680] [PMID: 36121671]

[22] Yoo JS, Ahn J, Karmarkar SS, Lamoutte EH, Singh K. The use of tranexamic acid in spine surgery. Ann Transl Med 2019; 7(S5) (Suppl. 5): S172.
[http://dx.doi.org/10.21037/atm.2019.05.36] [PMID: 31624738]

[23] Huec JCL, AlEissa S, Bowey AJ, *et al.* Hemostats in Spine Surgery: Literature Review and Expert Panel Recommendations. Neurospine 2022; 19(1): 1-12.
[http://dx.doi.org/10.14245/ns.2143196.598] [PMID: 35378578]

[24] Li S, Xing F, Cen Y, Zhang Z. The Efficacy and Safety of Epsilon-Aminocaproic Acid for Perioperative Blood Management in Spinal Fusion Surgery: A Systematic Review and Meta-Analysis. World Neurosurg 2021; 156: 12-21.
[http://dx.doi.org/10.1016/j.wneu.2021.08.113] [PMID: 34478888]

[25] Baker A, Widrich J. Somatosensory Evoked Potentials. 2023 Aug 14. In: StatPearls [Internet]. Treasure Island (FL): StatPearls Publishing; 2025.

[26] Sala F, Skrap B, Kothbauer KF, Deletis V. Intraoperative neurophysiology in intramedullary spinal cord tumor surgery. Handb Clin Neurol 2022; 186: 229-44.
[http://dx.doi.org/10.1016/B978-0-12-819826-1.00019-3] [PMID: 35772888]

[27] Scibilia A, Terranova C, Rizzo V, *et al.* Intraoperative neurophysiological mapping and monitoring in spinal tumor surgery: sirens or indispensable tools? Neurosurg Focus 2016; 41(2): E18.
[http://dx.doi.org/10.3171/2016.5.FOCUS16141] [PMID: 27476842]

[28] Buhl LK, Bastos AB, Pollard RJ, *et al.* Neurophysiologic Intraoperative Monitoring for Spine Surgery: A Practical Guide From Past to Present. J Intensive Care Med 2021; 36(11): 1237-49.
[http://dx.doi.org/10.1177/0885066620962453] [PMID: 32985340]

[29] Sala F, Bricolo A, Faccioli F, Lanteri P, Gerosa M. Surgery for intramedullary spinal cord tumors: the role of intraoperative (neurophysiological) monitoring. Eur Spine J 2007; 16(S2) (Suppl. 2): 130-9.
[http://dx.doi.org/10.1007/s00586-007-0423-x] [PMID: 17653776]

[30] Todd MM. Outcomes after neuroanesthesia and neurosurgery: what makes a difference. Anesthesiol Clin 2012; 30(2): 399-408.
[http://dx.doi.org/10.1016/j.anclin.2012.06.001] [PMID: 22901617]

[31] Li J, Gelb AW, Flexman AM, Ji F, Meng L. Definition, evaluation, and management of brain relaxation during craniotomy. Br J Anaesth 2016; 116(6): 759-69.
[http://dx.doi.org/10.1093/bja/aew096] [PMID: 27121854]

[32] Schmoch T, Jungk C, Bruckner T, *et al.* The anesthetist's choice of inhalational vs. intravenous anesthetics has no impact on survival of glioblastoma patients. Neurosurg Rev 2021; 44(5): 2707-15.
[http://dx.doi.org/10.1007/s10143-020-01452-7] [PMID: 33354749]

[33] Kumaria A, Hughes M, Fenner H, Moppett IK, Smith SJ. Total intravenous anaesthesia with propofol and remifentanil is associated with reduction in operative time in surgery for glioblastoma when compared with inhalational anaesthesia with sevoflurane. J Clin Neurosci 2024; 120: 191-5.
[http://dx.doi.org/10.1016/j.jocn.2024.01.022] [PMID: 38266592]

[34] Jiang Z, Wu Y, Liang F, *et al.* Brain relaxation using desflurane anesthesia and total intravenous anesthesia in patients undergoing craniotomy for supratentorial tumors: a randomized controlled study. BMC Anesthesiol 2023; 23(1): 15.
[http://dx.doi.org/10.1186/s12871-023-01970-z] [PMID: 36624384]

[35] Gopalakrishna KN, Dash PK, Chatterjee N, Easwer HV, Ganesamoorthi A. Dexmedetomidine as an Anesthetic Adjuvant in Patients Undergoing Transsphenoidal Resection of Pituitary Tumor. J Neurosurg Anesthesiol 2015; 27(3): 209-15.
[http://dx.doi.org/10.1097/ANA.0000000000000144] [PMID: 25493927]

[36] Potters JW, Klimek M. Local anesthetics for brain tumor resection: current perspectives. Local Reg Anesth 2018; 11: 1-8.
[http://dx.doi.org/10.2147/LRA.S135413] [PMID: 29440926]

[37] Batista S, Andreão FF, Palavani LB, *et al.* Enhancing meningioma resection: a comprehensive study on the safety and effectiveness of Onyx™ presurgical embolization. Neurosurg Rev 2023; 46(1): 299.
[http://dx.doi.org/10.1007/s10143-023-02200-3] [PMID: 37964033]

CHAPTER 13

Anesthetic Management of Major Cancer Surgical Procedures Part 2: Breast, Female Reproductive Organs, Prostate, Testicular, and Renal Cancers

Rajiv Lingaraju[1,*] and **Julie Mathew**[1]

[1] *Department of Anesthesiology, Cooper Medical School of Rowan University, Cooper University Health Care, Camden, NJ, USA*

Abstract: This chapter discusses the anesthetic management of major cancer surgeries involving the breast, female reproductive organs, prostate, testicle, and kidney. The focus will begin in the pre-operative area, addressing concerns for these patients prior to surgery. It will then explore the intraoperative anesthetic management of female and male cancers and their related surgeries. Finally, the chapter will examine the postoperative management of these patients.

Keywords: Breast cancer, Cervical cancer, Female reproductive organs, Intravenous access, Lumpectomy, Lymph node dissection, Mastectomy, Ovarian cancer, Prostate cancer, Trendelenburg.

INTRODUCTION

Surgical procedures can be performed in different settings - an office, an ambulatory surgery center, or a hospital operating room. The decision of where to perform a procedure involves quite a few variables, including the health status of the patient, the type of procedure or surgery, and what equipment is necessary.

The patient's health status is a very important factor in determining whether the procedure can be performed outside the operating room. For anesthesiologists, we evaluate the co-morbid conditions of the patient and classify the patient into the appropriate ASA classification. Usually, an ASA I or II can be safely cared for at an office or surgery center, if the appropriate equipment is available. ASA III patients can often be done at these locations; however, more vigilance needs to be taken to ensure the patient is appropriate for the site.

* **Corresponding author Rajiv Lingaraju:** Department of Anesthesiology, Cooper Medical School of Rowan University, Cooper University Health Care, Camden, NJ, USA; E-mail: lingaraju-rajiv@cooperhealth.edu

For most of the cancers discussed in this chapter, the first step typically involves a tissue sample for diagnosis. Most patients with ASA I or II can safely undergo tissue sampling in an ambulatory setting under mild to moderate sedation. Sometimes, they can even be done under local anesthesia only. General anesthesia is reserved for more complicated cases and would be used at discretion of both the anesthesiologist and surgeon performing the procedure. Patients who have an ASA status of III can also be treated at an ambulatory center but may require a higher level of vigilance, and expectations may need to be set pre-operatively that they may receive less anesthesia due to their medical history. If this is something the patient cannot tolerate, the case can be scheduled at a hospital with appropriate support.

Sometimes, the first professionals in the patient's cancer journey are the staff members who care for them during their initial procedure. Patients who come in for a procedure are often a little uneasy, but patients who come in for any type of procedure that may involve a cancer diagnosis are understandably anxious. Not only do they have fears involving the surgery or procedure itself, but also a real fear of what the diagnosis holds, so care should be taken to make each patient feel safe and comfortable. Patients may also benefit from anxiolytic medications.

Related to anxiolysis, the quickest way to deliver medication is through intravenous access. However, some of these patients, particularly as their cancer treatments progress, may have challenging venous access from genetic reasons or iatrogenic causes, such as chemotherapeutic side effects. Most of the time, the preoperative nursing staff can obtain intravenous access; however, sometimes they are unable to have intravenous access after multiple attempts. At that point, anesthesiologists may be asked to assist in this task and may need to perform ultrasound-guided intravenous insertion. Some patients who are very difficult or are undergoing chemotherapy may come in with a central access line, such as a port, that may be accessed in very difficult circumstances. Once intravenous access is achieved, an anxiolytic agent can be dosed if appropriate. Typically, in the perioperative setting, midazolam is used as the initial medication of choice to provide anxiolysis and amnesia.

Another consideration preoperatively is pre-emptive analgesia. This can be in the form of oral medications, possibly combined with a peripheral nerve block if indicated. There are not many nerve blocks that can be used, but some help mitigate post-operative pain and will be mentioned later in conjunction with the respective cancer discussions. Some of the nerve blocks that will be addressed are pectoralis blocks and transverse abdominus plane blocks, as well as local anesthetic injections by the surgeon. For cases with longer recovery times, some surgeons may place a pain pump that intermittently gives doses of local anesthetic for several days postoperatively.

Postoperative nausea and vomiting are of significant concern to patients and staff due to the discomfort and possible increased length of stay [1]. This can also be addressed preoperatively with topical patches like scopolamine and newer oral medications like Emend, which can help prevent nausea [1, 2].

Overall, there are several preoperative concerns for the anesthesiologist. From determining where the surgery is to occur, to developing an anesthetic plan that addresses safety, venous access, anxiety, analgesia, and postoperative nausea, there is an array of topics that both the anesthesiologist and patient will encounter related to cancer care.

SURGERIES FOR FEMALE CANCERS: BREAST AND FEMALE REPRODUCTIVE SYSTEMS

Breast surgery is a common surgical procedure for many indications, including biopsy of the breast, benign lump excision, breast cyst/abscess, and cosmetic procedures, but the most common reason is for breast cancer. The prevalence of breast cancer has been increasing, and continues to increase, in the United States, and is known to be one of the leading causes of death in females [3]. Breast cancer can be further classified into different histological and molecular subtypes that determine treatment and prognosis [4].

Types of Breast Surgery

Breast cancer surgery has made many advancements over the past several decades. Originally, total mastectomies were widely performed, but are now not as frequently done, thanks in part to landmark trials that have proven the efficacy of breast conserving treatment or BCT. Examples of BCT include wide local excision of the tumor, in addition to chemotherapy or radiation therapy, in comparison to full mastectomy alone. Wide local excision surgery requires histological confirmation that a minimum margin of typically 5mm of normal tissue has been excised around the tumor. There are contraindications to BCT, however, and these include inflammatory breast cancer, prior radiation to the breast, and multifocal disease [5]. Radical mastectomies are reserved for any tumor that invades the pectoral muscle. Some patients also choose to have a full mastectomy due to personal choice or not being a candidate for BCT. The patients who decide to have prophylactic mastectomies do so for risk reduction and can be simple, skin-sparing, or nipple-sparing mastectomies [6].

Sentinel Lymph Node Biopsy

The sentinel lymph node is the first node or group of nodes that drains from the primary cancer and is therefore most likely to contain metastatic disease. It has been found that sentinel lymph node biopsy is equally effective at predicting the status of axillary lymph nodes, with far fewer adverse effects than axillary lymph node dissection, such as upper limb sensory loss, increased length of hospital stay, lymphedema, and increased time to recovery of normal activities [7]. Sentinel lymph node biopsy has largely replaced axillary lymph node dissection in breast cancer staging, given that it is less invasive and equally effective. Sentinel lymph node mapping is typically carried out with a combination of radioisotopes and dye injected near the tumor during surgery involving the removal of the primary cancer. The lymph nodes with the highest radioactive signals will then be removed (usually up to four) [4].

Sentinel lymph node biopsy carries some risk, mostly associated with the dyes used during the procedure: Isosulfan blue and Patent Blue V. These two dyes have been associated with IgE-mediated anaphylactic reactions that can range from a urticarial rash to hypotension requiring vasopressor support and even cardiac arrest [8]. Anaphylaxis risk has been estimated to be 1% to 0.17% for more serious reactions. Methylene blue can be safer than other blue dyes, but problems such as interference with pulse oximetry and discoloration of the skin and body fluids, including urine, can cause confusion in both the intraoperative and postoperative settings [9]. Ultimately, the anesthesiologist should be aware of and consider anaphylaxis to dye as a cause if there is an acute cardiovascular event during sentinel lymph node biopsy surgery.

Reconstruction

Once the tumor is removed, breast reconstruction can take place immediately after or in a delayed fashion. Usually, tumors that are non-invasive can have immediate reconstruction for risk reduction, whereas more invasive tumors can be delayed for reconstructive surgery. The reconstructive surgery can be done with prosthetic or autologous material.

Prosthetic reconstruction can take place in one-stage or two-stage surgery. Tissue expanders are placed under the pectoral muscles and used to create space for a future prosthesis by gradually increasing in size. Silicone breast implants are typically used as prostheses.

Autologous reconstruction can take place by using a pedicle flap or free flaps. Pedicle or rotational flaps of tissue include skin, fat, and muscle with their original blood supplies, whereas free flaps are harvested from donor sites and transferred back to the breast for the reconstruction, requiring reattachment to new blood vessels.

The most used pedicle flap is the transverse rectus abdominis myocutanesous (TRAM) flap. Latisssimus dorsi (LD) flaps can be used when TRAM flaps are not adequate, mostly in patients at an increased risk for flap failure, likely due to smoking or diabetes history. Pedicled flaps can involve long surgical times, increased blood loss, and severe acute postoperative pain [6].

For the free flap breast reconstruction, the deep inferior epigastric perforator (DIEP) flap spares the rectus abdominis muscle and uses only skin and fat. The abdominal complications that are seen with the TRAM flaps are not seen with the free flaps. There is, however, a high risk of flap failure caused by microvascular thrombosis due to the microsurgical anastomosis that is required for this procedure. These procedures are usually done in specialist centers and are often long surgeries (more than 8 hours), and also present a challenge in the postoperative period, managing severe pain [6].

Anesthetic Management

Preoperative Assessment

Most patients who are coming in for breast cancer surgery have a very high level of anxiety, requiring an empathetic and sensitive approach to patient care. The patient's history, including any adverse effects from neoadjuvant, hormonal, chemotherapy, or radiotherapy, should be considered. Neoadjuvant therapy can be used to reduce the size of locally advanced tumors and make cancers that are at first thought to be inoperable more amenable to resection. It is also used in those with inflammatory breast cancers and those who may wish to delay surgery while pregnant. Adjuvant chemotherapy is best done within 90 days of surgery to improve outcomes [10].

Many anesthetic implications can come from the use of chemotherapeutic agents. Some agents, such as cyclophosphamide and doxorubicin, have cardiac side effects. These cardiotoxic agents can cause cardiomyopathy and QT prolongation, and can occur at any stage of treatment, including years after initiating chemotherapy. The patient should be assessed for any cardiac symptoms, and any testing (EKG, echocardiogram) should be performed prior to surgery [11].

There are also hematopoietic adverse effects from neoadjuvant therapy, including myelosuppression. These effects can manifest as perioperative anemia, an increased risk of bleeding from thrombocytopenia, and an increased risk of sepsis secondary to neutropenia. These potential factors should be identified and managed before surgery. The effects of myelosuppression usually reverse within 6 weeks of completion of chemotherapy [12].

Hormonal agents, such as aromatase inhibitors or tamoxifen, used in neoadjuvant treatment, may be continued in the perioperative period. Monoclonal antibody, trastuzumab (Herceptin), for human epidermal growth factor receptor 2-positive tumors is included and can be both cardiotoxic and increase the risk of perioperative venous thromboembolism.

Generally, patients should continue to take their regularly prescribed medications, including aspirin, even on the morning of the surgery day. Exceptions to this may be anticoagulants or antiplatelet therapy, in which case the risks should be weighed against the risk of a thrombotic event that may occur from holding these medications. Consultations with the prescribing specialists are always advised.

Regional anesthesia, usually combined with general anesthesia, has become common in the perioperative management of patients undergoing breast cancer surgery. Some of the commonly used blocks include thoracic paravertebral, pectoral nerve blocks (PECS) I and II, and serratus anterior (SA) plane blocks. Thoracic epidurals have also been employed as a neuraxial technique. Regional anesthesia provides excellent postoperative analgesia, decreases the need for opioids and the incidence of postoperative nausea and vomiting [4].

Intraoperative Management

Induction of anesthesia should proceed by using the standard monitors; medication options include using intravenous or inhalation methods, and maintenance anesthesia can be delivered using total intravenous anesthesia or a combination of inhalation and intravenous agents.

It is important to place the IV in the contralateral arm to the surgery, especially when axillary lymph nodes are involved, to avoid potential upper limb lymphedema while optimizing access to the breast and axilla. Large bore IVs should be used in longer cases to administer volume replacement and/or blood products. After surgery, guidelines suggest avoiding the use of the same side arm for IV and blood pressure readings, although the evidence is lacking to support this recommendation [13, 14].

If the patient has cardiac complications from neoadjuvant therapy or their own co-morbidities, invasive hemodynamic monitors, such as an arterial line, may be indicated.

Most procedures, unless they are short, will require tracheal intubation, especially if a different position is needed other than supine (*e.g.*, for LD flap reconstruction). In these longer procedures, attention should be paid to temperature monitoring and ensuring normothermia. This can be done with a convective forced-air warmer, warm fluids, and increased ambient room temperature [15].

For patients having flap surgery in particular, increased attention should be paid to avoiding hypothermia, hypovolemia, and vasoconstriction in order to optimize flap perfusion during surgery. Adequate ventilation of the lungs with normal PCO2 and PO2 will improve perfusion. It is also very important to avoid the excess administration of intravenous fluids to decrease the incidence of tissue edema postoperatively [16].

Positioning is also very important. Often, procedures for the breast are done supine with the arms abducted. It is important to ensure appropriate padding of the arms and to monitor throughout the case to prevent brachial plexus injuries that may be caused by overstretching and misalignment of the neck and shoulders. Patients who undergo LD reconstruction may start out in the lateral position, and then their position may be changed during the procedure. Towards the end of the procedure, the breast surgeon may request that the patient be placed in the sitting position to assess symmetry. This may cause hemodynamic changes that may necessitate the use of vasopressors and fluid boluses. With any of these positions, close and continuous vigilance is needed for the airway and intravenous access. Long procedures may also require the use of foam or jelly cushions to assist in relieving pressure over bony prominences. Compression stockings should be worn for shorter procedures, and for longer procedures sequential compression devices should be used to reduce the risk of venous thromboembolism [4].

Postoperative Considerations

Patients who undergo free flap procedures will require postoperative monitoring in an intermediate care or higher-level unit for at least 24 hours, with flap-specific monitoring during the first few postoperative days. The same principles that apply to intraoperative management should be employed postoperatively, such as adequate hydration and warm rooms to maintain flap perfusion.

Simple analgesics, such as acetaminophen and NSAIDs, can be used with or without regional anesthesia. Antiemetics should be dosed, and patients should try to mobilize early. A majority of patients undergoing minor procedures, including wide local excision with sentinel lymph node biopsy, can receive care at an ambulatory center with same-day discharge when criteria are met [4].

Gynecological Oncology Surgery

Gynecologic cancer surgery can be eventful for both the anesthesiologist and surgeon. Surgical access for pelvic malignancy can be difficult. Many gynecologic tumors may present late, have non-specific features, and can become an impressive size before any symptoms are noticed. Many tumors can be in close proximity to other abdominal structures, such as the kidneys or the rectum, and may require assistance from other surgical specialties. Neurovascular bundles and lymph nodes may be adherent to the pelvic sidewall, making dissection difficult. Cervical, endometrial, ovarian, vaginal, and vulvar cancers are all a part of cancers that may affect the female reproductive organs [17].

Types of Gynecologic Cancer

Endometrial cancer is the most common cancer of the female genital tract. Typically, a diagnosis is obtained by dilatation and curettage or biopsy, which can be done in both the office and operating room. Spread of this type of cancer is by local invasion, or *via* the fallopian tubes, which can lead to peritoneal metastasis, lymphatic, and hematogenous spread, which can then extend to the liver, lung, brain, and bone. Treatment consists of total abdominal hysterectomy and bilateral salpingo-oophorectomy with full pelvic lymphadenectomy [17].

Globally, cervical cancer is the second most common cancer to affect women. As a result of increased cancer screening, like the Pap smear, diagnosis has improved, as have management and ultimately prognosis. It is typically spread *via* vaginal mucosa, myometrium, and the paracervical lymphatics, but can also spread directly *via* the obturator fascia and involves other pelvic organs, such as the bladder and rectum. Hematogenous spread involves the lung, liver, and bone. In early occurrence with invasive disease, patients generally undergo simple hysterectomy. In contrast, those with later stage occurrence undergo radical hysterectomy, which involves the removal of the uterus, the uterosacral and uterovesical ligaments, parametrium, and pelvic node dissection [17].

The poorest survival is found in ovarian cancer, most likely due to the late-stage presentation in more than half of cases. Complete tumor removal improves survival but involves a highly invasive surgery. As a result of its spread that has no boundaries, surgical staging is required *via* an open or laparoscopic approach. Malignancy can travel easily along surfaces of the peritoneal cavity, often to the paracolic gutters, right hemidiaphragm, and intestinal mesentery. Lymphatic spread above the diaphragm can also occur. Hematogenous spread is to the lung parenchyma, skin nodules, pericardial effusion, central nervous system involvement, and bone metastasis [17].

The rarest female-specific cancer is vaginal cancer. These are often secondary to other pelvic cancers, particularly uterine, ovarian, or rectal. Spread occurs *via* a direct path to the pelvis or *via* lymphatics to the liver, lungs, and bones. Based on its staging, treatment involves partial vaginectomy and lymphadenectomy, followed by radiation therapy. Vulval cancer is also uncommon. Spread is *via* direct invasion of the vagina, urethra, and anal canal. Lymphatic spread is to the inguinal, pelvic, and femoral nodes, with distant spread to the bone, liver, and lungs. Treatment involves block dissection of the vulva, groin, and lymph nodes [17].

Anesthetic Management

Preoperative Assessment

Preoperative assessment should address general risk factors such as age, obesity, and co-morbid conditions, as well as cancer staging and what treatments the patients may have already received. Assessment of cardiac and pulmonary function is important, as some of these patients may experience dyspnea from an accumulation of ascites. Co-morbidities, such as severe ischemic heart disease, end-stage renal failure, advanced valvular lesions, or end-stage lung disease should also play a role in determing whether the surgeon chooses a laparoscopic or open procedure. Preoperative testing should include a full blood count (CBC), complete metabolic panel, coagulation studies, type and screen with crossmatch for the day of the surgery, depending on the amount of expected blood loss; chest x-ray and electrocardiogram should be ordered at a minimum for more invasive surgeries [17].

Some patients present after receiving neoadjuvant chemotherapy prior to surgery and may experience side effects from these medications. In addition, some patients with ovarian cancer may experience nausea, vomiting, or anorexia if omental spread is involved. They may also be given enemas for bowel involvement, and some electrolyte disturbances may occur. Appropriate intravenous access should be obtained in order to replete and hydrate these patients, if needed.

Patients with a significant history of chronic pain and or at risk for significant postoperative pain are given gabapentin, as well as other non-opioid medications.

Intraoperative Management

For biopsy and diagnostic purposes, sedation may potentially be used; however, most treatment procedures for gynecologic cancers require general anesthesia. Premedication with anxiolytic medications, such as midazolam, will help allay anxiety at the time of surgery. Standard induction of anesthesia with fentanyl, propofol, and a muscle relaxant should be followed by intubation. After induction and intubation, additional intravenous access may be obtained, as well as more invasive monitoring if the case and/or history warrant it. If there is a known amount of tumor invasion, preparation for significant blood loss should be considered with blood products available.

The trend in recent years has been to decrease the amount of opioids used and instead, to rely on multimodal analgesia. Epidural analgesia can be employed for radical hysterectomies and open procedures. Non-opioid intravenous medications, such as acetaminophen and NSAIDs, can be dosed and used in combination with long-acting local anesthetics, either infiltrated by the surgeon or delivered *via* a transversus abdominis plan (TAP) block.

Another factor to consider is obesity in the setting not only of anesthesia risk, but also for intraoperative positioning. Anti-slide sheets or bean bag devices should be employed to reduce the risk of sliding when in the Trendelenburg position, as is often necessary in laparoscopic or robotic procedures for gynecologic cancers. In addition, position changes and the combination of pneumoperitoneum can impair ventilation in morbidly obese patients or patients with severe lung disease. Padding the arms and ensuring access to intravenous lines and monitors while in position is very important, and care should be taken accordingly.

Upon emergence of anesthesia, there should be heightened vigilance of the airway, as prolonged Trendelenberg positioning can cause facial edema and airway swelling. Post-operative ventilation may be needed in these situations, or at the very least, close monitoring in an intensive care unit or high observation unit.

Postoperative Considerations

In the post-operative care unit (PACU), immediate anesthesia issues include pain management, nausea and vomiting, and surgical concerns or complications. Postoperative analgesia should be multimodal and, as mentioned earlier, can be started in the preoperative area and continued through the intraoperative and postoperative phases. Gynecological surgery is a risk factor for nausea and vomiting and should be addressed to optimize the patient's experience. Surgical complications can arise and be related to injury to pelvic structures or related to bleeding that will need to be monitored.

SURGERIES FOR MALE CANCERS: PROSTATE AND TESTICULAR

Prostate Cancer

Introduction

Prostate cancer is the most common cancer diagnosed in males in the United States, with an estimated 299,000 new cases in 2024, representing 29% of all male cancer diagnoses. Despite a five-year survival rate of 97%, prostate cancer is the second-leading cause of cancer-related mortality in males, causing an estimated 35,000 deaths in the United States in 2024. Age is a primary risk factor, with approximately one in eight men being diagnosed with prostate cancer during their lifetime [3]. Due to an aging global population, the number of new diagnoses of prostate cancer worldwide is expected to grow significantly, from 1.4 million cases annually in 2020 to 2.9 million in 2040. Prostate cancers vary significantly in clinical relevance, and many are considered slow-growing and may be subject to overtreatment and subsequent harm. However, diagnoses made in younger patients may nonetheless warrant intervention, while even aggressive subtypes in older males with comorbid conditions may be best left untreated [18].

Diagnosis

A diagnosis of prostate cancer is made through a combination of digital rectal exam, prostate-specific antigen laboratory testing, imaging, and tissue biopsy. Patients with physical exam, laboratory, and/or imaging results concerning prostate cancer are referred for prostate biopsy to a urologist.

Prostate Biopsy

Preoperative Concerns

Traditionally, the anesthesiologist will first encounter these patients at the time of ultrasound-guided prostate biopsy, which may be performed in an office setting or an operating room under monitored anesthesia care. If performed in an office setting, the patient should be screened by the anesthesiologist to determine if there are comorbid patient conditions, such as high BMI, severe obstructive sleep apnea, congestive heart failure, valvulopathies, or oxygen-dependent pulmonary diseases, that would suggest a hospital setting as more appropriate. As with most diagnostic procedures related to cancer diagnoses, patients will often present for prostate biopsy in a state of heightened anxiety, especially as a majority of prostate cancer diagnoses occur in asymptomatic patients. After intravenous line placement, anxiolysis with a benzodiazepine can be offered, as indicated.

Intraoperative Management

At the time of procedure, continuous electrocardiogram, pulse oximetry, end-tidal carbon dioxide, as well as intermittent noninvasive blood pressure monitors are applied, and supplemental oxygen is administered *via* nasal canula or facemask. The patient is asked to position himself into the left lateral position on the procedural table, with staff assistance as needed. Due to the quick nature of the procedure, an axillary roll for protection of the dependent-side brachial plexus is typically not required. Short-acting hypnotic medication is dosed intravenously, and the patient maintains spontaneous respirations. The urologist places a transrectal ultrasound probe, and a needle is positioned and directed through the rectum into the prostate to obtain prostate tissue. Enhanced patient comfort with anesthesia is thought to improve the tissue sampling obtained with the transrectal ultrasound method compared with local anesthetic administration alone [19].

Postoperative Considerations

Patients are discharged home after a brief PACU stay. Recent studies suggest that biopsies performed with MRI targeting for MRI-detectable lesions may be superior to transrectal ultrasound-guided biopsies – these are typically performed without systemic anesthesia [20].

Treatment

Patients meeting criteria for surgical intervention for prostate cancer will be referred for radical, or complete, prostatectomy. In the United States, a vast majority of these procedures are performed with robot assistance, which is associated with decreased bleeding, less postoperative pain, improved recovery, and shorter length of postoperative hospitalization. There are also improved surgical outcomes, including less biochemical recurrence, impotence, and urinary incontinence [21]. However, due to the high costs of robotic surgery, laparoscopic and open prostatectomies continue to be performed in other parts of the world.

Robot-Assisted Radical Prostatectomy

Preoperative Assessment

Preoperative testing is indicated based on patient history; often, it will include a complete blood count, basic metabolic panel, and electrocardiogram. Additional testing, such as cardiac echocardiography, stress testing, or pulmonary function testing, may be ordered depending on the patient's functional status and comorbid conditions.

Intraoperative Management

Intraoperatively, standard monitors are applied. General anesthesia is achieved with an intravenous induction, typically an opioid agonist, propofol, and a neuromuscular blocker. An endotracheal tube is placed. A second intravenous line is indicated, particularly with robot surgery, where the arms will be tucked and inaccessible once the robot is docked. An arterial line may be placed at the anesthesiologist's discretion, given patient factors, and if intraoperative lab work is anticipated. Central venous catheterization is not usually performed.

Surgical positioning is most commonly lithotomy with steep Trendelenburg, which has multiple known complications, ranging from mild to severe. Such positioning is associated with cardiopulmonary consequences, patient migration on the operating table, facial edema, increased intraocular pressure, and nerve palsies and compartment syndrome [22 - 24]. Steep Trendenburg positioning is associated with an increase in volume to the central circulation, subsequently increasing preload, and may precipitate congestive heart failure in susceptible individuals. The addition of abdominal insufflation can decrease mean arterial pressure and cardiac output, while increasing peak respiratory pressures [25]. Movement of abdominal viscera after insufflation, combined with gravitational force in the steep Trendelenburg position, can cause unintended mainstem bronchial intubation – bilateral breath sounds should be re-confirmed after positioning and insufflation. While high abdominal insufflation pressures were once the norm, recent studies utilizing ultra-low insufflation pressures in robotic-assisted radical prostatectomy have had encouraging results [26]. Devices, such as sticky pads and straps, must be used to prevent patients from sliding on the operating table once in steep Trendelenburg. Restrictive fluid management is preferred, as it reduces facial edema and also decreases surgical complications related to the urethral anastomosis [27]. Patients with known issues with increased intraocular pressure (IOP), such as glaucoma, were initially not offered robot-assisted prostatectomy due to known IOP increases with steep Trendelenburg that could be associated with postoperative visual loss. While those restrictions have been relaxed, anesthesiologists should be aware of the potential impact on vision in vulnerable patients [28, 29]. Pressure points should be well padded to prevent nerve and soft-tissue injury, and care must be taken to prevent inadvertent contact between the robot and the patient. Some surgeons are moving towards supine positioning for robot-assisted radical prostatectomy, eliminating the concerns specific to lithotomy position [24].

General anesthesia is maintained with a volatile or intravenous agent, per anesthesiologist preference, along with opioids and other analgesics. The degree of neuromuscular blockade should be monitored and maintained intraoperatively

– this is particularly important during robotic surgery while the robot is docked, as patient movement can cause patient injury. Significant bleeding is not typically associated with robot-assisted radical prostatectomy.

Postoperative Considerations

Many robot-assisted radical prostatectomies are now same-day procedures, with patients being discharged home after recovery in the post-anesthesia care unit, as long as they are free of complications and have assistance at home.

Testicular Cancer

Introduction

Testicular cancer is estimated to have been diagnosed in 10,000 males and is the cause of 500 deaths in the United States in 2024. It is the most frequently diagnosed solid organ tumor in males between the ages of 15 and 34 [30]. 95% of testicular cancers are germ cell tumors, and the overall prognosis is strong, with 10-year survival estimated at 98% [31]. Risk factors include a history of undescended testis and personal or family history of testicular cancer [30].

Diagnosis

Presenting symptoms of testicular cancer include painless scrotal mass, scrotal heaviness or swelling, dull scrotal ache, or acute testicular or scrotal pain. If testicular abnormalities are noted, patients are referred for scrotal ultrasound, which is highly sensitive and specific in diagnosing testicular cancer. Presence of a mass warrants serum laboratory studies, particularly alpha-fetoprotein, beta-human chorionic gonadotropin, and lactate dehydrogenase, which can help differentiate tumor type prior to orchiectomy. Imaging is used to assess for metastatic disease.

Treatment

Radical Inguinal Orchiectomy

Radical inguinal orchiectomy is indicated for malignant testicular masses and can be both diagnostic and, in non-metastatic cases, therapeutic as well. Radical orchiectomy alone is a relatively straightforward procedure with low risk of bleeding or other surgical complications; it is often performed with standard monitors under general anesthesia using a laryngeal mask airway and involves same-day discharge home.

Treatment of metastatic or potentially metastatic disease is more complex, potentially involving chemotherapy and retroperitoneal lymph node dissection (RPLND). RPLND may be indicated as a primary procedure for staging, or for the treatment of known metastases, and is a major intra-abdominal surgery that is often lengthy and is associated with a high risk of blood loss [32].

Retroperitoneal Lymph Node Dissection

Preoperative Concerns

Preoperative testing prior to RPLND includes a complete blood count, basic metabolic panel, and type and screen; additional studies may be indicated based on whether the patient received a chemotherapeutic regimen, as certain agents, such as bleomycin or cisplatin, have known cardiopulmonary effects. RPLND carries a significant risk of rapid and substantial surgical blood loss, given the position of the retroperitoneal lymph nodes in close proximity to the aorta and inferior vena cava. While RPLND has traditionally been performed with an open surgical approach, there has been a movement towards laparoscopic and robotic techniques [33].

Intraoperative Management

Intraoperatively, standard monitors are applied, and in the absence of significant comorbid conditions, general anesthesia can be induced in the usual fashion – typically opioid agonist, propofol, and a neuromuscular blocker. Post-induction, large-bore intravenous access is obtained, and an arterial line is placed for continuous blood pressure monitoring and serum sampling for intraoperative laboratory studies. If central venous pressure monitoring is desired or vasopressor administration is anticipated, a central venous catheter is placed. Active warming measures and continuous temperature monitoring should be employed, given the duration of surgery and the adverse impact of hypothermia on coagulation.

Fluid management during RPLND is goal-directed, maintaining normotension and adequate urine output in the setting of potential surgical bleeding and insensible losses from a large open incision. Episodes of hypotension may occur intraoperatively, not due to hypovolemia, but rather from surgical compression of the inferior vena cava, impeding venous return and reducing preload. Communication with the surgical team is essential to understand and appropriately manage intraoperative hemodynamics. In the setting of large volume surgical bleeding, consider resuscitation with a 1:1:1 transfusion ratio of packed red blood cells to fresh frozen plasma to platelets.

Surgical positioning is usually supine, with hyperextension of the back to improve surgical access. As RPLND can be a long surgery, averaging about six hours in duration, care must be taken to appropriately pad the patient's pressure points and maintain a neutral position as much as is feasible to avoid positioning injuries. It is important to note that patients who have received chemotherapy may be more susceptible to nerve injury, given the potential for pre-existing subclinical chemotherapy-induced nerve damage.

For open RPLND, regional anesthesia has a role in pain management, either *via* post-induction transverse abdominus plane blocks or other truncal blocks, or *via* a pre-induction low thoracic epidural catheter. If an epidural catheter is placed, a loading dose should not be administered until after the greatest risk of surgical bleeding has passed, to avoid creating a sympathectomy that can further complicate hemodynamic management. Opioids and multimodal analgesics are also dosed.

Postoperative Considerations

In the absence of complications, most patients are extubated at the completion of surgery and do not require intensive care unit admission. Postoperatively, epidural catheters can be dosed with dilute local anesthetic, with or without opioid, either by continuous infusion or by patient-controlled epidural analgesia. Breakthrough analgesics should be made available. The pain service should follow these patients postoperatively to ensure their comfort and to monitor for epidural catheter-related complications. These patients are often hospitalized for three to five days postoperatively.

Renal Cancer

Introduction

While not a male-specific cancer, tumors of the kidney are more than twice as likely to occur in males than in females; in the United States, there were an estimated 82,000 renal cancers diagnosed in 2024, with 52,000 of those diagnoses occurring in males [3]. About 90% of kidney tumors are renal cell carcinomas, and the median age of diagnosis is 65 years. The primary environmental risk factor is cigarette smoking, thought to contribute to 33% of cases. At the time of diagnosis, 66% of tumors will be confined to the kidney, while 25% will be associated with metastatic spread. Five-year survival is estimated at 76% [34].

Diagnosis

Symptomatic patients often have late-stage presentations, with hematuria, palpable mass, and weight loss. However, about 50% of diagnosed tumors are incidental findings on unrelated abdominal imaging [35]. CT imaging with contrast is the diagnostic modality of choice, as it identifies 90% of renal masses and can differentiate benign and malignant features. Up to 25% of cases are associated with tumor burden extending into the renal vein or inferior vena cava, with 10% having thrombus formation within the inferior vena cava [34].

Treatment

Radical or partial nephrectomy is indicated in most diagnoses of renal cell carcinoma, even in the presence of metastatic disease or tumor extension into the renal vein or inferior vena cava. Radical nephrectomy is the removal of the affected kidney plus perinephric fat, lymphatics, ipsilateral adrenal gland, and Gerota's fascia that encases the kidney and adrenal. Partial nephrectomy is planned for patients with small masses or in those with pre-existing renal disease where functional preservation of the affected kidney is prioritized [36]. Surgical options include open, laparoscopic, and robot-assisted procedures.

Radical and Partial Nephrectomy

Preoperative Concerns

Preoperative testing includes a complete blood count, a basic metabolic panel, and a type and screen. Additional cardiopulmonary testing may be warranted depending on the patient's comorbid conditions and functional capacity.

Intraoperative Management

Intraoperatively, standard monitors are applied, and general anesthesia is induced by the usual method – intravenous opioid agonist, propofol, and neuromuscular blocker. An endotracheal tube is placed. Post-induction, large-bore intravenous access and an arterial line are obtained. Central venous cannulation is typically not indicated. The patient is placed in the lateral position with the surgical side up, and the operating table is manipulated to create lateral flexion at the waist. Care is taken to pad pressure points, protect the brachial plexus, and maintain neutral anatomical positioning as much as possible. Some degree of Trendelenburg positioning is often requested by the urologist.

Anesthesia is maintained with a volatile agent or an intravenous anesthetic, opioids, and neuromuscular blockade. Temperature is managed with a forced air warming blanket and continuous monitoring. Intravenous fluids are administered to maintain euvolemia and appropriate urine output, ensuring adequate perfusion of the unaffected kidney. Blood products are not always administered, but given as indicated by surgical bleeding. Pain management is multimodal; typically, nonsteroidal anti-inflammatory drugs are avoided, given their impact on renal blood flow. Open nephrectomy may warrant placement of a pre-induction thoracic epidural catheter [34]. Regional anesthetic techniques are less frequently required in robotic and laparoscopic procedures.

Postoperative Considerations

In the absence of complications, most patients are extubated at the completion of surgery and do not require intensive care unit admission. Most patients stay in the hospital for one to two nights.

CONCLUSION

Individuals undergoing surgery for cancers involving the breast, female pelvic organs, prostate and testicles involve a wide range of individuals. Each case has a specific anesthetic management that should be tailored to that individual, but also throughout the perioperative period. In this chapter, we have discussed the guidelines specific to these surgeries and the concerns in the preoperative area, which is managed in the intraoperative period and followed into the postoperative period.

REFERENCES

[1] Gan TJ, Belani KG, Bergese S, *et al.* Fourth Consensus Guidelines for the Management of Postoperative Nausea and Vomiting. Anesth Analg 2020; 131(2): 411-48. [http://dx.doi.org/10.1213/ANE.0000000000004833] [PMID: 32467512]

[2] Liu Y, Chen X, Wang X, *et al.* The efficacy of aprepitant for the prevention of postoperative nausea and vomiting: A meta-analysis. Medicine (Baltimore) 2023; 102(29): e34385. [http://dx.doi.org/10.1097/MD.0000000000034385] [PMID: 37478247]

[3] Siegel RL, Giaquinto AN, Jemal A. Cancer statistics, 2024. CA Cancer J Clin 2024; 74(1): 12-49. [http://dx.doi.org/10.3322/caac.21820] [PMID: 38230766]

[4] Sherwin A, Buggy DJ. Anaesthesia for breast surgery. BJA Educ 2018; 18(11): 342-8. [http://dx.doi.org/10.1016/j.bjae.2018.08.002] [PMID: 33456800]

[5] McLaughlin SA. Surgical management of the breast: breast conservation therapy and mastectomy. Surg Clin North Am 2013; 93(2): 411-28. [http://dx.doi.org/10.1016/j.suc.2012.12.006] [PMID: 23464693]

[6] Petit JY, Rietjens M, Lohsiriwat V, *et al.* Update on breast reconstruction techniques and indications. World J Surg 2012; 36(7): 1486-97. [http://dx.doi.org/10.1007/s00268-012-1486-3] [PMID: 22395342]

[7] Motomura K. Sentinel node biopsy for breast cancer: past, present, and future. Breast Cancer 2015; 22(3): 212-20. [http://dx.doi.org/10.1007/s12282-012-0421-7] [PMID: 23250812]

[8] White V, Harvey JR, Griffith CDM, Youssef M, Carr M. Sentinel lymph node biopsy in early breast cancer surgery – Working with the risks of vital blue dye to reap the benefits. Eur J Surg Oncol 2011; 37(2): 101-8.
[http://dx.doi.org/10.1016/j.ejso.2010.12.007] [PMID: 21195576]

[9] Ramin S, Azar FP, Malihe H. Methylene blue as the safest blue dye for sentinel node mapping: Emphasis on anaphylaxis reaction. Acta Oncol 2011; 50(5): 729-31.
[http://dx.doi.org/10.3109/0284186X.2011.562918] [PMID: 21413854]

[10] Chavez-MacGregor M, Clarke CA, Lichtensztajn DY, Giordano SH. Delayed Initiation of Adjuvant Chemotherapy Among Patients With Breast Cancer. JAMA Oncol 2016; 2(3): 322-9.
[http://dx.doi.org/10.1001/jamaoncol.2015.3856] [PMID: 26659132]

[11] Shakir D, Rasul KI. Chemotherapy induced cardiomyopathy: pathogenesis, monitoring and management. J Clin Med Res 2009; 1(1): 8-12.
[http://dx.doi.org/10.4021/jocmr2009.02.1225] [PMID: 22505958]

[12] Allan N, Siller C, Breen A. Anaesthetic implications of chemotherapy. Contin Educ Anaesth Crit Care Pain 2012; 12(2): 52-6.
[http://dx.doi.org/10.1093/bjaceaccp/mkr055]

[13] Cemal Y, Pusic A, Mehrara BJ. Preventative measures for lymphedema: separating fact from fiction. J Am Coll Surg 2011; 213(4): 543-51.
[http://dx.doi.org/10.1016/j.jamcollsurg.2011.07.001] [PMID: 21802319]

[14] Bodenham A. Vascular access after axillary lymph node surgery – a reply. Anaesthesia 2017; 72(1): 128-9.
[http://dx.doi.org/10.1111/anae.13778] [PMID: 27988959]

[15] Hart SR, Bordes B, Hart J, Corsino D, Harmon D. Unintended perioperative hypothermia. Ochsner J 2011; 11(3): 259-70.
[PMID: 21960760]

[16] Nimalan N, Branford OA, Stocks G. Anaesthesia for free flap breast reconstruction. BJA Educ 2016; 16(5): 162-6.
[http://dx.doi.org/10.1093/bjaed/mkv036]

[17] Morosan M, Popham P. Anaesthesia for gynaecological oncological surgery. Contin Educ Anaesth Crit Care Pain 2014; 14(2): 63-8.
[http://dx.doi.org/10.1093/bjaceaccp/mkt035]

[18] James ND, Tannock I, N'Dow J, *et al.* The Lancet Commission on prostate cancer: planning for the surge in cases. Lancet 2024; 403(10437): 1683-722.
[http://dx.doi.org/10.1016/S0140-6736(24)00651-2] [PMID: 38583453]

[19] Kim HY, Choi YH, Lee SJ. Effect of Sedation Anesthesia With Intravenous Propofol on Transrectal Ultrasound-Guided Prostate Biopsy Outcomes. J Korean Med Sci 2022; 37(15): e115.
[http://dx.doi.org/10.3346/jkms.2022.37.e115] [PMID: 35437964]

[20] Kasivisvanathan V, Rannikko AS, Borghi M, *et al.* MRI-Targeted or Standard Biopsy for Prostate-Cancer Diagnosis. N Engl J Med 2018; 378(19): 1767-77.
[http://dx.doi.org/10.1056/NEJMoa1801993] [PMID: 29552975]

[21] Carbonara U, Srinath M, Crocerossa F, *et al.* Robot-assisted radical prostatectomy versus standard laparoscopic radical prostatectomy: an evidence-based analysis of comparative outcomes. World J Urol 2021; 39(10): 3721-32.
[http://dx.doi.org/10.1007/s00345-021-03687-5] [PMID: 33843016]

[22] Bačak Kocman I, Mihaljević S, Goluža E, *et al.* Anesthesia for robot-assisted radical prostatectomy - a challenge for anaesthesiologist. Acta Clin Croat 2022; 61 (Suppl. 3): 76-80.
[http://dx.doi.org/10.20471/acc.2022.61.s3.11] [PMID: 36938550]

[23] Kaye AD, Vadivelu N, Ahuja N, Mitra S, Silasi D, Urman RD. Anesthetic considerations in robotic-assisted gynecologic surgery. Ochsner J 2013; 13(4): 517-24.
[PMID: 24358000]

[24] Wayne G, Wei J, Atri E, *et al.* Trends in Positioning for Robotic Prostatectomy: Results From a Survey of the Endourological Society. Cureus 2021; 13(1): e12628.
[http://dx.doi.org/10.7759/cureus.12628] [PMID: 33585117]

[25] Danic MJ, Chow M, Alexander G, Bhandari A, Menon M, Brown M. Anesthesia considerations for robotic-assisted laparoscopic prostatectomy: a review of 1,500 cases. J Robot Surg 2007; 1(2): 119-23.
[http://dx.doi.org/10.1007/s11701-007-0024-z] [PMID: 25484947]

[26] Johnstone C, Hammond J, Hanchanale V. Is the use of ultra-low insufflation pressure safe and feasible in robot assisted radical prostatectomy. Turk J Urol 2021; 47(3): 199-204.
[http://dx.doi.org/10.5152/tud.2021.20568] [PMID: 35929873]

[27] Chiumello D, Fratti I, Coppola S. The intraoperative management of robotic-assisted laparoscopic prostatectomy. Curr Opin Anaesthesiol 2023; 36(6): 657-65.
[http://dx.doi.org/10.1097/ACO.0000000000001309] [PMID: 37724574]

[28] Khan A, Wang S, Saeedi O, Ryan A, Siddiqui MM. The Impact of Abdominal Insufflation on the Intraocular Pressure During Robot-Assisted Radical Prostatectomy. J Endourol 2025; Online ahead of print.
[http://dx.doi.org/10.1089/end.2024.0509] [PMID: 39925307]

[29] Taketani Y, Mayama C, Suzuki N, *et al.* Transient but significant visual field defects after robot-assisted laparoscopic radical prostatectomy in deep tRendelenburg position. PLoS One 2015; 10(4): e0123361.
[http://dx.doi.org/10.1371/journal.pone.0123361] [PMID: 25906167]

[30] Baird DC, Meyers GJ, Hu JS. Testicular cancer: Diagnosis and treatment. Am Fam Physician 2018; 97(4): 261-8.
[PMID: 29671528]

[31] Stephens M, Murphy T, Hendry D. Anaesthesia for retroperitoneal lymph node dissection in the treatment of testicular cancer. BJA Educ 2019; 19(9): 283-9.
[http://dx.doi.org/10.1016/j.bjae.2019.04.003] [PMID: 33456904]

[32] Tran V, Gibson L, Sengupta S. Retroperitoneal lymph node dissection for germ cell tumour. Transl Androl Urol 2020; 9(6): 3103-11.
[http://dx.doi.org/10.21037/tau-2019-suc-18] [PMID: 33457283]

[33] Chavarriaga J, Atenafu EG, Mousa A, *et al.* Propensity-matched analysis of open versus robotic primary retroperitoneal lymph node dissection for clinical stage II testicular cancer. Eur Urol Oncol 2024; 7(5): 1034-41.
[http://dx.doi.org/10.1016/j.euo.2024.01.006] [PMID: 38278693]

[34] Chapman E, Pichel AC. Anaesthesia for nephrectomy. BJA Educ 2016; 16(3): 98-101.
[http://dx.doi.org/10.1093/bjaceaccp/mkv022]

[35] Gray RE, Harris GT. Renal Cell Carcinoma: Diagnosis and Management. Am Fam Physician 2019; 99(3): 179-84.
[PMID: 30702258]

[36] Krabbe LM, Bagrodia A, Margulis V, Wood C. Surgical management of renal cell carcinoma. Semin Intervent Radiol 2014; 31(1): 027-32.
[http://dx.doi.org/10.1055/s-0033-1363840] [PMID: 24596437]

CHAPTER 14

Anesthetic Management of Major Cancer Surgical Procedures Part 3: Musculoskeletal, Head and Neck, Hematological, and Endocrine Malignancies

Crystal Adams[1] and **Akhil Patel**[1,*]

[1] *Department of Anesthesiology, George Washington School of Medicine and Health Sciences, Washington, DC, USA*

Abstract: Major oncologic surgeries present unique challenges for anesthesiologists, requiring a deep understanding of the pathophysiology of malignancy, the physiological impact of extensive surgical procedures, and the complexities of perioperative care. The anesthetic management involves a multidisciplinary approach between the surgical team and anesthesia providers. Methodical planning and advanced techniques can lead to optimal management of patients.

Keywords: Adrenalectomies, Airway fire, Amputation, Bone marrow biopsies, Laryngectomy, Limb sparing surgery, Parathyroidectomies, Thyroidectomies, Tracheostomy.

INTRODUCTION

Oncologic surgeries present unique challenges for anesthesiologists, requiring careful consideration of both the underlying malignancy and the physiological demands of complex surgical procedures. This chapter explores the specific nuances associated with musculoskeletal, head and neck, hematological, and endocrine malignancies, focusing on the anesthetic considerations relevant to surgical interventions in each system. Each of these cancer types poses distinct perioperative concerns that must be thoughtfully integrated into the anesthetic plan. The following sections will highlight these challenges and provide guidance for their effective management.

* **Corresponding author Akhil Patel:** Department of Anesthesiology, George Washington School of Medicine and Health Sciences, Washington, DC, USA; E-mail: ap1189@gmail.com

Bharathi Gourkanti, Irwin Gratz, William Marion, Rajiv Lingaraju & Grace Abramian (Eds.)

MUSCULOSKELETAL CANCERS AND ANESTHETIC CONSIDERATIONS

Musculoskeletal cancers involve the bones and soft tissues of the body, which create the musculoskeletal system. These cancers typically produce pain and limit functionality. As surgical management and surgical techniques have been refined, perioperative management has evolved to meet patient needs. In this section, we will discuss the anesthetic management of patients undergoing surgery for musculoskeletal cancers, more specifically, primary bone sarcoma including osteosarcoma, chondosarcoma, and ewing sarcoma, and soft tissue sarcoma.

Primary Bone Sarcoma

Osteosarcoma is the most common primary bone sarcoma [1]. Most patients are diagnosed between the ages of 10 and 19; however, there has been an increase in the diagnosis of patients over the age of 40 associated with Paget's disease. Together with Ewing's sarcoma, these two cancers account for most primary bone cancers in patients under the age of 20. The incidence was the highest in long bones, but the face, skull, and other parts of the skeleton can also be involved [1]. Ewing Sarcoma is an aggressive tumor mostly diagnosed in adolescence. It presents with pain at a local site and typically involves the pelvis, axial skeleton, and femur [2]. Although most diagnoses occur with local infiltration, subclinical metastasis is often present, increasing the chances for relapse.

Chondrosarcoma accounts for the majority of primary bone sarcomas in patients over the age of 40. Unlike osteosarcoma and Ewing's sarcoma, chondrosarcoma involves cartilage, much like the name insinuates. Chondrosarcoma typically involves the central axial skeleton, including the sternum, pelvis, and ribs, but can often be found within the proximal humerus and femur [3].

Limb-Sparing Surgery

The primary surgical intervention for patients with primary bone sarcoma is limb-sparing surgery. The goal is to allow for local resection of the primary tumor and maintain full functionality. The anesthetic plan for these patients can be very complex and does involve discussions with the patient and surgeon for optimal management. A primary focus for these patients is adequate pain management and volume resuscitation. Pre-operative consultation and introduction of regional and neuraxial anesthesia prior to the day of surgery can ease the patient's anxiety. Effective pain management is crucial for early rehabilitation and overall functional recovery [4, 5].

Limb-sparing surgery is determined by anatomical findings on initial imaging. Reconstruction is often avoided, but must be considered based on tumor growth and invasion. The popular reconstruction methods include endoprosthesis, allograft-prosthetic, and biological reconstructions [4]. The final decision lies in the hands of the surgeon, but many factors, including financial cost, durability, infection risk, and evaluation of limb length disparities, help decide the final reconstruction graft type [4].

The type of anesthetic used for limb-sparing surgery depends on the location of the tumor, size of the resection, concern for local vascular involvement and hemodynamic instability, and optimization for post-operative pain. General anesthesia is often considered for complex procedures and those with large fluid shifts. With prolonged procedures, general anesthesia appears to be the safest route to maintain ventilatory support. Neuraxial anesthesia can be considered for shorter procedures, especially for lower extremity surgeries. Due to the large sympathetic blockage that occurs with spinal anesthesia, it may be avoided for concerns of hemodynamic instability. Epidural anesthesia will likely not be sufficient for surgical purposes, but it is optimal for intra-operative and post-operative pain control. Of note, epidural analgesia has the potential effect of causing motor weakness, which may complicate post-operative rehabilitation. Many institutions also prevent patients from getting out of the hospital bed with epidurals in place, further complicating early rehabilitation efforts [4, 5].

In place of epidural analgesia for pain control, regional anesthesia is an effective method to reduce intraoperative pain and enhance postoperative recovery. Various nerve blocks can be utilized for upper and lower extremities [6, 7]. Brachial plexus nerve blocks are utilized for upper extremity procedures, whereas femoral nerve, adductor canal, sciatic nerve (sub-gluteal and popliteal approaches), lateral cutaneous femoral nerve, fascia iliaca, and quadratus lumborum nerve blocks are among the most common lower extremity nerve blocks [6, 7]. Single-shot nerve blocks with ropivacaine or bupivacaine have been effective for pain control but only have significant effects for up to 16 hours. Adjuncts such as dexamethasone, dexmedetomidine, clonidine, phenylephrine, and epinephrine have been used to extend the duration of action to about 24 hours [8]. To achieve longer pain control, nerve catheters have been used for continuous administration of low-concentration ropivacaine. Other options include the use of Exparel, a liposomal bupivacaine, which has been reported to increase the duration to up to 72 hours but does not require a catheter for continuous infusion [9]. There are contradictory studies on the use and efficacy of Exparel with no clear guidelines. Other pain modalities include patient-controlled analgesia, allowing patients to trigger a bolus of opioids intravenously.

Large-bore IV access should be considered for all cases due to the high risk for bleeding. Fluid resuscitation must be judicious based on other comorbidities such as congestive heart failure, pulmonary hypertension, and renal failure [4, 5]. In that scenario, the use of appropriate vasopressors would be required to maintain adequate perfusion. For prolonged surgeries and for patients with cardiopulmonary co-morbidities, an arterial line can be utilized for beat-to-beat blood pressure monitoring as well as frequent lab draws. Overhydration with crystalloids may cause poor surgical site closure and wound healing from peripheral edema and third-spacing [4, 5]. This can be prevented with the use of an arterial line. Frequent lab testing of lactate, base excess, and hemoglobin levels, combined with systolic pressure variation and pulse pressure variation from the arterial line assessment on the monitor, can help reduce excessive crystalloid administration and ensure appropriate transfusion of blood products.

Amputation Surgery

Prior to the advent of limb-salvaging surgery, amputations were considered the gold standard. Amputations are now less likely to occur and are necessitated based on tumor morphology and invasion [10]. As compared to limb-salvaging surgery, the risk for bleeding and hemodynamic instability is higher. Amputations involve the removal of all or part of a limb. To minimize blood loss, a tourniquet is placed, but it is limited to distal limb amputations. Once a portion of the limb is amputated, the blood within that limb is not returned to the patient, and a large unaccounted blood loss occurs, which is evidenced by compensatory tachycardia from hypotension and a decrease in hemoglobin [11]. Two large-bore IVs can be utilized for blood product administration. IVs can be used for venous blood draws and routine point-of-care assessment; an arterial line would be more accurate. As mentioned above, the use of systolic pressure variation and pulse pressure variation can show beat-to-beat trends and assist in volume resuscitation [11].

Skin flaps are utilized to close the amputation site. These flaps must have adequate blood flow to decrease the risk of wound necrosis and breakdown. Nutrition has an important role in the healing of the incision and can be factored into anesthetic management. Malnourished patients will have less available protein to bind to medications and allow for higher plasma levels, potentiating the effect of medications [12]. Nutrition also plays a key role in the development of various clotting factors [13]. Due to the high risk of bleeding, appropriate factors are necessary to avoid hemorrhage. The administration of fresh frozen plasma and cryoprecipitate can be used to assist with coagulopathy, and the use of viscoelastic testing can direct the administration of these products [13]. Antifibrinolytic agents such as amino-caproic acid or tranexamic acid can be used to prevent clot breakdown.

Pain control is as important for amputation surgery as limb-salvaging surgery. The use of epidural anesthesia and regional anesthesia is strongly encouraged for amputation surgery. One of the largest risks is phantom limb syndrome, a psychological pain condition that occurs with having pain in the amputated limb. Several studies have found that the administration of an epidural or nerve block within 24 hours of the procedure, lasting for 24 hours post-operatively, has decreased the incidence of phantom limb syndrome [6, 7]. The use of regional and epidural anesthesia can treat phantom limb syndrome, intraoperative pain, and postoperative pain [6, 7]. Use of non-opioids for pain control can decrease overall opioid pain administration and possible complications, including nausea, vomiting, constipation, change in mental status, and respiratory decompensation [14].

Soft Tissue Sarcoma

Soft tissue sarcomas are a complex combination of relatively rare cancers involving connective tissue that affect individuals at the extremes of age. Over 100 subtypes of soft tissue sarcoma have been identified as per the World Health Organization. The most common subtypes include benign lesions, such as lipomas, to more malignant angiosarcoma and leiomyosarcoma. The mainstay of treatment remains surgery with chemotherapy [15].

The location of soft tissue tumors can have variable effects on anesthetic considerations. Tumors within the integumentary system are less likely to cause large vessel compression, but may be close to nerves, causing compression or injury. In this case, an evaluation for potential nerve injury may preclude patients from regional anesthesia. Whereas retroperitoneal masses have the risk of compressing major vessels or invading into the vessels, requiring reconstruction [15]. Chest wall tumors may create large hemodynamic shifts, cardiac abnormalities, or pulmonary complications necessitating advanced intubation or resuscitative measures [16]. Positioning for surgical optimization can be difficult due to all these concerns, skin breakdown, ulcerations, and nerve damage. Padding of the soft tissues and bone areas to support the arms, head, legs, and torso must be considered to prevent skin injuries during long surgical procedures. If the legs are placed in lithotomy, special considerations should be considered to reduce time in stirrups to avoid rhabdomyolysis, allow for normal blood flow to decrease the risk for deep vein thrombosis, and prevent nerve injury [17].

As noted above, perioperative risk for major cardiovascular complications varies based on patient co-morbidities and location of surgery. For masses within the retroperitoneum, invasion of the large vessels can lead to prolonged surgery and an increased risk of bleeding; therefore, large-bore IV and central line placement should be considered. Arterial line placement would also be indicated to assess for proper fluid resuscitation and for frequent lab draws to assess for electrolyte abnormalities and blood product administration. Chest wall masses or those involving the neck can be concerning for airway and great vessel compression. Examination of the patient's airway and assessment of the patient's ability to lie flat are crucial to identify airway compression. In this case, it would be necessary to intubate *via* fiberoptic awake intubation, having a surgical team available for emergency tracheostomy, and discussing with the cardiovascular team for pre-emptive veno-venous or veno-arterial extracorporeal membrane oxygenation (VV or VA ECMO). VV ECMO can be utilized to support the pulmonary system with a fully functional cardiac system. If there is or will potentially be a collapse of the cardiac system, VA ECMO can be utilized to support both organ systems [18].

Regional and neuraxial anesthesia can be considered for pain management. The use of local anesthetics will decrease the overall need for opioids and thereby decrease complications associated with opioid use. Some of these procedures may be completed with the use of neuraxial and regional anesthesia with sedation rather than utilizing general anesthesia. The location, duration of surgery, and surgical preference are key variables in determining the method of anesthesia.

HEAD AND NECK CANCERS AND ANESTHETIC CONSIDERATIONS

Head and neck cancers are malignancies found within the mucosal lining of the mouth, nasal cavity, nasopharynx, oropharynx, and hypopharynx. It also includes the tongue, paranasal sinuses, salivary glands, and larynx [19]. Increasing usage of tobacco and alcohol has shown a simultaneous rise in head and neck cancer [20]. Oropharyngeal and tongue-based cancer has been specifically linked to increasing human papillomavirus infections [20]. Patients typically present with growths of the mucosa, tongue, or jaw, trouble breathing or changing voice, ear pain, or sinus congestion [19]. Surgical planning is typically done in conjunction with the patient's oncologist, radiation oncologist, and oncological otolaryngologist. Although only presenting 4% of all cancers in the United States, head and neck cancers present specific anesthetic considerations that must be addressed cautiously [20]. In this section, various pre-operative, intra-operative, and post-operative considerations will be discussed, including airway management, neurological monitoring, volume resuscitation and perfusion goals, airway fire, and neck hematoma.

Airway Management

Airway management is the most important anesthetic consideration. The airway may be altered due to prior chemotherapy and radiation exposure. Anatomical difficulties can arise from tumor growth and mouth opening restrictions. A detailed airway examination and discussion with the surgeon on the preferred airway is necessary. General anesthesia is required for these procedures; however, the method of airway protection may vary. Nasal intubations are required for tonsillar and tongue surgeries [19]. Oral Rae tubes may be necessary for nasal surgeries to better allow surgical exposure [19]. Salivary tumors and neck dissections may be completed with regular oral endotracheal intubations [19]. However, due to the complexity of the cancer, video laryngoscopy or fiberoptic assistance may be required to overcome changes in the airway. Otolaryngology reports may also include nasopharyngeal video examinations, which can assist with intubation technique and examine for subglottic stenosis. In reconstruction procedures, intubation will be required, but an airway will be required for long-term care and therefore a tracheostomy will be created prior to the initiation of the resection and reconstruction [21].

In patients undergoing complete laryngectomies, the entire anatomy of the airway is altered. In these patients, intubation is required to begin the procedure, but, like reconstruction procedures, a definitive airway is needed, and therefore, a laryngectomy is created. It is important to be able to distinguish a laryngectomy from a tracheostomy. In the case of an airway emergency, it is not possible to intubate from the oropharynx and through the vocal cords after a laryngectomy. However, is it possible to intubate *via* the larynx in patients with a tracheostomy [22].

Neurological Monitoring

Many of these procedures, such as neck dissections and salivary gland resections, require neurological monitoring intraoperatively. These procedures are completed near nerve plexuses of great importance. Neck dissections are particularly concerning for the proximity to the carotid artery, internal jugular, and brachial plexus. Salivary gland procedures are near the facial nerve and its branches [23]. Local neurological stimulation and monitoring are used by otolaryngologists to assess nerve branches and patients who cannot be paralyzed [23]. Typically, succinylcholine is utilized for intubation, and higher levels of sedation are required to reduce the likelihood of patient response to surgical stimulus. If a long-acting paralytic is used for intubation, reversal may be needed to allow for proper monitoring.

Volume Resuscitation

Head and neck resection and reconstruction procedures are intricate surgeries that require diligent volume resuscitation [24]. Arterial lines can be utilized for adequate blood pressure monitoring and volume assessment. The use of devices such as FloTrac and the evaluation of systolic pressure variation and pulse pressure variation can assist with overall volume resuscitation. With the advent of Enhanced Recovery after Surgery, or ERAS programs, patients are now presenting to the operating room hydrated, allowing for lower fluid administration during the procedure. In a prolonged procedure, a significant amount of volume would be required to overcome insensible volume loss. However, the continued administration of crystalloid will result in edema, most notably at the surgical site, due to the increased inflammation [24]. The use of vasopressors to support the patient's blood pressure may also be frowned upon. Vasoconstriction is a concern for decreasing blood supply to the new graft that was created, increasing the risk for necrosis [24]. A discussion with the surgical team prior to the procedure creates guidelines for the teams to further discuss intra-operatively, providing optimal care in the operating room.

Airway Fire

Airway fires are an operating room emergency. In any procedure in which the airway may be manipulated, the surgical, anesthesia, and OR nursing team must be aware of the risk, causes, and management of an airway fire. Airway fires have three components: ignition source, fuel, and oxidizers. The most common igniters for an airway fire in these surgeries include the use of electrocautery and laser within the airway. The fire is fueled by the alcohol preparation to sterilize the skin, the drapers covering the patient, gauze and sponges in the field, and the endotracheal tube. The oxidizer continuing the fire would be the oxygen supplied *via* the endotracheal tube [25].

Prevention of fires requires minimizing all three components of the airway fire and a coordinated effort from surgery, anesthesia, and the nursing team. Constant communication between the surgical team and anesthesia team is needed to decrease the oxygen requirements to maintain a safe oxygen level. Electrocautery usage should be minimized within the trachea and only used if needed. Surgical communication with the anesthesia team is necessary for oxygen circulation to be minimized or even turned off. To minimize fuel sources, 3 minutes are required between alcohol usage for sterilization and draping of the surgical field. Minimize the use of gauze in the airway and ensure moist sponges are near the surgical field. Finally, laser-resistant endotracheal tubes should be used for laser surgery [25].

In the case of an airway fire, the oxygen source should be eradicated first by disconnecting the circuit from the endotracheal tube and removing the endotracheal tube from the patient. Saline should be poured into the airway, and all other debris, including sponges and drapes, should be removed from the field. Once the fire has been extinguished, ventilation should be reestablished.

Minimize supplemental oxygen, and if needed, the patient may need to be intubated. Bronchoscopy should be completed to remove any debris. The endotracheal tube should be inspected for any fragments that may need to be retrieved [25].

Neck Hematoma

Patients with head and neck cancer may undergo neck dissections for lymph node involvement. When obtaining biopsies and making diagnosis, lymph node diagnosis can assist with staging and further treatment. Extensive neck dissections may include visualization of the internal jugular vein and the carotid artery. Due to the highly vascular area, these procedures may have small tributaries that may become disrupted either during the exploration or upon closure of the fascia and skin. In the recovery room, patients are monitored for hematoma formation at the site of the dissection. In this life-threatening condition, patients will describe a fullness and pain at the surgical site, which may lead to compression of the airway with stridor and difficulty breathing. As the hematoma expands, it continues to deviate from the airway, worsening the shortness of breath. Intubation for these patients may become difficult if it is not intervened upon too late. Video laryngoscopy may be necessary in order to overcome the deviation. Definitive treatment is to open the surgical incision at the bedside to allow for decompression of the hematoma. Although a surgical complication, if there is concern for airway compression, anesthesia providers should feel confident in their ability to incise the suture line and complete hematoma evacuation [26, 27].

HEMATOLOGICAL CANCERS AND ANESTHETIC CONSIDERATIONS

Hematological cancers involve malignancies within the blood, bone marrow, and lymphatic system, disrupting the proliferation and function of normal cell lines. Although the only major surgical intervention for these cancers involves bone marrow biopsies, these cancers can affect the anesthetic management for patients undergoing non-cancer-related surgery. Hematological cancers account for 9% of all cancers worldwide. These cancers include lymphomas, leukemias, myeloma, myeloproliferative syndrome, and myelodysplastic syndrome. A patient's initial presentation includes a constellation of nonspecific symptoms and irregular lab work. Treatment is managed by an oncologist and consists of chemotherapy, radiation, bone marrow transplantation, immunotherapy, and targeted therapies [28].

Patients are at high risk for infection due to the disruption of plasma cell function and the administration of chemotherapy. Although prophylactic antibiotics are given to treat opportunistic infections, maintaining sterile procedure and administering appropriate antibiotics for surgical incisions is paramount to prevent sepsis. Patients are routinely monitored for their cell counts and concern for developing neutropenic fever, which can be devastating, resulting in an ICU admission [29].

Tumor lysis syndrome is a life-threatening condition resulting from the rapid cellular lysis of tumor cells, which releases potassium, uric acid, and phosphate into the bloodstream, causing a cascade of electrolyte imbalances that affect the renal and cardiac systems, among others. Although difficult to diagnose without lab work, the risk is noted to be higher in patients who have a large tumor burden and have recently initiated chemotherapy [30].

Bone Marrow Biopsy

Bone marrow biopsies are integral for the diagnosis and treatment of those suffering from hematological malignancies. Although most procedures do not require anesthesia assistance, conscious sedation is typically administered with the focus on pain control. Local anesthesia is administered at the side of the biopsy; however, additional opioids and pain medications may be necessary to complete the procedure. Bone marrow biopsies typically occur at the pelvis and are an outpatient procedure. Anesthesia may be necessary for patients suffering from chronic pain and experiencing high levels of anxiety [31].

ENDOCRINE CANCERS AND ANESTHETIC CONSIDERATIONS

Endocrine-related cancers are noted to be found within the thyroid, parathyroid, and adrenal glands [32]. Although rare, thyroid cancer is the most common of the three types. These cancers can be delineated as functional, hormone-producing, or non-functional, non-hormone-producing. Patients may need medical interventions to decrease overall hormone levels circulating in the bloodstream to maintain normal function [32]. Other treatments include chemotherapy, radiation, and surgical resection of the mass. If a total resection is indicated, replacement hormone therapy may be indicated.

Thyroidectomy and Parathyroidectomy

These surgeries carry similar anesthetic considerations; however, they do have their differences. Due to the location of the glands, the surgical exposure and techniques have similar approaches, resulting in comparable anesthetic considerations. The airway is typically secured with an oral endotracheal tube. Due to the proximity of the glands to critical nerves that affect the function of the vocal cords, neuromonitoring is utilized for the procedure [33]. The monitoring requires the use of the neural integrity monitor (NIM) tube, which has electromyography electrodes at a specific place that can measure electrical activity of the laryngeal muscles with direct stimulation of the recurrent laryngeal nerve. The recurrent laryngeal nerve passes posterior to the thyroid gland and innervates all the laryngeal muscles except the cricothyroid muscle and is responsible for abduction of the vocal cords [34]. The superior laryngeal muscle innervates the cricothyroid muscle. Injury to the recurrent laryngeal nerve results in adduction of the afflicted side [34]. Damage bilaterally resulted in the adduction of the vocal cords and inability to ventilate, leading to an emergency airway.

To utilize electromyography, long-acting paralytics are avoided, and succinylcholine is typically used for induction. Intubation is completed *via* video laryngoscopy to ensure proper placement of the NIM tube, with the electrodes correlating to the correct side [33]. During the procedure, the surgeon can then test tissue in the surgical field to assess for the nerve and ensure no damage is done [33]. The use of volatile agents does not affect the electromyography and may be utilized for maintenance of general anesthesia. Higher levels of sedation will be required to prevent any response to surgical stimuli.

Airway intubation may be difficult depending on the size of the malignancy. The use of video laryngoscopy is required for the appropriate placement of the NIM tube [33]. However, if a patient is unable to lie flat due to airway compression from tumor burden, an awake fiberoptic intubation should be considered. In this scenario, a patient may require topical anesthesia of the oral airway and vocal cords. Once anesthetized, with the patient spontaneously breathing, a fiberoptic camera with the NIM tube loaded on can be advanced into the airway beyond the vocal cords. The NIM tube can be advanced over the fiberoptic camera beyond the level of the cords, after which the patient can be induced safely and ventilated with the anesthesia machine.

The size of the goiter may also cause compression of the superior vena cava. This can become a medical emergency and require immediate intervention. Obstruction of the superior vena cava can lead to decreased venous return from the head, neck, heart, and upper extremities. A more detailed discussion can be found in Chapter 11 [35].

A smooth emergence should be planned. Coughing and bucking may result in excess pressure at the site of incision and resection. To minimize bleeding and injury to the incision, deep extubation or extubating while on low levels of dexmedetomidine and remifentanil are utilized. Decreasing the risk of bleeding will reduce the risk of a neck hematoma, which, as discussed above, is a life-threatening complication [35].

After a total resection, thyroid replacement therapy is required for thyroidectomies, and parathyroid replacement therapy is required for parathyroidectomies. If there is damage to the nonoperative gland during surgery, hormone replacement therapy may be indicated based on symptomology [35].

Thyroid Specific Considerations

Patients presenting with a functional goiter may experience a thyroid storm with manipulation. Symptoms of thyroid storm include tachycardia, hypertension, hyperthermia, and elevated levels of end tidal carbon dioxide. Beta blockers should be readily available to treat tachycardia and hypertension. Due to the administration of hormone regulation therapy, the incidence of this has decreased significantly [35].

Corneal abrasions are a common side effect of general anesthesia, which should be discussed with patients during the consenting process. Although the incidence is low, patients with hyperthyroid states may present with exophthalmos. It is important to attempt to completely shut the patient's eyes and cover them from any possible trauma. General anesthesia increases the risk of dryness and therefore the closure of the eyelids helps prevent abrasions [35].

Parathyroid Specific Considerations

Hyperparathyroidism results in the elevation of calcium levels. A pre-operative electrocardiogram and lab work assessing the calcium level should be completed. Intravenous fluid administration and diuretics can be administered to immediately address hypercalcemia. If there is an arrhythmia on the electrocardiogram, it may be beneficial to decrease the calcium level to a normal level and to reassess the cardiac arrhythmia for resolution [36].

Intra-operatively, the removal of the parathyroid gland is measured *via* multiple lab tests. An arterial line can be placed to reduce venipuncture. A baseline parathyroid hormone level can be drawn prior to resection and then followed by repeat checks after resection, with repeat frequencies every 5 to 10 minutes based on surgeon preference. A decrease by 50% or return to normal levels within 10 minutes is evidence of a successful resection [37].

Postoperatively, hypocalcemia may be a complication of the surgery. This may not be present until 24-48 hours post-operative. Patients should be monitored for signs of hypocalcemia, which include paresthesia, perioral numbness, and tetany [36].

Adrenal Gland Surgery

The adrenal gland produces three types of hormones, each with its own function within the human body. It produces mineralocorticoids, glucocorticoids, and androgens. Overproduction of mineralocorticoids, such as aldosterone in Conn's syndrome, clinically presents with metabolic alkalosis, hypertension, and fatigue. Cushing's syndrome is caused by an increased level of cortisol from secretion from the adrenal gland or exogenous glucocorticoid therapy. When the medulla overproduces androgens, namely norepinephrine and epinephrine, it results in tachycardia and hypertension. Three of these diseases are indications for surgical intervention, each with its specific anesthetic considerations [38, 39].

With resection of the adrenal gland, there are several unique considerations that must be incorporated within the anesthetic plan, regardless of the disease process affecting the adrenal gland. Airway management is completed with oral endotracheal intubation. Adequate pain control should be considered with a multimodal approach. Regional anesthesia with a transverse abdominal plane block or a quadratus lumborum block can be utilized [38, 39]. If neuraxial anesthesia is preferred, an epidural is another adequate option for pain control, which minimizes opioid administration. Antihypertensives and vasoactives should be available for rapid shifts in blood pressure readings due to manipulation of the adrenal gland. Large-bore IV access is necessary for operative blood loss and resuscitation, with central line placement as an acceptable alternative. Invasive monitoring with an arterial line is recommended for frequent lab draws and beat-to-beat blood pressure monitoring [39]. Volume status assessments can be ascertained from the arterial line to maintain euvolemia. Insulin should be used for close glucose correction, aiming for a target of less than 180 mg/dL [39].

Cushing's Syndrome

Cushing syndrome is caused by an inappropriate level of cortisol and other glucocorticoids. Patients present with central obesity, hypertension, hyperglycemia, metabolic alkalosis, hypokalemia, a moon face, and buffalo hump, among other symptoms. Lab testing will be positive for 17-hydroxycorticosteroids and excessive ACTH [39]. To diagnose pituitary-driven Cushing's disease, a dexamethasone test can be completed with repeat imaging. If both the cortisol and 17-hydroxycorticosteroids are found to decrease, it is likely Cushing syndrome, meaning the pituitary is the cause rather than Cushing syndrome [39]. Imaging can also be utilized to see tumor growth in the pituitary *versus* the adrenal gland [39].

Patients are usually hypervolemic and need diuresis. Spironolactone is the diuretic of choice as it will prevent further diuresis of potassium [38, 39]. Due to the musculoskeletal effects of cortisol and the duration of the procedure, padding and positioning are important to prevent skin breakdown. As the adrenal gland is removed, hemodynamic instability may be due to a sudden decrease in glucocorticoids [39]. Hydrocortisone should be readily available. Of note, due to central obesity, preoxygenation and preparation for a difficult airway are part of the initial anesthesia plan. Rapid deoxygenation may occur due to a decreased functional residual capacity, hypoventilation, and atelectasis [39].

Conn's Syndrome

Inappropriate aldosterone production from the adrenal gland is called Conn's syndrome. Secondary hyperaldosteronism is due to increased renin production. Patients present with hypertension, hypokalemia, and skeletal muscle weakness. Generally, management is similar to Cushing's syndrome, with patients appearing hypervolemic due to increased water absorption, and so diuresis with spironolactone is indicated [38, 39]. Metabolic alkalosis should be monitored with repeat arterial blood gases, and hyperventilation should be avoided. Vasoactives and anti-hypertensives should be available for rapid changes in blood pressure from adrenal manipulation. Hydrocortisone should be readily available for possible hemodynamic instability post resection [38, 39].

Pheochromocytoma

Pheochromocytoma is a disease of excess androgens, norepinephrine, and epinephrine. Preoperative management is predicated upon blood pressure control. Initial administration of a beta blocker would result in uncontrolled alpha activation, leading to profound hypertension. For this reason, beta blockers are not the first-line agent for blood pressure control, and initial therapy is based on alpha blocking agents such as doxazosin and phenoxybenzamine. Doxazosin is the medication of choice due to the short duration of action, allowing more stability after adrenal resection [39]. Phenoxybenzamine has been found to have profound hypotension postoperatively because of the prolonged duration of action. Clonidine and calcium channel blockers are other medications that are safe to use to normalize blood pressure [38, 39].

Along with the general considerations of adrenal surgery, patients undergoing pheochromocytoma surgery must be closely monitored. All sympathetic responses should be blunted with deep sedation and appropriate multimodal pain control [39]. Patients are typically hypovolemic and require a large amount of volume resuscitation. Sympathetic-stimulating medications such as ketamine and rapid administration of volatiles such as desflurane should be avoided [39]. Facilitation of a smooth induction with significant blunting of the sympathetic response to intubation should be planned. Short-acting anti-hypertensives, such as bolus and infusions, should be readily available for large increases in blood pressure. Vasopressors and inotropes may be needed once the adrenal gland is removed [38, 39].

CONCLUSION

Oncological malignancies affecting the musculoskeletal, head and neck, hematological, and endocrine systems have unique considerations that an anesthesiologist must address prior to initiation of care in the operating room. Decisions and plans created in the pre-operative setting can lead to better intra-operative and post-operative outcomes. With surgery being part of curative therapy, it is imperative to understand the change in normal physiology that these cancers cause. This leads to an informed conversation with all teams involved, improves team dynamics within the operating room and patient care.

REFERENCES

[1] Pullan JE, Lotfollahzadeh S. Primary Bone Cancer. [Updated 2024 Mar 20]. In: StatPearls [Internet]. Treasure Island (FL): StatPearls Publishing; 2025. Available from: https://www.ncbi.nlm.nih.gov/books/NBK560830/

[2] Gaspar N, Hawkins DS, Dirksen U, *et al.* Ewing sarcoma: current management and future approaches through collaboration. J Clin Oncol. 2015; 33(27): 3036-3046. [PMID: 26304893]

[3] Van Oosterwijk JG, Anninga JK, Gelderblom H, *et al.* Update on targets and novel treatment options for high-grade chondrosarcoma. Expert Opin Ther Targets. 2016; 20(10): 1239-1251. [PMID: 27384366]

[4] Howard A, Kolodzie K. Anesthetic Considerations for Orthopedic Amputation Surgery. Curr Anesthesiol Rep 2025; 15(1): 34. [http://dx.doi.org/10.1007/s40140-025-00692-x]

[5] Weinbroum A, Marouani N, Lang E, Niv D, Wittig J, Rudick V. Anesthesia and Perioperative Pain Management for Limb-sparing Surgery. Musculoskeletal Cancer Surgery. Dordrecht: Springer 2004. [http://dx.doi.org/10.1007/0-306-48407-2_35]

[6] Tran DQ, Salinas FV, Benzon HT, *et al.* Lower extremity regional anesthesia: essentials of our current understandingRegional Anesthesia &. Pain Med 2019; 44: 143-80.

[7] Mirza, Farheen, and Anthony R. Brown. "Ultrasound-Guided Regional Anesthesia for Procedures of the Upper Extremity." Anesthesiology research and practice 2011.1 (2011): 579824. [http://dx.doi.org/10.1155/2011/579824]

[8] Desai N, Kirkham KR, Albrecht E. Local anaesthetic adjuncts for peripheral regional anaesthesia: a narrative review. Anaesthesia 2021; 76(S1) (Suppl. 1): 100-9. [http://dx.doi.org/10.1111/anae.15245] [PMID: 33426668]

[9] Kaye AD, Armstead-Williams C, Hyatali F, *et al.* Exparel for postoperative pain management: a comprehensive review. Curr Pain Headache Rep 2020; 24(11): 73. [http://dx.doi.org/10.1007/s11916-020-00905-4] [PMID: 33098008]

[10] Zhu Y, Wu X, Zhang W, Zhang H. Limb-salvage surgery *versus* extremity amputation for early-stage bone cancer in the extremities: a population-based study. Front Surg 2023; 10: 1147372. [http://dx.doi.org/10.3389/fsurg.2023.1147372] [PMID: 37325420]

[11] Payne WG, Naidu DK, Wheeler CK, *et al.* Wound healing in patients with cancer. Eplasty 2008; 8: e9 Howard A, Kolodzie K. Anesthetic Considerations for Orthopedic Amputation Surgery. Curr Anesthesiol Rep 2025; 15(1): 34.
[http://dx.doi.org/10.1007/s40140-025-00692-x] [PMID: 18264518]

[12] Payne WG, Naidu DK, Wheeler CK, *et al.* Wound healing in patients with cancer. Eplasty 2008; 8: e9. [PMID: 18264518]

[13] Miller GJ. Effects of diet composition on coagulation pathways. Am J Clin Nutr 1998; 67(3) (Suppl.): 542S-5S.
[http://dx.doi.org/10.1093/ajcn/67.3.542S] [PMID: 9497167]

[14] Paice JA, Bohlke K, Barton D, *et al.* Use of Opioids for Adults With Pain From Cancer or Cancer Treatment: ASCO Guideline. J Clin Oncol 2023; 41(4): 914-30.
[http://dx.doi.org/10.1200/JCO.22.02198] [PMID: 36469839]

[15] Hoang NT, Acevedo LA, Mann MJ, Tolani B. A review of soft-tissue sarcomas: translation of biological advances into treatment measures. Cancer Manag Res 2018; 10: 1089-114.
[http://dx.doi.org/10.2147/CMAR.S159641] [PMID: 29785138]

[16] Li WWL, van Boven WJP, Annema JT, Eberl S, Klomp HM, de Mol BAJM. Management of large mediastinal masses: surgical and anesthesiological considerations. J Thorac Dis 2016; 8(3): E175-84.
[http://dx.doi.org/10.21037/jtd.2016.02.55] [PMID: 27076967]

[17] Armstrong M, Moore RA. Anatomy, Patient Positioning. [Updated 2022 Oct 31]. In: StatPearls [Internet]. Treasure Island (FL): StatPearls Publishing; 2025 Jan-. Available from: https://www.ncbi.nlm.nih.gov/books/NBK513320/

[18] Dhamrait RS, Tumber SS. Anesthetic Considerations for Chest Wall Surgery. In: Raff G, Hirose S, Eds. Surgery for Chest Wall Deformities. Cham: Springer 2017.
[http://dx.doi.org/10.1007/978-3-319-43926-6_5]

[19] Khan, Muhammad Jaffar, *et al.* "Principles of anesthesia and airway management in head and neck surgery." Surgical Management of Head and Neck Pathologies. IntechOpen, 2020.

[20] Thompson-Harvey A, Yetukuri M, Hansen AR, *et al.* Rising incidence of late-stage head and neck cancer in the United States. Cancer 2020; 126(5): 1090-101.
[http://dx.doi.org/10.1002/cncr.32583] [PMID: 31722124]

[21] Anehosur VS, Karadiguddi P, Joshi VK, Lakkundi BC, Ghosh R, Krishnan G. Elective Tracheostomy in Head and Neck Surgery: Our Experience. J Clin Diagn Res 2017; 11(5): ZC36-9.
[http://dx.doi.org/10.7860/JCDR/2017/24117.9854] [PMID: 28658904]

[22] Manoucherian N, Arman P, Rahmati Torkashvand P, Barazesh Y. Challenges of airway management in patients with a history af total laryngectomy: A case report. Arch Anesth & Crit Care 2025; 11(4): 599-602.

[23] Cirignaco G, Monarchi G, Betti E, *et al.* Outcome of Facial Nerve Integrity After Parotid Gland Surgery With and Without Intraoperative Monitoring: A Ten-Year Retrospective Study. Journal of clinical medicine 2025; 14(4): 1156.
[http://dx.doi.org/10.3390/jcm14041156]

[24] Le JM, Ponto J, Yedeh YP, Morlandt AB. Perioperative management for microvascular free tissue transfer for head and neck reconstruction – commentary. J Diagn Treat Oral Maxillofac Pathol 2024; 8(9): 100287.

[25] Jones TS, Black IH, Robinson TN, Jones EL. Operating Room Fires. Anesthesiology 2019; 130(3): 492-501.
[http://dx.doi.org/10.1097/ALN.0000000000002598] [PMID: 30664060]

[26] Gerasimov M, Lee B, Bittner EA. Postoperative anterior neck hematoma (ANH): timely intervention is vital. The Official Journal of the Anesthesia Patient Safety Foundation 2021; 36(1): 44.

[27] Thomas SA, Moideen SP, George SM, Ipe S, Menon DG. Management of Spontaneous Neck Hematoma in Patients on Anticoagulant Therapy: Our Experience from a Tertiary Care Center. Indian J Otolaryngol Head Neck Surg 2022; 74(S3) (Suppl. 3): 6362-6.
[http://dx.doi.org/10.1007/s12070-021-02990-2] [PMID: 35437479]

[28] Smith-Graziani D, Flowers CR. Understanding and Addressing Disparities in Patients With Hematologic Malignancies: Approaches for Clinicians. Am Soc Clin Oncol Educ Book 2021; 41(41): 351-7.
[http://dx.doi.org/10.1200/EDBK_320079] [PMID: 33793311]

[29] Chen Y, Ma T. Hematologic cancers and infections: how to detect infections in advance and determine the type? Front Cell Infect Microbiol 2024; 14: 1476543.
[http://dx.doi.org/10.3389/fcimb.2024.1476543] [PMID: 39559703]

[30] Adeyinka A, Kaur A, Bashir K. Tumor Lysis Syndrome. [Updated 2024 Oct 5]. In: StatPearls [Internet]. Treasure Island (FL): StatPearls Publishing; 2025 Jan-. Available from: https://www.ncbi.nlm.nih.gov/books/NBK518985/

[31] Tomasian A, Jennings JW. Bone marrow aspiration and biopsy: techniques and practice implications. Skeletal Radiol 2022; 51(1): 81-8.
[http://dx.doi.org/10.1007/s00256-021-03882-w] [PMID: 34398308]

[32] Moini J, Badolato C, Ahangari R. Epidemiology of endocrine tumors. Elsevier, 2021: p. 568.

[33] Jung JY. Intraoperative Nerve Monitoring in Thyroid Surgery: A Comprehensive Review of Technical Principles, Anesthetic Considerations, and Clinical Applications. J Clin Med 2025; 14(9): 3259.
[http://dx.doi.org/10.3390/jcm14093259] [PMID: 40364290]

[34] Mahyoub, Abdullatif, *et al.* "Recurrent and superior laryngeal nerve injury in thyroid surgery: literature review." International Journal of Community Medicine and Public Health 8.2 (2021): 862.
[http://dx.doi.org/10.18203/2394-6040.ijcmph20210002]

[35] Russell T, Cooper RM. Anesthesia for thyroid and parathyroid surgery. Anesthesia for Otolaryngologic Surgery 2012; p. 163.

[36] Perrier ND, Dickson PV, Figueroa AS. Parathyroid exploration for primary hyperparathyroidism. In: Post T, Ed. UpToDate. 2022.

[37] Kazaure H, Lin D, Lorenzo J, Mihm F. Endocrine surgery: Parathyroidectomy. In: Jaffe R, Schmiesing C, Golianu B. Anesthesiologist's Manual of Surgical Procedures. 6th edition. Philadelphia; Wolters Kluwer; 2020: 753-8

[38] Memtsoudis SG, Swamidoss C, Psoma M. Anesthesia for Adrenal Surgery. In: Linos D, van Heerden JA, Eds. Adrenal Glands. Berlin, Heidelberg: Springer 2005.
[http://dx.doi.org/10.1007/3-540-26861-8_28]

[39] Domi R, Sula H, Kaci M, Paparisto S, Bodeci A, Xhemali A. Anesthetic considerations on adrenal gland surgery. J Clin Med Res 2015; 7(1): 1-7.
[http://dx.doi.org/10.14740/jocmr1960w] [PMID: 25368694]

CHAPTER 15

Anesthetic Management for Major Surgical Procedures Part 4 – Gastrointestinal Oncology

Aakash Patel[1] and **Bharathi Gourkanti**[1,*]

[1] *Department of Anesthesiology, Cooper Medical School of Rowan University, Cooper University Health Care, Camden, NJ, USA*

Abstract: Gastrointestinal (GI) oncology presents a uniquely complex and evolving landscape for anesthesiologists, requiring a thorough understanding of tumor biology, surgical approaches, and perioperative physiology. This chapter provides a comprehensive overview of anesthetic management in patients undergoing surgery for GI malignancies, including esophageal, gastric, colorectal, hepatobiliary, pancreatic, and stromal tumors. The discussion emphasizes the interplay between anatomical considerations and surgical demands, as well as the anesthetic implications of cancer-related physiological derangements such as cachexia, malnutrition, anemia, and immunosuppression.

A focused approach to preoperative optimization, including Enhanced Recovery After Surgery (ERAS) protocols and prehabilitation strategies, is presented alongside a detailed review of anesthetic techniques—ranging from total intravenous anesthesia (TIVA) to regional modalities—and pharmacological considerations unique to oncologic surgery. Procedure-specific challenges are analyzed in the context of esophagectomy, gastrectomy, hepatectomy, pancreaticoduodenectomy, and carcinoid tumor resection, with particular attention to fluid management, pain control, and intraoperative monitoring.

Additionally, the chapter addresses the growing evidence linking anesthetic management to long-term oncologic outcomes, including tumor recurrence and immune modulation. It concludes with a forward-looking discussion on emerging practices in immunomodulatory anesthesia, ERAS innovations, and the role of anesthesiology in optimizing return to intended oncologic therapy (RIOT). This chapter aims to serve as a practical and evidence-based reference for anesthesiologists managing patients with GI cancers in high-acuity surgical settings.

Keywords: Blood transfusion, Enhanced Recovery After Surgery (ERAS), GI oncology anesthesia, Multimodal analgesia, Opioid-sparing, Regional anesthesia.

* **Corresponding author Bharathi Gourkanti:** Department of Anesthesiology, Cooper Medical School of Rowan University, Cooper University Health Care, Camden, NJ, USA; E-mail: gourkanti-bharathi@cooperhealth.edu

Bharathi Gourkanti, Irwin Gratz, William Marion, Rajiv Lingaraju & Grace Abramian (Eds.)

INTRODUCTION TO GASTROINTESTINAL ANESTHESIA

Gastrointestinal (GI) cancer surgeries present significant anesthetic challenges due to the complexity of the operations and the often fragile condition of oncology patients. These surgeries involve extensive anatomy – from the esophagus and stomach to the intestines, liver, and pancreas and may require large incisions, retraction, and occasionally thoracic components (*e.g.*, esophagectomies), all contributing to physiological stress. A thorough understanding of GI anatomy and tumor biology is essential, and anesthesiologists must be familiar with the anatomical considerations and clinical course of common GI malignancies (such as esophageal, gastric, colorectal, hepatobiliary, pancreatic cancers, and gastrointestinal stromal tumors) in order to optimally plan perioperative care [1]. GI tumors are among the leading causes of cancer morbidity, and their resection can be curative but is associated with high perioperative risk due to factors like tumor bleeding, nutritional derangements, and the potential for major fluid shifts or blood loss.

Patient-Specific Factors: Patients with GI cancers frequently present with cachexia, anemia, and malnutrition. Tumor-related anorexia and metabolic changes (cancer cachexia) lead to loss of lean body mass and hypoalbuminemia, which in turn alter drug pharmacokinetics and reduce physiologic reserve. Malnutrition is a well-known predictor of poor surgical outcomes; for example, in esophageal cancer surgery, poor preoperative nutritional status correlates with significantly higher postoperative complication rates [2]. Anemia is common (due to chronic blood loss or bone marrow suppression from cancer or chemotherapy) and can exacerbate tissue hypoxia; it should be optimized preoperatively (*e.g.*, with iron therapy or erythropoietin) to reduce the need for transfusions. Additionally, many cancer patients are immunosuppressed from the malignancy or prior treatments, increasing their infection risk. The anesthesiologist's preoperative assessment should thus include a careful evaluation of nutritional and volume status, end-organ function, and performance status. Often, a multidisciplinary optimization is needed, such as dietary counseling or feeding tube placement for severe malnutrition, or hematologic optimization for anemia.

Preoperative Risk Assessment and Optimization: Careful risk stratification is critical in GI oncology cases. Standard cardiopulmonary evaluation must be tailored to the patient's oncologic history – for instance, identifying cardiotoxic effects of chemotherapy or reduced pulmonary reserve from prior thoracic radiation. Objective measures like cardiopulmonary exercise testing or frailty indices can help quantify risk, aligning with the updated 2024 AHA Guidelines.

Optimization strategies are implemented whenever possible: treatment of anemia, aggressive nutritional support, physiotherapy for deconditioned patients, glycemic control in diabetics (pancreatic cancer patients may have diabetes), and abstinence from smoking and alcohol. Evidence suggests that interventions such as smoking cessation at least several weeks before surgery reduce postoperative pulmonary and wound complications [3]. In summary, the aim is to have the patient optimized as much as possible prior to undergoing these large operations.

Perioperative Goals: The overarching anesthetic goals for GI cancer surgery are maintaining hemodynamic stability, attenuating the surgical stress response, and providing effective analgesia (often *via* multimodal strategies) to facilitate recovery. Hemodynamic stability can be challenging to maintain during phases like induction (due to hypovolemia in dehydrated or bowel-prepped patients) or during large fluid shifts (*e.g.*, during liver resection or when the abdomen is open and exposed). Invasive arterial monitoring is commonly used for blood pressure management, and central venous access is often indicated for major cases for vasopressor infusions or rapid volume shifts. Close communication with the surgical team is important to anticipate stages of the operation that may require blood conservation (such as hepatic vascular clamping). Attenuating the surgical stress response is another key goal: major surgery triggers a surge of catecholamines and inflammatory cytokines, leading to immunosuppression in the perioperative period [4, 5].

This immunosuppressive (characterized by high levels of stress hormones and prostaglandins) can potentially promote tumor cell dissemination and impair wound healing [4]. Anesthetic techniques that blunt this response, such as epidural analgesia, regional blocks, and depth of anesthesia sufficient to prevent excessive sympathetic surges, are therefore desirable. Finally, multimodal analgesia, combining regional anesthesia, non-opioid analgesics, and other adjuncts to minimize opioid requirements, is very important. Effective pain control not only improves patient comfort but also enables early mobilization, deep breathing exercises, and faster return of bowel function, all of which are critical in ERAS (Enhanced Recovery After Surgery) protocols.

Preoperative Considerations in GI Oncology Surgery

Enhanced Recovery After Surgery (ERAS) Protocols: ERAS principles have become the standard of care in many GI oncology centers, with protocols specifically developed for colorectal, pancreatic, gastric, and esophagectomy surgeries. ERAS is a multimodal perioperative care pathway designed to reduce the surgical stress response and expedite recovery. Key ERAS elements begin preoperatively: patient education, optimization of medical comorbidities, minimization of preoperative fasting (with carbohydrate drinks up to a few hours before surgery), and preemptive analgesia plans.

Studies have demonstrated that ERAS pathways in major abdominal surgery significantly reduce postoperative morbidity and shorten hospital length of stay [6]. For example, one meta-analysis in colorectal surgery showed ERAS reduced complications and accelerated the return of bowel function compared to traditional care. Anesthesiologists play a central role in ERAS implementation [7, 8], since many protocol elements are anesthetic-related: maintaining normothermia, avoiding excess IVF (intravenous fluids), using opioid-sparing analgesia, preventing nausea, and ensuring full reversal of neuromuscular blockade to allow early extubation. ERAS guidelines for GI surgery emphasize goal-directed fluid therapy (to avoid both dehydration and overload), active warming, and avoiding drains/tubes that impede mobilization (*e.g*., early removal of nasogastric tubes and urinary catheters). By adhering to ERAS protocols, the anesthesiologist helps attenuate the stress response and supports faster recovery. For instance, maintaining intraoperative euvolemia and normothermia has been shown to reduce ileus and improve wound healing [9, 10].

Prehabilitation Strategies: In recent years, the concept of prehabilitation has gained traction for oncology patients. Prehabilitation involves improving a patient's physical fitness, nutritional status, and mental well-being in the weeks leading up to surgery, thereby building a "reserve" that can be drawn upon during the stress of surgery and recovery. GI cancer patients often have a window between diagnosis (or completion of neoadjuvant therapy) and surgery during which prehab can be implemented. Multimodal prehabilitation programs typically include exercise training (aerobic and resistance exercises to improve cardiopulmonary fitness and muscle strength), nutritional supplementation (to address protein-calorie malnutrition or specific deficiencies), and psychological support or stress-reduction techniques [11].

Evidence suggests that prehabilitation can reduce postoperative complications and speed up functional recovery. For example, in colorectal cancer surgery, patients who underwent an exercise and nutrition prehabilitation program had improved 6-minute walk distances pre-surgery and a reduction in hospital length of stay by ~2 days [12, 13]. Even a short-duration intervention (2–4 weeks) can be beneficial. It is worth noting that a large proportion of GI surgery patients (30–45% in some series) experience major postoperative complications [14], which often delay or even preclude adjuvant therapies. By improving baseline fitness and nutrition, prehabilitation aims to reduce this complication rate and thereby improve not just surgical outcomes but also long-term oncologic outcomes. As part of preoperative planning, anesthesiologists should advocate for and participate in prehab programs when available – for example, guiding patients on inspiratory muscle training for those at risk of pulmonary complications, or referring to dietitians for immune-nutrition supplements (formulas enriched with arginine or omega-3 fatty acids, which may improve immune function).

Effects of Neoadjuvant Therapies: Many GI oncology patients receive neoadjuvant chemotherapy, chemoradiation, or newer immunotherapies (such as immune checkpoint inhibitors) before surgery to shrink tumors and improve resectability. These treatments carry implications for anesthetic management that must be assessed in the preoperative evaluation. Chemotherapy agents often have organ-specific toxicities [15]. For instance, platinum-based drugs (like cisplatin, oxaliplatin) can cause peripheral neuropathy and renal impairment; anthracyclines (doxorubicin, epirubicin) can lead to cardiomyopathy; bleomycin (sometimes used for squamous esophageal cancers) may cause pulmonary fibrosis.

These effects can persist long after chemotherapy is completed [16]. Therefore, a patient with prior anthracycline exposure should have a cardiac evaluation (*e.g.*, echocardiogram to assess ejection fraction) to screen for cardiomyopathy, and high fractions of inspired oxygen should be used cautiously in a patient with a history of bleomycin (to minimize the risk of oxygen-related pulmonary injury) [17]. Bone marrow suppression from chemotherapy can result in thrombocytopenia or leukopenia, affecting bleeding risk and infection risk; a complete blood count should be checked, and any severe cytopenia corrected or planned for (*e.g.*, platelet transfusion if necessary).

Immune checkpoint inhibitors (such as nivolumab and pembrolizumab, used in some metastatic GI cancers or trials) introduce unique considerations as well. These drugs can cause immune-related adverse events in virtually any organ system, including pneumonitis, colitis, hepatitis, myocarditis, nephritis, and various endocrinopathies (secondary adrenal insufficiency, or thyroiditis) are among the most common. Anesthesiologists should inquire about any history of autoimmune side effects from immunotherapy and ensure they are optimally treated. For example, a patient on immunotherapy may require a stress-dose steroid plan if they have adrenal insufficiency. Even if immunotherapy has been discontinued, residual autoimmune effects can persist and necessitate ongoing steroid/immunosuppressant therapy. Coordination with the oncology team is important to determine whether immunotherapy will be held around the time of surgery (often it is paused a few weeks before and after major surgery to reduce overlapping toxicity and infection risk). In summary, the preoperative period for a GI oncology patient must include a detailed treatment history and targeted work-up: cardiopulmonary testing for chemo/radiation toxicity, lab tests for hepatic/renal function, and potentially endocrinologic evaluation (*e.g.*, morning cortisol levels if immunotherapy-induced adrenal insufficiency is a concern). The anesthetic plan and drugs can then be tailored (for instance, avoiding agents predominantly metabolized by a chemo-damaged liver, or ensuring extra lung-protective ventilation strategies for a bleomycin-exposed patient).

Anesthetic Techniques and Pharmacological Considerations

Choice of Anesthetic Technique: General *vs.* Regional: Most GI oncology surgeries are performed under general anesthesia (GA), often in combination with regional anesthesia for analgesia. Within GA, an important consideration is whether to use inhalational (volatile) anesthetics or total intravenous anesthesia (TIVA) with propofol for maintenance. In recent years, a growing body of laboratory and clinical research has investigated the impact of anesthetic technique on cancer outcomes. Volatile anesthetics (*e.g.*, sevoflurane, isoflurane) have been shown in some in-vitro models to impair immune cell function and upregulate pro-tumorigenic pathways such as hypoxia-inducible factor 1-alpha (HIF-1α), potentially promoting tumor growth and metastasis [4, 18].

Propofol, by contrast, may have anti-inflammatory and antioxidant properties and has been shown to reduce HIF-1α and other tumor growth signals in laboratory studies [19]. These findings led to the hypothesis that TIVA with propofol might confer an oncologic benefit over volatile anesthesia. Retrospective clinical studies have indeed reported associations between propofol-based TIVA and improved recurrence-free survival in certain cancers (*e.g.*, some studies in breast, colon, and esophageal cancer surgeries) [20]. A pooled meta-analysis by Yap and colleagues (2019) of 10 nonrandomized studies found a lower risk of recurrence (pooled hazard ratio ~0.78) and improved overall survival in patients who received propofol TIVA compared to inhalational anesthesia [21].

However, it is critical to note that these data are retrospective and subject to confounding; to date, no large randomized controlled trial has definitively shown that anesthetic choice alters oncologic outcomes [18, 22]. Several prospective trials are underway (*e.g.*, the international VAPOR-C and others) to address this question [22]. For now, the selection of TIVA *vs.* volatile should be based on patient and surgical factors (and perhaps institutional ERAS protocols or clinician preference), rather than on unproven cancer outcome benefits. That said, many centers favor propofol TIVA in long oncologic cases due to additional advantages (less postoperative nausea and vomiting, faster early recovery, and avoidance of the immunosuppressive effects of volatile anesthetics on neutrophils and natural killer cells).

Regional anesthesia and analgesia techniques are heavily utilized in GI cancer surgery – both for their superior pain control and their potential modulatory effect on the stress response. Thoracic epidural analgesia has long been the gold standard for open abdominal procedures such as esophagectomy, open gastrectomy, pancreaticoduodenectomy (Whipple procedure), and open liver resections. By delivering local anesthetic (often combined with low-dose opioid) directly to the thoracic nerves, epidurals provide dense analgesia that blunts afferent pain signaling and attenuates the neuroendocrine stress response to surgery. This can in turn mitigate the perioperative immunosuppression and theoretically could improve oncologic surveillance by the immune system [23, 24]

Early retrospective data suggested that regional anesthesia (epidurals or nerve blocks) might reduce cancer recurrence or metastasis, possibly by both reducing surgical stress and decreasing opioid requirements. However, more recent evidence – including several randomized trials – has not shown a clear recurrence or survival benefit from regional techniques in cancer surgery [25, 26]. For example, a large RCT in breast cancer patients comparing paravertebral block + GA versus GA alone found no significant difference in cancer outcomes at long-term follow-up [27]. Similarly, a multicenter trial in patients undergoing intra-abdominal cancer surgery with or without epidural did not demonstrate an improvement in recurrence-free survival with epidural use (though one subset analysis suggested a possible survival benefit in a certain subgroup, this finding is not yet definitive) [28, 29].

Therefore, while regional anesthesia is highly recommended for GI oncology surgeries to improve analgesia and enhance recovery, it should be employed primarily for those reasons, with any potential tumor-related benefits considered unproven. Common regional techniques in GI surgery include: thoracic epidurals (often placed at T7–T10 level for upper abdominal coverage) for open laparotomy pain control; transverse abdominis plane (TAP) blocks or rectus sheath blocks for abdominal wall analgesia (useful in laparoscopic or open cases, especially if epidural is contraindicated); paravertebral blocks (in lieu of epidural in some esophagectomies); and intrathecal morphine (single-shot spinal analgesia, sometimes used in major laparoscopic cases). The choice depends on surgical approach and patient factors (coagulation status, *etc.*). In summary, a balanced anesthesia plan is typically employed: GA (TIVA or inhalational) for unconsciousness and reflex suppression, combined with regional anesthesia for analgesia and stress attenuation. This not only provides excellent pain relief and may reduce opioid needs but also aligns with ERAS goals of facilitating early mobilization and recovery.

Multimodal Anesthesia and Opioid-Sparing Strategies

Given the deleterious effects of both surgical stress and excessive opioids on the immune system, multimodal anesthesia/analgesia has become a cornerstone of anesthesia practice. Multimodal analgesia refers to using a combination of analgesic drug classes and techniques to provide pain relief through different mechanisms, thereby reducing reliance on any single class (particularly opioids). By minimizing opioids, we aim to reduce opioid-related side effects (respiratory depression, ileus, sedation) and potentially avoid opioid-induced immune suppression and tumor-promoting effects. Opioids, while potent analgesics, can suppress natural killer cell activity and other immune functions, and in some preclinical studies, morphine has been shown to promote angiogenesis and tumor cell proliferation *via* μ- opioid receptors on cancer cells [24, 30].

Clinically, it remains inconclusive whether perioperative opioid use at typical doses influences cancer recurrence, as current evidence does not definitively link intraoperative opioids to worse oncologic outcomes [30].

Non-Opioid Analgesics: Non-steroidal anti-inflammatory drugs (NSAIDs) and acetaminophen are first-line adjuncts. NSAIDs (*e.g.*, ketorolac, ibuprofen, celecoxib) not only provide analgesia and opioid-sparing effects but also inhibit cyclooxygenase and prostaglandin E2, which are mediators that are part of the inflammation-induced immunosuppressive pathway.

Some data even suggest NSAIDs or COX-2 inhibitors could have direct anti-tumor effects (for example, aspirin and other NSAIDs have been associated with reduced colorectal polyp formation and possibly improved cancer-specific survival in colorectal cancer patients). Of course, NSAIDs must be used with caution due to risks of bleeding (inhibiting platelet function) and anastomotic ulceration or renal impairment; many surgeons avoid NSAIDs in the immediate post-colorectal resection period due to concern for anastomotic leak, although evidence on this is mixed. Acetaminophen is routinely given as part of multimodal analgesia (often 1g IV intraoperatively and continued post-op) for its opioid-sparing effect.

Local Anesthetics: In addition to epidurals and nerve blocks, another important application of local anesthetics is the use of intravenous lidocaine infusion. IV lidocaine infusion during and after surgery has been shown to reduce postoperative pain scores, opioid consumption, and ileus duration in abdominal surgery patients. Lidocaine's systemic anti-inflammatory and analgesic properties are leveraged here, and it can directly modulate the stress response and inflammatory cascade [26].

Some studies suggest lidocaine infusions also improve the return of bowel function (hence their inclusion in many colorectal ERAS protocols). From an oncologic perspective, local anesthetics in the periphery or circulation may exert immunomodulatory effects that are being investigated for potential anti-metastatic influence [26]. In practice, a lidocaine infusion (*e.g.*, 1–2 mg/min after a bolus of 1.5 mg/kg) is often started after induction and continued until the end of surgery (or up to a few hours post-op) in major GI cases if no contraindications (like heart block or arrhythmia history).

Alpha-2 Agonists: Adjuncts such as dexmedetomidine (an alpha-2 adrenergic agonist) can provide sedation, sympathetic blockade, and some analgesic-sparing effect. Dexmedetomidine infusions during GI cancer surgery may help blunt the stress response by reducing circulating catecholamines, and they can decrease opioid requirements by providing a component of analgesia while sparing major respiratory depression.

However, the impact of dexmedetomidine on cancer outcomes is complex. Animal studies have yielded conflicting results: some have reported that dexmedetomidine can promote tumor metastasis in certain models (perhaps by suppressing NK cell activity or promoting angiogenesis), whereas other studies suggest dexmedetomidine might have neutral or even anti-tumor immune effects in different contexts [23]. The clinical literature is limited and has not shown any clear harm or benefit of intraoperative dexmedetomidine on cancer recurrence [23]. Thus, dexmedetomidine should be used for its anesthetic merits (analgesia, anxiolysis, hemodynamic stability) and titrated carefully (watching for bradycardia or hypotension), but not withheld solely out of concern for theoretical tumor effects. If a patient is hemodynamically fragile (common in cachectic patients), low-dose dexmedetomidine can be very useful to reduce anesthetic requirements and provide postoperative ICU sedation if needed.

Other Adjuncts: Low-dose ketamine (*e.g.*, 0.25–0.5 mg/kg bolus, then 2–5 μg/kg/min infusion) is another multimodal component that can reduce opioid use and is particularly helpful in opioid-tolerant patients. There is no strong evidence linking ketamine to cancer outcomes, positive or negative. Magnesium sulfate infusions have analgesic and NMDA-antagonist effects and can be included (taking care to monitor levels if renal function is impaired). Gabapentin or pregabalin are sometimes given preoperatively to reduce post-op pain and opioid use, but sedative side effects must be considered, especially in frail patients (these are used more cautiously in ERAS now due to the risk of prolonged sedation and respiratory depression in combination with opioids).

Blood Transfusion Considerations: GI oncology surgeries often carry a risk of substantial blood loss (*e.g.*, liver resections or Whipple procedures can involve several liters of loss). Transfusion thresholds should be carefully considered, as emerging evidence links allogeneic blood transfusions to worse cancer outcomes. Mechanistically, transfusions can induce immunomodulation (transfusion-related immunosuppression) that might impair the body's anti-tumor immune surveillance and may supply growth factors that help any residual tumor cells survive [12, 13].

Meta-analyses in colorectal and gastric cancer have found that patients receiving blood transfusions during surgery have higher rates of cancer recurrence and poorer overall survival [12, 13]. Thus, judicious blood conservation is important: techniques include acute normovolemic hemodilution, cell-saver autotransfusion (with caution in oncologic cases – cell salvage is often avoided if the surgical field is grossly contaminated with tumor cells, to prevent reintroduction; however, some centers use leukocyte filters when salvaging blood in cancer cases), and permissive hypotension or low central venous pressure techniques in liver surgery to reduce hemorrhage.

Of course, patient safety comes first – transfusions should not be withheld when needed for oxygen delivery and hemostasis. The goal is to optimize patients preoperatively (correct anemia, iron supplements) and use meticulous surgical and anesthetic techniques to minimize blood loss so that transfusion can be avoided or minimized. If transfusion is required, leukoreduced blood is preferred (to lessen immunogenic load), and some studies suggest that autologous blood transfusion (if available) might carry less immunosuppressive risk than allogeneic transfusion [12, 13].

In summary, an anesthetic plan for a GI cancer case typically involves GA combined with regional anesthesia, and a host of adjunct medications to implement an opioid-sparing, hemodynamically stable course. This might look like: induction with propofol (TIVA maintenance if chosen) or volatile agent, plus epidural placed pre-induction; maintenance infusions of lidocaine, low-dose ketamine, and dexmedetomidine as appropriate; NSAID and acetaminophen given; active warming; low tidal volume ventilation (especially in colorectal laparoscopic cases with Trendelenburg); and vigilant fluid and transfusion management. Each component is directed at a specific goal and together, they maintain stability, provide analgesia, and potentially modulate the perioperative environment in favor of better short-term recovery and possibly long-term outcomes.

Procedure-Specific Considerations

While general principles apply to all GI oncology surgeries, there are important procedure-specific anesthetic considerations for different tumor types and operations. Below, we address key points for major GI cancer surgeries:

Esophageal Cancer (Esophagectomy)

Anesthetic and Surgical Overview: Esophagectomy for esophageal cancer is one of the most invasive GI surgical procedures, associated with significant morbidity and mortality. It typically involves resection of the esophagus and reconstruction using a gastric or colonic conduit. Common approaches include the transthoracic (*e.g.*, Ivor Lewis esophagectomy, requiring a thoracotomy or thoracoscopic phase and laparotomy) or transhiatal approach (through the abdomen and neck without formal thoracotomy). Newer minimally invasive and robotic techniques are increasingly employed to reduce surgical trauma, but even these minimally invasive esophagectomies can last many hours and pose challenges such as one-lung ventilation and difficult patient positioning. One-lung ventilation (OLV) is required for thoracic exposure in transthoracic approaches, and OLV in esophagectomy can lead to hypoxemia or high airway pressures, so protective lung strategies (low tidal volume, judicious use of PEEP on the dependent lung, intermittent recruitment) are important.

Hemodynamic and Monitoring Considerations: These patients are often older and may have significant weight loss and poor baseline cardiopulmonary reserve. Intra-arterial blood pressure monitoring is recommended. A central line is often placed for vasopressors and volume management, especially given the potential adjunct of epidural analgesia (which can cause sympathectomy and hypotension). Major fluid shifts can occur as the abdomen is opened (third-space losses), and the thoracic phase can also cause fluid losses and changes in venous return. Goal-directed fluid therapy is recommended to avoid both under-resuscitation (risking organ hypoperfusion and anastomotic ischemia) and over-resuscitation (which can contribute to pulmonary edema and anastomotic leak). Esophagectomy patients are particularly prone to pulmonary complications; fluid overload can exacerbate postoperative acute lung injury and potentially compromise the new esophagogastric anastomosis by causing tissue edema [24].

Analgesia: A thoracic epidural (usually mid-thoracic, T5–T10 coverage) is recommended for open esophagectomy for superior analgesia of both the chest and abdominal incisions. Epidurals have been shown to improve pulmonary outcomes by facilitating better pain control for breathing exercises, thereby reducing respiratory complications. If an epidural is contraindicated or if the approach is minimally invasive (with smaller incisions), alternatives can include paravertebral blocks. During surgery, anesthesiologists should carefully titrate vasopressors if an epidural is running to maintain perfusion to the gastric conduit, which will be used for anastomosis, as prolonged hypotension can risk poor gastric perfusion and contribute to anastomotic leak.

Complication Risk Mitigation: Anastomotic leak at the esophagogastric anastomosis is one of the most feared complications, occurring in 5-15% (or up to 30% in some series) of cases and carries high mortality. While surgical technique and perfusion are the primary determinants of leak, anesthetic management can contribute by ensuring adequate oxygenation and perfusion of the gastric tube. Avoiding excessive vasoconstriction in the graft (which is often reliant on marginal blood supply) is key. Thus, if possible, maintaining mean arterial pressure with fluids and moderate-dose vasopressors while avoiding profound hypertension or hypoperfusion episodes is advisable. Postoperatively, early identification of a leak (*e.g.*, *via* swallow study or clinical signs) is critical, and these patients often require intensive care observation.

Respiratory Complications: Due to the combination of thoracic surgery, one-lung ventilation, and a frequent history of smoking or radiation, esophagectomy patients have a high incidence of respiratory complications (atelectasis, pneumonia, ARDS). Protective ventilation and aggressive postoperative pulmonary care (incentive spirometry, early ambulation) are important. If a patient has borderline pulmonary function (*e.g.*, low DLCO or COPD), planning for staged weaning or even postoperative ventilation in the ICU may be prudent. Enhanced Recovery pathways for esophagectomy encourage early extubation in the operating room when feasible, as prolonged intubation can increase pneumonia risk. Extubation criteria should be carefully evaluated after these long cases, considering airway swelling (from prone or lateral positions and large fluid volumes), which could complicate re-intubation if needed.

In summary, esophagectomy requires meticulous planning: double-lumen tube management, likely thoracic epidural analgesia, invasive monitoring, careful fluid and vasopressor titration, and a vigilant eye on oxygenation and ventilation parameters. The anesthesiologist must be prepared for sudden hemodynamic changes (*e.g.*, during mediastinal manipulation or if a vagal response is elicited) and have vasopressors and antidysrhythmic drugs readily available. Coordination with the surgical team is essential, especially during critical moments like gastric conduit pull-up (the surgeon may request hypotension or ventilation strategies).

Gastric Cancer (Gastrectomy)

Overview: Anesthesia for gastrectomy (partial or total) in gastric cancer is generally focused on managing an upper abdominal surgery that can be done either open or laparoscopically. Total gastrectomy involves the removal of the entire stomach and construction of an esophagojejunostomy, whereas subtotal or distal gastrectomy removes part of the stomach and anastomoses the remainder to the small intestine. Key issues in gastric cancer patients include malnutrition (many have weight loss, hypoalbuminemia, and vitamin deficiencies like B12 if long-standing obstruction or prior partial gastrectomy) and risk of aspiration (if there is gastric outlet obstruction or large tumor causing delayed gastric emptying).

Aspiration Prophylaxis: Preoperatively, a gastric cancer patient, especially with a proximal tumor or outlet obstruction, should be considered for full stomach. Even if they have been fasting, retained food or fluid can be present. A period of nasogastric decompression before induction may be warranted in cases of symptomatic obstruction. Rapid-sequence induction with cricoid pressure is often indicated to mitigate aspiration risk.

Monitoring and Access: Standard monitors and at least two IV lines (one large bore) are typically used. An arterial line is considered if it is an open gastrectomy (moderate risk of blood loss and fluid shifts) or if the patient has significant comorbidities. Laparoscopic gastrectomy may have less hemodynamic fluctuation, but if the case is oncologic (with extensive lymph node dissection), it can still last many hours and involve significant blood loss, so an atrial line is reasonable. Central venous access is not routinely required for gastrectomy unless the patient is high-risk or TPN-dependent (total parenteral nutrition *via* central line preoperatively).

Analgesia: For open gastrectomy, a thoracic epidural (around T6–T9 dermatomes) provides excellent analgesia, improves postoperative pain and pulmonary function. For laparoscopic cases, an epidural can still be used, especially if conversion to open is possible, but some prefer transverse abdominis plane (TAP) blocks or intraperitoneal local anesthetic infiltration instead. An increasingly common approach for laparoscopic subtotal gastrectomy is a TAP block (subcostal approach to cover the upper abdominal wall) combined with non-opioid analgesics and a low-dose opioid PCA if needed. Early feeding is a goal in ERAS for gastric surgery, so minimizing systemic opioids is beneficial to prevent ileus or nausea.

Nutritional Considerations: Total gastrectomy patients will lose intrinsic factor production (leading to B12 deficiency over time) and have altered GI transit (risk of dumping syndrome, where rapid transit of food into the small bowel causes vasomotor and hypoglycemic symptoms). While these issues manifest postoperatively rather than intraoperatively, the anesthesiologist should ensure the patient has had nutritional optimization pre-surgery (some may come in on preoperative enteral feeding *via* jejunostomy if malnourished). Intraoperatively, because many gastric cancer patients are volume-depleted (from chronic vomiting or poor intake), careful fluid management is needed, and they often require fluid replacement, but one should avoid over-resuscitation that could contribute to bowel edema and delayed recovery of gut function.

Surgical Considerations: Surgeons may request certain maneuvers, such as a leak test of the anastomosis (requiring inflation of the stomach remnant or endoscope insufflation of air to check for bubbles in submerged anastomosis). The anesthesiologist coordinates this by either manually ventilating to increase pressure or assisting with an endoscope if needed. If the tumor is large and vascular, there might be brisk bleeding on resection; be prepared with blood availability. However, in general, gastrectomies are not as hemorrhage-prone as liver or pelvic surgeries, with estimated blood losses often <500 mL for partial and <1000 mL for total gastrectomy unless complicated.

ERAS for Gastrectomy: A noteworthy element is early oral feeding. Traditional management kept patients NPO until flatus or bowel sounds returned, but modern ERAS protocols encourage starting fluids and a soft diet within the first 24 hours if tolerated. Studies confirm that early oral feeding after gastrectomy is feasible, safe, and associated with faster recovery of bowel function and shorter hospital stays. For the anesthesiologist, this means ensuring any postoperative nausea is well controlled (aggressive prophylaxis with antiemetics like aprepitant, ondansetron, and dexamethasone is recommended) and that analgesia is optimized to allow eating (epidural functioning well so the patient can sit up and take liquids). If a total gastrectomy patient has a postoperative enteral feeding tube (jejunostomy), anesthesiologists in the ICU or PACU should ensure feeds are started as per protocol.

In summary, anesthesia for gastrectomy focuses on preventing aspiration, providing good analgesia (epidural or blocks), and careful fluid/blood management. These patients often do well if ERAS pathways are followed, with ambulation and feeding soon after surgery. The anesthesiologist's role in facilitating that (through opioid-sparing and nausea prevention) is crucial.

Colorectal Cancer (Colon and Rectal Resections)

Overview: Colorectal cancer surgeries range from right or left hemicolectomies to low anterior resections of the rectum, sometimes with stoma formation. Many of these are done laparoscopically or robotically, especially for colon lesions, while rectal cancers often require pelvic dissection that can be done open, laparoscopic, or robotic. Key anesthetic considerations include bowel preparation status (many patients undergo a cathartic prep the day before, which can cause dehydration and electrolyte imbalances, patient positioning (often lithotomy with steep Trendelenburg for low pelvic work in rectal cases), and measures to prevent postoperative ileus.

ERAS and Fluid Management: Colorectal surgery is where ERAS protocols were first widely adopted and studied. A major focus is avoiding excessive IV fluids, as liberal fluids historically contributed to bowel wall edema and anastomotic issues, as well as prolonged ileus. Current practice is often "zero-balance" fluid therapy or very restricted crystalloid with early transition to oral intake. Goal-directed fluid therapy using stroke volume variation or similar monitors can help titrate fluids to actual needs, improving outcomes by optimizing perfusion without overload.[10] Anesthetic management thus often involves the use of advanced hemodynamic monitors (*e.g.*, esophageal Doppler, arterial pressure waveform analysis) to guide fluid boluses versus vasopressors. Colorectal ERAS protocols also call for avoidance of drains and NG tubes post-op, early removal of Foley catheters, and ambulation on day 0 or 1, all of which require that the patient is awake, not orthostatic, and free of severe pain or sedation.

Analgesia: Thoracic epidural analgesia has been shown to reduce ileus and improve recovery in open colorectal surgery by blocking afferent pain and sympathetic fibers that innervate the colon. Epidurals can hasten the return of bowel function and allow earlier mobilization, as well as reduce opioid consumption. In laparoscopic colon resections, epidurals are not always used due to reports of urinary retention and hypotension; instead, transverse abdominis plane blocks (including bilateral TAP or quadratus lumborum blocks for broader coverage) can be alternatives. A multimodal pain approach (acetaminophen, NSAIDs if not contraindicated, ketamine, lidocaine infusion) is particularly beneficial in colorectal cases to minimize opioids, since opioid-induced ileus is a major concern. The difference in recovery can be significant: patients in opioid-sparing pathways often tolerate diet and have bowel movements earlier, facilitating discharge.

Surgical Technique Impacts: The presence of an epidural can influence the surgical field; for example, an epidural may cause vasodilation that could slightly increase mesenteric blood flow (potentially beneficial for anastomotic perfusion), but also can contribute to venous pooling that might obscure the field in low pelvic cases. Most surgeons and anesthesiologists coordinate epidural dosing so as not to cause profound hypotension during critical portions of surgery (*e.g.*, pelvic dissection, where excessive bleeding is a risk if veins are engorged). Low thoracic epidurals (around T10) might be used primarily for lower abdominal incisions.

Positioning and Nerve Injuries: In rectal cancer cases done in lithotomy and steep Trendelenburg (especially robotic-assisted surgeries), anesthesiologists must pad pressure points carefully and monitor for compartment syndrome risk in legs (long cases in lithotomy). The steep head-down position can increase intraocular pressure and facial edema; caution is needed in patients with glaucoma or intracranial pressure issues. Securing the airway well (taping and bite blocks) is important as well, given the shift in position.

Preventing Complications: Antibiotic prophylaxis is critical in colorectal surgery due to the clean-contaminated nature of entering the bowel; ensure appropriate broad-spectrum antibiotics (often cefazolin plus metronidazole, or a carbapenem in high-risk) are given timely and re-dosed during long cases. Thromboembolism prophylaxis is also crucial as cancer and pelvic surgery both increase risk (patients will often be started on heparin or enoxaparin soon after surgery, which the anesthesiologist should remember if considering neuraxial catheter removal timing). Postoperatively, common complications include ileus, anastomotic leak, and wound infection.The anesthesiologist can help reduce ileus by avoiding excess opioids and fluids, as described. If an epidural is in place, it may be continued 2–3 days for analgesia, which also coincides with the typical time frame for ileus resolution; epidural local anesthetics have a pro-motility effect by blocking sympathetic drive to the gut.

In essence, colorectal anesthesia aligns closely with ERAS principles: focus on euvolemia, excellent analgesia without heavy opioids, normothermia, and expeditious emergence (patients are often extubated deep in Trendelenburg at the end of the case to prevent coughing, which could stress fresh anastomoses in the pelvis). Proper coordination ensures the patient can participate in recovery activities (early diet, walking), which in turn reduces complications like pneumonia and venous thromboembolism.

Pancreatic and Hepatobiliary Cancers (Whipple Procedure, Liver Resections)

Pancreatic (Whipple) Surgery: Pancreaticoduodenectomy, or the Whipple procedure, performed for pancreatic head tumors (and some periampullary tumors), is one of the most extensive abdominal operations. It involves resection of the pancreatic head, duodenum, gallbladder, and part of the bile duct, with a complex reconstruction (pancreaticojejunostomy, hepaticojejunostomy, gastrojejunostomy). These cases often last 6-10 hours and can have large fluid shifts and blood loss. Anesthetic management for Whipple is demanding in terms of monitoring, fluid/blood management, and analgesia.

A thoracic epidural is commonly employed in open Whipple surgeries because it provides superior pain relief and helps attenuate the massive stress response to this surgery. Epidural analgesia in Whipple patients has been associated with improved postoperative pain control and possibly fewer pulmonary complications, though it requires careful intraoperative management to avoid hypotension.

One consideration: large fluid shifts and insensible losses occur (open abdominal cavity for many hours, evaporation, third-spacing due to extensive retroperitoneal dissection). The anesthesiologist should use goal-directed techniques (*e.g.*, cardiac output monitoring or stroke volume variation) to judiciously replace fluid. Pancreatic surgery teams often aim to avoid excessive crystalloids because fluid overload has been linked to higher rates of pancreatic anastomotic leak (pancreatic fistula). Some studies suggest that very liberal fluid administration may contribute to pancreatic edema and leak formation.

Therefore, maintaining a neutral fluid balance (avoiding unnecessary positive balance) is a strategy, sometimes combined with low-dose vasopressors to maintain perfusion rather than fluid boluses. Blood loss in a Whipple can be moderate (several hundred mL) to major (especially if the tumor involves vasculature and requires vein resection). Cross-matched blood should be available. Cell salvage can be considered, but is not universally used in oncologic surgery due to theoretical spread of tumor cells, though for pancreatic cancer, which rarely has gross tumor rupture, some centers do use cell salvage with a leukocyte filter.

Metabolic issues: If the patient has obstructive jaundice preoperatively (common in pancreatic head cancer), they may have impaired hepatic function and coagulopathy (vitamin K malabsorption). Often, these patients are stented preoperatively to relieve jaundice. But anesthesiologists should be mindful of liver function and, if possible, correct any coagulopathy beforehand (vitamin K administration, FFP if INR is significantly elevated).

Jaundice also increases the risk of renal failure (hepatorenal syndrome-like physiology), so maintain good renal perfusion (avoid hypotension, use vasopressors early if needed). Glucose management is important: the pancreas is manipulated and partly removed, so insulin/glucagon balance is disrupted. These patients may have significant intraoperative hyperglycemia; frequent glucose checks and an insulin infusion may be needed. Conversely, if a long procedure and a patient was kept NPO plus an epidural causing sympathectomy, they could become hypoglycemic, so close monitoring is advised.

Emergence and Disposition: After a Whipple, given the duration and fluid shifts, patients often go to the ICU intubated or at least for close monitoring. However, with ERAS, some centers extubate Whipple patients in the OR if they are stable and warm, to avoid ventilator-associated complications. The decision should be individualized based on blood loss, fluid status (severe edema or not), and pulmonary function. If extubated, a well-functioning epidural is invaluable for pain control to allow breathing and coughing.

Postoperative Concerns: Pancreatic fistula (leak from the pancreatic anastomosis) is a dreaded complication that can cause sepsis. There is some evidence (though not conclusive) that epidural analgesia might improve perfusion at the anastomosis by blocking splanchnic vasoconstriction, potentially reducing fistula rates – but data are limited. Pain from a pancreatic resection is significant; inadequate analgesia can contribute to splinting, atelectasis, and pneumonia, so multimodal analgesia is critical (epidural + IV acetaminophen, NSAIDs if renal function allows, *etc.*). Enhanced recovery protocols for Whipple also encourage early feeding (often *via* a jejunostomy tube) and mobilization by POD 1 or 2, which requires the anesthesiologist's efforts in minimizing opioids and preventing ileus.

Hepatobiliary (Liver Resections): Liver resections (for hepatocellular carcinoma or metastatic colorectal cancer to the liver, *etc.*) present a different set of challenges. The major intraoperative risks are hemorrhage and hemodynamic instability during manipulation of the liver (especially if inflow occlusion techniques are used). Anesthetic management often includes a strategy of low central venous pressure (CVP) during parenchymal transection to minimize venous bleeding from the hepatic veins [28]. This may involve limiting fluid administration and even giving diuretics or nitroglycerin to reduce CVP to a target (*e.g.*, <5 mmHg) when the surgeons are transecting the liver. The trade-off is that a low CVP can reduce preload and blood pressure, so one must carefully balance perfusion of vital organs. It requires close monitoring – invasive arterial pressure and often central venous pressure monitoring are used. An anesthesiologist may use a combination of phlebotomy, positioning (reverse Trendelenburg), and IV nitroglycerin to transiently lower CVP, while using vasopressors like norepinephrine to maintain arterial pressure to perfuse organs. As soon as the liver resection is done and hemostasis is achieved, volume is usually given to restore normal volume status.

Coagulation management is crucial: liver patients may have baseline coagulopathy if there is cirrhosis or cholestasis (vitamin K-dependent factors are low). During resection, bleeding can be rapid and massive, requiring the availability of blood products (packed RBCs, FFP, platelets). Rapid infusion systems and cell savers can be very useful here (though, again, tumor considerations apply; for primary liver tumors like HCC, cell salvage is sometimes avoided due to the risk of tumor spread if malignant cells were in the field). Thromboelastography (TEG/ROTEM) can guide blood product therapy during liver cases, as routine lab coagulation tests often lag.

Another consideration is post-resection physiology: removal of a large portion of the liver (especially >50%) can lead to a post-hepatectomy syndrome of coagulopathy, fluid shifts, and metabolic disturbances. These patients often require ICU care. Maintaining normothermia and normoglycemia is important – the liver is key in heat production and glucose homeostasis, and large resections can result in hypothermia and hypoglycemia intraoperatively. Frequent blood glucose checks are indicated.

Analgesia: Thoracic epidural analgesia in liver resection is debated. Many centers use epidurals for open liver resections because of the clear analgesic benefits. However, coagulopathy concerns are significant – if a patient has existing coagulopathy or is likely to get coagulopathic during surgery, an epidural could pose a bleeding risk upon removal. Some clinicians opt for alternative analgesia, like TAP blocks, to avoid an indwelling epidural in this context. If an epidural is placed, careful attention to the correction of coagulopathy before catheter removal is mandatory. For laparoscopic liver resections, regional blocks (TAP or paravertebral) plus systemic non-opioids can suffice since the incisions are smaller.

Special Situations: For cirrhotic patients undergoing liver resection, portal hypertension can cause large collateral vessels – bleeding risk is higher, and they may have severe ascites (which should be drained preoperatively to reduce respiratory compromise). Cirrhotics are very sensitive to anesthetic agents (with reduced hepatic metabolism, higher volume of distribution due to ascites and low albumin), so dosing should be cautious. Also, these patients often have esophageal varices; an NG tube should be placed with care (or avoided) not to rupture varices.

In conclusion, **major liver and pancreatic surgeries** demand an anesthesiologist who is vigilant and proactive: expecting rapid swings in volume status, using advanced monitoring (arterial line, CVP, possibly cardiac output monitoring), and coordinating with the surgical team on maneuvers like low CVP technique and clamping sequences. The emphasis is on maintaining end-organ perfusion while minimizing bleeding. Pain control is balanced with coagulopathy considerations, and often the postoperative phase is in the ICU. Enhanced recovery for these surgeries is still evolving but includes epidural use (if safe), early mobilization, and sometimes early oral intake (for liver resection, early feeding is usually fine; for Whipple, they might start tube feeds early).

Neuroendocrine Tumors and GISTs

Neuroendocrine Tumors (Carcinoid Syndrome): GI neuroendocrine tumors (NETs) – often arising in the small intestine, appendix, or pancreas – can produce a spectrum of hormones. The classic syndrome is carcinoid syndrome, usually from metastatic midgut carcinoid tumors that secrete serotonin and vasoactive substances. These patients present a unique intraoperative challenge: carcinoid crisis – a sudden release of massive amounts of tumor mediators – can be precipitated by stress, anesthesia induction, or tumor manipulation [29].

A carcinoid crisis is characterized by severe flushing, bronchospasm, tachycardia or bradycardia, and extreme blood pressure fluctuations (often profound hypotension that is resistant to conventional vasopressors) [29]. The primary prophylactic and therapeutic measure is the use of **somatostatin analogues**, namely octreotide. Octreotide binds to somatostatin receptors on the tumor and inhibits the release of serotonin and other vasoactive peptides [29]. Patients with known carcinoid syndrome are usually optimized before surgery with octreotide (*e.g.*, they may be on monthly long-acting octreotide injections). On the day of surgery, a continuous infusion of octreotide is typically run (*e.g.*, 50 μg/ hour) starting before induction and continued through the procedure. Additional boluses (50–100 μg IV) should be immediately available if signs of a carcinoid crisis appear.

Anesthetic management includes avoiding drugs or events that could trigger mediator release. Things to avoid or use carefully: histamine-releasing drugs (like morphine, atracurium – better to use fentanyl and cisatracurium instead), sympathetic stimulants (epinephrine can paradoxically cause the tumor to release more hormone; if needed, direct-acting vasopressors like phenylephrine or vasopressin are generally preferred over epinephrine). Induction should be smooth with adequate depth to prevent hypotension or bronchospasm on intubation. If a carcinoid crisis occurs (manifesting as sudden

hypotension and flushing/bronchospasm), the treatment is an IV octreotide bolus and aggressive supportive care. Conventional vasopressors alone often fail until octreotide is given. Thus, having a syringe of octreotide (100 μg/mL) at the bedside is critical.

Monitoring for these cases should be standard, plus an arterial line due to potential rapid hemodynamic swings. Volume status should be maintained; some carcinoid patients have chronic diarrhea and may be volume-depleted. They can also have cardiac involvement – carcinoid syndrome often leads to fibrotic plaques on the right side of the heart (tricuspid regurgitation and pulmonary stenosis are common), so a preoperative echocardiogram is indicated. If significant cardiac carcinoid disease is present (*e.g.*, heart failure), invasive monitoring like a central line and PA catheter could be considered, but often octreotide management suffices.

Gastrointestinal Stromal Tumors (GISTs): GISTs are mesenchymal tumors of the GI tract, often in the stomach or small intestine, driven by c-kit mutations. They typically do not cause carcinoid syndrome or hormone issues; the main concerns are related to their size and location. Large GISTs can be very vascular and prone to hemorrhage during resection. They can also undergo necrosis and bleeding preoperatively, so some patients might present with anemia. From an anesthesia perspective, having blood available for large GIST resections is wise. If the GIST is in a challenging location (like the gastric fundus requiring possibly a large incision), plan monitors and lines accordingly for a major case. Some patients may be on tyrosine kinase inhibitor therapy (imatinib) preoperatively to shrink the GIST. Imatinib's side effects include hepatic toxicity and cytopenia, so check liver function and blood counts.

Unlike carcinoids, GISTs generally do not cause intraoperative hemodynamic crises beyond what any large tumor resection might cause (bleeding, *etc.*). Therefore, management is similar to a standard gastric or intestinal resection with attention to volume and hemodynamics. Pain control can be *via* an epidural or an open approach.

Pheochromocytomas and Pancreatic NETs: It is worth noting that some pancreatic neuroendocrine tumors (*e.g.*, insulinomas, gastrinomas) or adrenal pheochromocytomas may be encountered; each has specific considerations (*e.g.*, insulinomas risk hypoglycemia during handling; pheochromocytomas require alpha-blockade preop and careful adrenergic management). If any functional tumor is present, appropriate preoperative medical optimization and intraoperative monitoring should be guided by the tumor's profile.

Pheochromocytomas, though arising from the adrenal medulla, may also occur in paraganglia throughout the abdomen and may be discovered incidentally during imaging or resection of GI malignancies. These tumors secrete excessive catecholamines, resulting in severe labile hypertension, tachyarrhythmias, and multi-system complications if not adequately blocked. The cornerstone of perioperative management is preoperative alpha-adrenergic blockade (typically with phenoxybenzamine or selective alpha-1 agents such as doxazosin) for at least 10–14 days prior to surgery to control blood pressure and reduce intraoperative catecholamine surges. Adequate alpha-blockade is assessed clinically by the absence of orthostatic hypotension and normalization of blood pressure. Beta-blockade may be added after alpha-blockade to control reflex tachycardia, but should never precede alpha-blockade to avoid unopposed vasoconstriction.

Intraoperatively, meticulous hemodynamic monitoring is critical. An arterial line should be in place prior to induction, and large-bore intravenous access or central line access is recommended. Induction and tumor manipulation are periods of high risk for hypertensive crises, which must be anticipated with vasodilators (nitroprusside, nicardipine, clevidipine) and short-acting beta-blockers (esmolol) readily available. Volatile anesthetics, propofol, and remifentanil are all appropriate; agents that release histamine (*e.g.*, morphine, atracurium) should be avoided. Post-resection, a sudden drop in catecholamine levels can precipitate hypotension, which may require aggressive volume resuscitation and vasopressor support. Continuous invasive monitoring should be maintained postoperatively in an ICU setting until hemodynamics stabilize. Optimal perioperative management of pheochromocytomas not only reduces cardiovascular complications but also minimizes delays in recovery and return to cancer therapy.

Perioperative Management and Complications

The perioperative period for a GI oncology surgery extends from intraoperative management into the postoperative recovery phase. Thoughtful anesthetic management can significantly influence the incidence of complications and the speed of recovery.

Intraoperative Monitoring and Goal-Directed Fluid Therapy: As discussed in procedure-specific sections, appropriate monitoring is essential; most major GI cancer surgeries warrant an arterial line for blood pressure monitoring and frequent labs (arterial blood gases, lactate, glucose). Central venous pressure monitoring is used selectively (commonly in liver cases or if large fluid shifts are expected). Additionally, many centers employ advanced hemodynamic monitors or point-of-care ultrasound to guide fluid and vasoactive management. Goal-directed fluid therapy (GDFT) involves titrating fluid administration to dynamic indices of volume responsiveness (such as stroke volume variation, pulse pressure variation, or fluid challenge responses) rather than giving large, empirically determined fixed volumes. GDFT in major abdominal surgery has been associated with improved tissue perfusion (measured by markers like lactate) and better organ function, such as improved gastrointestinal motility and earlier return of bowel function, as well as reduced postoperative complications like pulmonary edema [10].

The anesthesiologist should use a combination of crystalloids, colloids, and vasoactive drugs to maintain an adequate circulating volume and blood pressure that ensures end-organ perfusion (especially to the liver and kidneys, which are critical in these surgeries) without causing edema. A common approach is a relatively restrictive crystalloid strategy (to avoid salt and water overload) combined with small boluses given when hypoperfusion signs appear (guided by monitors). In lengthy cases, measuring hourly urine output (*via* a Foley catheter) and blood loss gives additional guidance. Near-infrared spectroscopy (NIRS) of cerebral or tissue oximetry can sometimes be used as a surrogate for perfusion adequacy, though not routinely.

Another intraoperative focus is **temperature management**. All abdominal cancer surgeries expose the patient to large open cavities or insufflation gases, leading to heat loss. Hypothermia contributes to coagulopathy, wound infection, and shivering (which raises oxygen consumption). Thus, active warming (forced-air warmers, fluid warmers) from the start is necessary. Normothermia is one of the components of ERAS that improves outcomes [9].

Postoperative Complications and their Management: Patients undergoing GI cancer surgery are at risk for various complications, and anesthetic management plays a role in both prevention and early recognition:

- **Respiratory Complications:** Atelectasis and pneumonia are common, particularly after upper abdominal or thoracic incisions (esophagectomy, gastrectomy). Good pain control (so the patient can cough and breathe deeply) is the main preventative measure – hence the emphasis on neuraxial analgesia. Incentive spirometry should be initiated as soon as the patient is awake. If high epidural blocks cause intercostal muscle weakness that might impair coughing, adjustments in epidural dosing may be needed (reducing local anesthetic concentration while retaining opioid for analgesia). Patients with pre-existing lung disease or smokers benefit from preoperative pulmonary rehabilitation (incentive spirometry training, bronchodilators) and should be extubated only when fully able to protect their airway. In some cases, short-term postoperative ventilation in the ICU is elected to stabilize respiratory status (for example, after a lengthy esophagectomy in a smoker with marginal pulmonary function).
- **Cardiovascular Instability:** Hypotension in the immediate postoperative period can result from epidural analgesia (sympathectomy), ongoing third-space losses, or bleeding. The anesthesiologist should ensure adequate intravascular volume before leaving the OR (using parameters like lactate clearance, hemodynamic monitor readings). Unrecognized internal bleeding (such as an anastomotic site hemorrhage or spleen injury) should always be in the differential for persistent hypotension; this underscores the importance of monitoring trends in heart rate, blood pressure, abdominal drain outputs, and hemoglobin levels post-op. Patients at high risk (post liver resection) will have frequent lab checks and ICU

monitoring for this reason.

- **Ileus:** Postoperative ileus (delayed return of bowel motility) plagues many abdominal surgeries. It can lead to abdominal distension, discomfort, inability to tolerate oral intake, and risk of pulmonary complications. Anesthetic contributions to minimizing ileus include limiting intraoperative opioids (as emphasized earlier), using epidural local anesthetic (which encourages gut motility *via* sympathetic blockade) and maintaining euvolemia (neither dry nor overloaded, as both extremes can affect gut perfusion and motility). When ileus does occur, supportive management with IV fluids, sometimes nasogastric decompression, and minimizing opioids will continue. Alvimopan, a peripheral opioid antagonist, is used in some institutions to accelerate GI recovery if opioids were used.
- **Anastomotic Leak:** Leaks after GI anastomoses (esophageal, gastric, colorectal, pancreatic, *etc.*) are serious complications causing sepsis. While primarily surgical in origin, anesthetic management can influence factors like tissue perfusion (through blood pressure management, oxygenation), as mentioned. The anesthesiologist should maintain adequate mean arterial pressure (MAP >65 mmHg or higher, depending on the patient's baseline) throughout surgery to ensure organ perfusion. Postoperatively, signs of a possible leak may include tachycardia, fever, abdominal pain, or drainage of succus/pus from drains. In the PACU or ICU, any such signs should prompt immediate communication with the surgical team and possibly imaging (like a CT scan with contrast) to diagnose a leak early.
- **Venous Thromboembolism (VTE):** Cancer and major surgery both confer a high risk for VTE (deep vein thrombosis, pulmonary embolism). While mechanical prophylaxis (compression boots) is started intraoperatively, pharmacologic prophylaxis with low-molecular-weight heparin is usually started 6–12 hours after surgery if bleeding risk allows. Anesthesiologists need to coordinate the timing of neuraxial catheter removal with these anticoagulants. Many GI cancer patients will remain on prophylactic anticoagulation for weeks after surgery. High suspicion for VTE should be maintained if a patient has unexplained tachycardia or hypoxia post-op; a prompt workup for PE might be warranted.
- **Pain and Delirium:** Uncontrolled pain can lead to tachycardia, hypertension, and delirium, which can then precipitate other complications (cardiac ischemia, poor respiratory effort). Thus, ensuring the analgesic plan is effective is a core responsibility. Conversely, overly deep sedation from analgesics can also cause delirium or respiratory depression. Achieving the right balance with multimodal analgesia and frequent reassessment is key. In older patients, the use of dexmedetomidine for ICU sedation can sometimes reduce delirium compared to benzodiazepines.

Return to Intended Oncologic Therapy (RIOT): A critical concept in oncology and anesthesia is facilitating the patient's timely return to any adjuvant therapy (chemotherapy, radiation) that is indicated after surgery. Delays in starting or resuming systemic therapy due to surgical complications can adversely impact long-term survival.Perioperative care is thus not only about the surgery itself, but also about enabling the patient to continue their cancer treatment trajectory. An example metric that has been proposed is RIOT – the time from surgery to the resumption of intended oncologic therapy. Anesthesiologists can influence RIOT by reducing complications (through all the measures described) and proactively managing issues that do arise, so they resolve faster. For instance, a study found that improving postoperative analgesia with intraperitoneal local anesthetic in ovarian cancer debulking surgery allowed chemotherapy to begin earlier than in controls. Early mobilization (to build strength), excellent pain control, and prevention of infections and respiratory complications all contribute to a shorter convalescence period. This underscores that the goals of anesthesia in cancer surgery extend beyond the immediate operative survival – they include setting the patient up for the best chance at oncologic success by optimizing recovery.

In practical terms, during the immediate post-op phase in the PACU or ICU, the anesthesiologist or intensivist should diligently address each recovery pillar: pain, hydration/nutrition, pulmonary toileting, and mental status. If a patient can be extubated early, ambulates on day 1, has minimal ileus with early feeding, and suffers no major complications, they are likely to start adjuvant chemotherapy on schedule (usually 4–6 weeks post-op for many regimens). Each deviation (an infection requiring antibiotics, a readmission for dehydration) could delay therapy. Thus, anesthesia's role in fast-tracking recovery cannot be overstated, it is a direct contributor to long-term cancer outcomes.

FUTURE DIRECTIONS AND ADVANCES IN GI ONCO-ANESTHESIA

The field of onco-anesthesia is rapidly evolving, with a strong emphasis on integrating perioperative care into the overall cancer care pathway. Several future directions and innovations are on the horizon:

Enhanced Recovery and Beyond: ERAS protocols will continue to be refined and expanded. One future direction is tailoring ERAS to specific populations – for instance, developing geriatric-specific ERAS pathways for older cancer patients or "precision ERAS" where fluid and analgesia strategies are personalized to an individual's risk profile. Additionally, the ERAS concept is extending into prehabilitation (as discussed) and even into the postoperative long-term care (sometimes termed Enhanced Recovery After Cancer Treatment, ERAC). Anesthesiologists will increasingly be involved not just in the immediate perioperative period but also in survivorship optimization, such as managing chronic pain syndromes from surgery or neuropathies from chemotherapy.

Minimally Invasive and Robotic Surgery: The advent of robotic-assisted surgery, especially for colorectal and esophageal cancers, has implications for anesthesia. Robotic surgeries often mean longer operative times (especially during the learning curve) and require specific patient positioning (steep Trendelenburg for pelvic cases, or lateral/prone for some esophagectomies) that can affect physiology. As robotic techniques become standard, anesthesiologists are adapting strategies to manage the associated challenges, including prolonged steep Trendelenburg, which increases intracranial pressure and facial edema. Strategies like slight head elevation when feasible, careful fluid restriction, and using shorter-acting anesthetics to allow prompt emergence are used.

Robotic thoraco-laparoscopic esophagectomy may require the patient to be repositioned mid-surgery (from supine to prone or lateral, for example), which necessitates secure airway management and vigilant pressure point padding. The future will see even less invasive approaches (natural orifice transluminal surgery, more endoscopic tumor resections), which might shift some traditionally surgical patients into procedural sedation cases (*e.g.*, advanced endoscopic resections of early tumors). Anesthesiology will need to cover these with non-operating room anesthesia expertise. Overall, minimally invasive surgery has the benefit of reduced pain and quicker recovery, which aligns with anesthesia goals of minimal opioids and fast-tracking. We may see more ambulatory cancer surgeries for select cases (for instance, some colon cancer surgeries are now done with a 1-night stay or even same-day discharge in ERAS superfast-track programs), which challenges anesthesiologists to provide surgical anesthesia that wears off quickly and postoperative analgesia that is robust yet allows discharge.

Novel Immunomodulatory Techniques: Research is ongoing into drugs that might favorably modulate the perioperative immune environment. Some areas of interest include: perioperative beta-blockade (as mentioned) to reduce stress; α-2 agonists like dexmedetomidine, not just for sedation but for their potential to preserve Th1/Th2 immune balance (though results have been mixed as noted); Intravenous lidocaine for its anti-inflammatory effect; and even agents like tranexamic acid, which aside from reducing bleeding, might have anti-inflammatory benefits. On the horizon, we might see trials of administering checkpoint inhibitor therapy or cancer vaccines around the time of surgery. For example, one could envision a protocol where, a day after surgery, the patient receives an immunotherapy dose to capitalize on the release of tumor antigens during surgery – essentially turning surgery into an immune "vaccine" event. Anesthesiologists will collaborate in these trials to ensure patients are stable and to monitor for immune-related adverse events if such therapies are given in the perioperative setting.

Another area is pharmacogenomics and precision medicine in anesthesia – perhaps identifying patients who are more susceptible to immunosuppression from opioids or volatiles and tailoring anesthetic drugs accordingly. Research into biomarkers of immune function (like measuring circulating NK cell activity perioperatively) could guide how aggressively to pursue certain techniques for a given patient.

In summary, the next phase of GI onco-anesthesia is characterized by innovation and integration: integrating anesthetic care with surgical oncology and medical oncology and innovating with new techniques and drugs to improve patient outcomes not just in the OR, but months and years after. The hope is that by refining anesthetic techniques, we can contribute to the goal of oncology care, not only a successful surgery but also a cure or prolonged survival.

CONCLUSION

GI oncology patients require a meticulous, evidence-based anesthetic approach that addresses their unique challenges. We have reviewed how patient factors like malnutrition or neoadjuvant therapy effects must be optimized preoperatively, and how intraoperative management should prioritize hemodynamic stability, adequate oxygenation, and pain control while minimizing stress responses. Anesthesiologists play a pivotal role in Enhanced Recovery After Surgery protocols for GI cancer – by employing multimodal analgesia (epidurals, blocks, non-opioid adjuncts) and goal-directed fluid therapy with fewer complications and faster recovery [9, 10]. Procedure-specific nuances, from one-lung ventilation in esophagectomies to low CVP techniques in liver resections, must be mastered to ensure patient safety and optimal outcomes. Postoperatively, vigilant management aimed at preventing and treating complications (respiratory issues, ileus, *etc.*) can make the difference in a patient's ability to resume chemotherapy or other treatments on schedule.

Throughout, a common theme is the integration of anesthetic care with the broader oncologic treatment plan. Every decision, choice of anesthetic agent, analgesic technique, and transfusion threshold is made not only for immediate surgical success but also considering potential impacts on tumor biology and the patient's long-term prognosis. While definitive evidence is still emerging regarding anesthesia's influence on cancer recurrence, we have adopted practices that are theoretically beneficial and, at a minimum, do no harm: *e.g.*, using regional anesthesia and TIVA when appropriate, avoiding excessive opioids and transfusions, and tightly controlling perioperative physiology [20].

As research advances, anesthesiology may become an even more active partner in cancer care, possibly administering targeted therapies perioperatively or customizing anesthesia based on tumor immunology.

In conclusion, the care of GI oncology patients exemplifies the need for precision, vigilance, and a multimodal strategy in anesthesiology. By adhering to ERAS protocols, leveraging regional anesthesia, and staying attuned to oncologic considerations, anesthesiologists significantly improve patient outcomes, not only reducing surgical stress and complications but also potentially impacting long-term survival. Ongoing and future studies will further clarify how we can modulate the perioperative period to enhance cancer care. In the meantime, our focus remains on providing safe, effective anesthesia that aligns with oncologic goals: extubating a well-analgesic, hemodynamically stable patient who can recover swiftly and continue the fight against cancer with minimal delay. This integration of innovation with evidence-based practice is at the heart of anesthesia for GI oncology, ultimately striving to improve both perioperative and oncologic results for our patients.

REFERENCES

[1] Hariharan U, Garg R. Anesthesia for Gastrointestinal Cancer Surgeries. In: Garg R, Bhatnagar S, Eds. Textbook of Onco-Anesthesiology. Singapore: Springer 2021; pp. 217-25. [http://dx.doi.org/10.1007/978-981-16-0006-7_14]

[2] Keane E, Nestor C. Implications of Anaesthesia on Cancer Surgery. Anaesthesia Tutorial of the Week 487, World Federation of Societies of Anaesthesiologists (WFSA); Dec 20, 2022.

[3] Feldheiser A, Aziz O, Baldini G, *et al.* Enhanced Recovery After Surgery (ERAS) for gastrointestinal surgery, part 2: consensus statement for anaesthesia practice. Acta Anaesthesiol Scand 2016; 60(3): 289-334. [http://dx.doi.org/10.1111/aas.12651] [PMID: 26514824]

[4] Chan A, *et al.* Prehabilitation in gastrointestinal cancer surgery: results from the PREHAB-GI study. Support Care Cancer in press

[5] Allan N, Siller C, Breen A. Anaesthetic implications of chemotherapy. Contin Educ Anaesth Crit Care Pain 2012; 12(2): 52-6. [http://dx.doi.org/10.1093/bjaceaccp/mkr055]

[6] Evans MT, Wigmore T, Kelliher LJS. The impact of anaesthetic technique upon outcome in oncological surgery. BJA Educ 2019; 19(1): 14-20. [http://dx.doi.org/10.1016/j.bjae.2018.09.008] [PMID: 33456849]

[7] Wigmore TJ, Mohammed K, Jhanji S. Long-term survival for patients undergoing volatile versus IV anesthesia for cancer surgery: a retrospective analysis. Anesthesiology 2016; 124(1): 69-79. [http://dx.doi.org/10.1097/ALN.0000000000000936] [PMID: 26556730]

[8] Yap A, Lopez-Olivo MA, Dubowitz J, *et al.* Anesthetic technique and cancer outcomes: a meta-analysis of total intravenous versus volatile anesthesia. Can J Anaesth 2019; 66(5): 546-61. [http://dx.doi.org/10.1007/s12630-019-01330-x] [PMID: 30834506]

[9] Sessler DI, Pei L, Huang Y, *et al.* Recurrence of breast cancer after regional or general anaesthesia: a randomised controlled trial. Lancet 2019; 394(10211): 1807-15. [http://dx.doi.org/10.1016/S0140-6736(19)32313-X] [PMID: 31645288]

[10] Du YT, Li YW, Zhao BJ, *et al.* Long-term survival after combined epidural-general anesthesia or general anesthesia alone: follow-up of a randomized trial. Anesthesiology 2021; 135(2): 233-45. [http://dx.doi.org/10.1097/ALN.0000000000003835] [PMID: 34195784]

[11] Grandhi RK, Lee S, Abd-Elsayed A. The relationship between regional anesthesia and cancer: a meta-analysis. Ochsner J 2017; 17(4): 345-61. [PMID: 29230120]

[12] Amato A, Pescatori M. Perioperative blood transfusions and recurrence of colorectal cancer. Cochrane Libr 2006; 2011(2): CD005033. [http://dx.doi.org/10.1002/14651858.CD005033.pub2] [PMID: 16437512]

[13] Agnes A, *et al.* Prognostic role of perioperative blood transfusions in gastric cancer surgery: systematic review and meta-analysis. Eur J Surg Oncol 2018; 44(4): 404-19. [http://dx.doi.org/10.1016/j.ejso.2018.01.006] [PMID: 29398320]

[14] Kinney MAO, Warner ME, Nagorney DM, *et al.* Perianaesthetic risks and outcomes of abdominal surgery for metastatic carcinoid tumours. Br J Anaesth 2001; 87(3): 447-52. [http://dx.doi.org/10.1093/bja/87.3.447] [PMID: 11517130]

[15] Cata JP, *et al.* Effects of anesthetic agents and techniques on oncologic outcomes: a narrative review. Br J Anaesth 2019; 123(2): 135-50. [http://dx.doi.org/10.1016/j.bja.2019.04.062] [PMID: 31255291]

[16] Hariharan U, Garg R. Anesthesia for Gastrointestinal Cancer Surgeries. SpringerLink: https://link.springer.com/chapter/10.1007/978-981-16-0006-7_14 [http://dx.doi.org/10.1007/978-981-16-0006-7_14]

[17] Hariharan U, Garg R. Anesthesia for Esophageal Surgery. SpringerLink: https://link.springer.com/chapter/10.1007/978-3-031-39086-9_11

[18] WFSA. Implications of Anaesthesia on Cancer Surgery. Available from: https://resources.wfsahq.org/atotw/implications-of-anaesthesia-on-cancer-surgery/

[19] Feldheiser A, Aziz O, Baldini G, *et al.* Enhanced Recovery After Surgery (ERAS) for gastrointestinal surgery, part 2: consensus statement for anaesthesia practice. Acta anaesthesiologica Scandinavica 2016; 60(3): 289–334. [http://dx.doi.org/10.1111/aas.12651]

[20] Gao M, Chen M, Dai G, Zhu D Cai Y. Clinical study: the impact of goal-directed fluid therapy on volume management during enhanced recovery after surgery in gastrointestinal procedures. Acta Biochim 2024; Pol 71: 12377. [http://dx.doi.org/10.3389/abp.2024.12377]

[21] Raso KL, Suen M, Egger S. *et al.* Moving from theory to practice: implementing a prehabilitation program before gastrointestinal cancer surgery (PREHAB-GI). Support Care Cancer 2025; 33: 458. [http://dx.doi.org/10.1007/s00520-025-09496-5]

[22] Allan N, Siller C, Breen A, Anaesthetic implications of chemotherapy, Continuing Education in Anaesthesia Critical Care & Pain 2012; 12(2): 52–6. [http://dx.doi.org/10.1093/bjaceaccp/mkr055]

[23] Cai Q, Liu G, Huang L, *et al.* The Role of Dexmedetomidine in Tumor-Progressive Factors in the Perioperative Period and Cancer Recurrence: A Narrative Review. Drug Des Devel Ther 2022; 16: 2161-75. [http://dx.doi.org/10.2147/DDDT.S358042]

[24] Triantafyllou A, Mela E, Theodoropoulos C, *et al.* Addressing Anastomotic Leak After Esophagectomy: Insights from a Specialized Unit. J Clin Med 2025; 14(11): 3694. [http://dx.doi.org/10.3390/jcm14113694] [PMID: 40507455] [PMCID: PMC12156875]

[25] Desiderio J, Trastulli S, D'Andrea V, Parisi A. Enhanced recovery after surgery for gastric cancer

(ERAS-GC): optimizing patient outcome. Transl Gastroenterol Hepatol 2020; 5: 11.
[http://dx.doi.org/10.21037/tgh.2019.10.04]

[26] De Pietri L, Montalti R, Begliomini B. Anaesthetic perioperative management of patients with pancreatic cancer. World J Gastroenterol 2014; 20(9): 2304-20.
[http://dx.doi.org/10.3748/wjg.v20.i9.2304] [PMID: 24605028] [PMCID: PMC3942834]

[27] Linares A, Pabloa J Quiroz E, *et al.* Analysis of complications after Whipple's procedure using ERAS protocols. Colombian Journal of Anesthesiology 2019; 47(4): 219-25.
[http://dx.doi.org/10.1097/CJ9.0000000000000140]

[28] Goal Directed Fluid Therapy During Pancreatico-Duodenectomy. Available from: https://www.menoufia-med-j.com/cgi/viewcontent.cgi?article=1139&context=journal

[29] Carcinoid Syndrome. OpenAnesthesia. Available from: https://www.openanesthesia.org/keywords/carcinoid-syndrome/

[30] Wu H, Liu Q, Zhang N, *et al.* Road of recovery in gastrointestinal surgery: From ERAS to FRAS. Gastroenterology & Endoscopy 2024; 2(2): 84-9.

CHAPTER 16

Management and Treatment of Pain in Cancer Patients

Kingsuk Ganguly[1,*]

[1] *Department of Anesthesiology, Cooper Medical School of Rowan University, Cooper University Health Care, Camden, NJ, USA*

Abstract: Cancer pain is a complex condition that significantly impacts the quality of life in patients at all stages of disease. Effective pain management requires a nuanced understanding of the underlying causes of pain. This chapter provides a comprehensive review of cancer pain management strategies, with evidence-based approaches to assessment and treatment.

Keywords: Adjuvant analgesics, Breakthrough pain, Cancer pain, Chemotherapy-induced peripheral neuropathy, Cognitive-behavioral therapy, Epidural injections, Gene therapy, Intrathecal drug delivery, Interventional pain management, Multidisciplinary care.

INTRODUCTION

Pain secondary to malignancy is a prevalent symptom experienced by cancer patients. Chronic pain is defined as pain that persists or recurs for more than three months. Along with the distressing symptoms already faced by a cancer patient, pain on top can further exacerbate complications and the treatment process. It can arise at any stage of the disease, due to the tumor itself, treatments, or other medical factors related to the patient's condition. Effective pain management is essential for reducing suffering but also plays a crucial role in enhancing the patient's functional ability and psychological state. Despite advances in medical therapies, pain in cancer patients remains under-treated in many cases, often due to misconceptions about opioid use, inadequate assessment, or challenges in managing complex pain syndromes. It is important for the clinician to employ a comprehensive, multidisciplinary approach that includes both pharmacological and non-pharmacological methods to help optimize pain control and improve quality of life for cancer patients at every stage.

* **Corresponding author Kingsuk Ganguly:** Department of Anesthesiology, Cooper Medical School of Rowan University, Cooper University Health Care, Camden, NJ, USA; E-mail: ganguly-kingsuk@cooperhealth.edu

Bharathi Gourkanti, Irwin Gratz, William Marion, Rajiv Lingaraju & Grace Abramian (Eds.)

Pathophysiology of Cancer Pain

Cancer pain arises from multiple mechanisms, each contributing to the complexity of pain perception in oncology patients [1]. Pain can be broadly classified into two main categories: 1. nociceptive pain and 2. neuropathic pain. The additional diagnosis of cancer leads to tumor and treatment-related factors, which also play a role [2].

Nociceptive pain is a type of pain that occurs due to tissue damage or inflammation, leading to activation of peripheral nociceptors that transmit pain signals throughout the nervous system [3]. Nociceptive pain can be broadly divided into two sources:

1. Somatic pain originates from bones, muscles, joints, or connective tissues. Somatic pain is well-localized and can be characterized as aching, sharp, or throbbing in nature and can often exacerbate with mobility. With regard to cancer pain, bone metastases can be a common cause [4].
2. Visceral pain originates from internal organs such as the intestines, liver, or pancreas. This pain is characterized as diffuse and dull and can be accompanied by referred pain. Tumors encapsulating the gastrointestinal tract or liver can lead to this type of pain [5].

Neuropathic pain occurs due to nerve damage, either due to the tumor itself or as a result of treatment [6]. It is characterized by burning, shooting, sharp, tingling, or electrical shock-like sensations. Nociceptive pain is usually more responsive to conventional analgesics as opposed to neuropathic pain [7]. A tumor can infiltrate the nerves, leading to direct compression and severe symptoms.

Cancer itself can be a source of pain, arising from various mechanisms [8].Tumors invade and compress nerves, bones, and soft tissues, leading to inflammatory and neuropathic pain. Metastatic disease due to the bone leads to pathologic fractures and inflammatory cytokine release [9]. Tumors can obstruct organs and tracts in the gastrointestinal and genitourinary system, causing colicky visceral pain secondary to distension [10]. Vascular compression from tumors induces ischemic pain. Metastatic disease from breast cancer, lung cancer, melanoma, and lymphoma can lead to Leptomeningeal carcinomatosis, a condition where infiltration of the meninges causes headaches, nausea, vomiting, as well as sensory and motor deficits [11].

Treatment modalities such as chemotherapy can induce chronic peripheral neuropathy [12]. Chemotherapy-induced peripheral neuropathy (CIPN) agents, such as platinum-based drugs, taxanes, and vinca alkaloids, are known culprits that can damage peripheral nerves during treatment [13]. Furthermore, post-surgical nerve injury can introduce trauma in cancer-related surgeries, and Radiation-induced nerve damage can cause fibrosis and scarring, resulting in neuropathic pain syndromes [14]. The table below summarizes common causes of treatment-related pain (Table **1**).

Table 1. Common causes of cancer-treatment related pain.

Cause	Examples
Chemotherapy-related pain	Peripheral neuropathy (*e.g.*, platinum-based drugs, taxanes)
-	Mucositis and stomatitis (*e.g.*, methotrexate, fluorouracil)
-	Myalgia and arthralgia (*e.g.*, paclitaxel, aromatase inhibitors)
Radiation therapy-induced pain	Fibrosis and scarring cause chronic pain
-	Brachial plexopathy from radiation exposure in breast cancer
-	Osteoradionecrosis leading to bone pain
Surgical pain	Post-mastectomy pain syndrome
-	Phantom limb pain following amputation
-	Post-thoracotomy pain syndrome due to intercostal nerve damage

Effective cancer pain management involves a thorough understanding of these pathophysiological mechanisms, allowing clinicians to tailor multimodal treatment strategies that address the underlying cause of pain and improve patient outcomes [15]. Pain in cancer patients can be acute, chronic, or breakthrough pain. Acute pain arises immediately and is usually self-limited [16]. This can be secondary to acute post-operative surgical procedures or tumor growth. Chronic pain persists 3-6 months beyond the normal course of expected healing and can arise from cancer progression or treatment-related effects [17]. Breakthrough pain is a transient event that can result in intermittent exacerbations despite ongoing analgesia treatment [18].

Pain Assessment in Cancer Patients

A comprehensive pain assessment in cancer patients should include a detailed history and physical examination, a quantifying pain scale, psychological assessment, and pertinent diagnostic imaging to identify underlying causes and guide treatment [15].

History should include the character, onset, location, duration, intensity, exacerbation, and relieving factors [15]. Impact on activities of daily living (ADLs), level of function, and sleep must be documented. A patient's history of response to previous pain treatments is important to help guide what treatments are more likely to be effective [19].

Physical examination should evaluate the location of pain and any associated neuropathic signs such as numbness, tingling, allodynia, or hyperalgesia to palpation [1]. Musculoskeletal tenderness and neurological reflexes must be checked. Tumor related burden of disease may also be palpated and can serve as pressure points of pain [20].

The use of pain scales helps quantify pain using standardized assessment tools [21]. A Numerical Rating Scale (NRS) is the most commonly used, with patients rating their pain on a scale from 0 (no pain) to 10 (worst pain). The Visual Analog Scale involves a 10 cm line where the patient marks their pain level [22]. Inventories and questionnaires are routinely provided to patients prior to assessment, which can help patients document the severity of the pain and its impact on daily activities as well as evaluate sensory and affective pain dimensions. The Brief Pain Inventory (BPI) [23] and McGill Pain Questionnaire [24] are two such examples, respectively.

Psychological assessment of pain perception should also be assessed as multiple factors, such as preexisting depression or anxiety, are known to exacerbate pain [25]. Depression and anxiety screening includes PHQ-9 and GAD-7 [26]. Cognitive behavioral screening can help a clinician understand what pain coping mechanisms a patient uses [27]. It is important to incorporate a patient's personal beliefs about pain, such as opioid use, elective interventions, and social support.

The role of diagnostic imaging can help further elucidate the causes of pain [28]. Plain film x-rays are able to assess bone fractures secondary to tumors and metastatic disease. Advanced imaging, such as CT and MRI, evaluates soft tissue and nerve involvement [29]. Clinicians routinely use bone and PET scans as surveillance studies to detect metastases, lesions, and systemic tumor burden [30]. Patients undergoing chemotherapy are known to suffer from peripheral neuropathies, which can be confirmed by electromyography (EMG) and nerve conduction studies [31].

Effective pain assessment ensures targeted and individualized treatment strategies, optimizing patient comfort and quality of life [15].

Pharmacological Pain Management

The World Health Organization (WHO) Pain Ladder is a guideline for managing cancer pain, advocating a stepwise approach to analgesia [32]:

1. Mild pain → Non-opioid analgesics (*e.g.*, NSAIDs, acetaminophen).
2. Moderate pain → Weak opioids (*e.g.*, codeine, tramadol) ± non-opioids.
3. Severe pain → Strong opioids (*e.g.*, morphine, fentanyl) ± non-opioids ± adjuvants.

This structured approach ensures appropriate pain relief while minimizing opioid-related side effects [33].

Non-Opioid Analgesics

Non-opioid medications are the first-line treatment for mild to moderate cancer pain and can be used in combination with others for multimodal analgesia [17]. Non-steroidal anti-inflammatory drugs (NSAIDs) and Acetaminophen can be effective for mild to moderate pain relief [34]. Some formulations are available over the counter, while others are prescribed as first-line agents for pain (Table **2**).

Table 2. First line agents for mild to moderate pain.

Class	Examples	Mechanism & Use
NSAIDs	Ibuprofen, Naproxen, Celecoxib	Effective for bone metastases and inflammatory pain due to anti-inflammatory properties□4□.
Acetaminophen (Paracetamol)	Acetaminophen	Preferred for mild pain due to lower gastrointestinal and renal toxicity but lacks anti-inflammatory effects □34□.

Adjuvant analgesics are useful for neuropathic pain [35]. Antidepressants such as amitriptyline, duloxetine, and anticonvulsants such as gabapentin and pregabalin are the most commonly used [36, 37]. Duloxetine is a serotonin-norepinephrine reuptake inhibitor (SNRI) that has been shown to be effective for chemotherapy-induced peripheral neuropathy and other neuropathic pain syndromes [38]. Steroids reduce inflammation-related pain, particularly in cases of spinal cord compression or peritumoral edema [39]. The table below summarizes common adjuvants used for cancer pain (Table **3**).

Table 3. Adjuvant agents for cancer-related pain.

Adjuvant Agent	Drug Class	Mechanism of Action	Indications	Common Side Effects
Amitriptyline	Tricyclic antidepressant (TCA)	Inhibits reuptake of serotonin and norepinephrine; anticholinergic effects	Neuropathic pain, insomnia	Dry mouth, sedation, orthostatic hypotension

(Table 3) cont.....

Adjuvant Agent	Drug Class	Mechanism of Action	Indications	Common Side Effects
Duloxetine	SNRI	Serotonin-norepinephrine reuptake inhibition	Chemotherapy-induced peripheral neuropathy (CIPN)	Nausea, fatigue, and sexual dysfunction
Gabapentin	Anticonvulsant	Inhibits voltage-gated calcium channels in the CNS	Neuropathic pain, CIPN	Drowsiness, dizziness, peripheral edema
Pregabalin	Anticonvulsant	Similar to gabapentin, more predictable absorption	Neuropathic pain, fibromyalgia, CIPN	Weight gain, somnolence, blurred vision
Lidocaine (topical)	Local anesthetic	Blocks sodium channels to inhibit peripheral nerve signaling	Localized neuropathic pain	Skin irritation, systemic toxicity (rare)
Dexamethasone	Corticosteroid	Anti-inflammatory, and reduces peritumoral edema	Bone pain, liver capsule distension, CNS metastases	Hyperglycemia, insomnia, immunosuppression

Muscle Relaxants

Muscle relaxants can be beneficial in cancer pain patients experiencing spasticity, muscle tension, or secondary musculoskeletal pain [40]. Common agents include Baclofen, a GABA-B receptor agonist that reduces muscle spasticity and can help with neuropathic pain. Tizanidine, methocarbamol, and cyclobenzaprine are also popular choices. The table below summarizes the most commonly used muscle relaxants (Table **4**).

Table 4. Muscle relaxants used for cancer-related pain.

Muscle Relaxant	Mechanism of Action	Indications	Common Side Effects
Baclofen	GABA-B receptor agonist	Spasticity, neuropathic pain	Sedation, dizziness; use with caution in renal impairment
Tizanidine	Alpha-2 adrenergic agonist	Muscle spasm, mild analgesia.	Hypotension, dry mouth, liver enzyme elevation.
Methocarbamol	Central depressant action, exact mechanism unknown.	Musculoskeletal pain, cancer-related fatigue.	Drowsiness, dizziness
Cyclobenzaprine	Centrally acting skeletal muscle relaxant, structurally related to TCAs.	Muscle spasm, tension-related pain.	Dry mouth, drowsiness, confusion; avoid in the elderly.

Novel Agents

Several novel pharmacological agents are being explored for cancer pain management, particularly for refractory pain (Table **5**). This includes cannabinoids, lidocaine infusions, and ketamine, an NMDA receptor antagonist used in general anesthesia for patients with high opioid tolerance [41].

Table 5. Novel agents for cancer-related pain.

Novel Agents	Mechanism of Action	Indications	Common Side Effects
Cannabinoids	Modulate the endocannabinoid system.	Neuropathic pain, chemotherapy-induced nausea.	Drowsiness, dizziness, cognitive changes, dry mouth.
Ketamine	NMDA receptor antagonist.	Opioid-resistant pain, severe neuropathic pain.	Hallucinations, elevated BP/HR, nausea, dissociation.
Lidocaine Infusion	Sodium channel blocker.	Refractory neuropathic pain syndromes.	Perioral numbness, tinnitus, dizziness, cardiac arrhythmias.

Opioids

Opioids remain the mainstay for moderate to severe cancer pain [42]. Opioids act primarily on mu, kappa, and delta opioid receptors to inhibit nociceptive transmission at both spinal and supraspinal levels [43]. The choice of opioid is guided by individual patient response, renal and hepatic function, and history of prior opioid exposure. With chronic cancer pain, consideration of opioid rotation is necessary when efficacy wanes or side effects become intolerable [44]. Equianalgesic dosing and careful cross-titration are essential to avoid withdrawal and overdose, respectively [45].

Common agents include morphine, fentanyl, oxycodone, hydromorphone, methadone, and buprenorphine (Table **6**). Dosing strategies of these medications must ensure careful titration for optimal pain relief while minimizing adverse effects. The table below summarizes commonly used opioids in cancer pain management:

Table 6. Commonly used opioids for cancer-related pain.

Opioid	Mechanism of Action	Onset of Action	Duration of Action	Common Side Effects
Morphine	Mu-opioid receptor agonist	15–30 min (oral)	3–6 hours (IR)	Constipation, nausea, sedation, pruritus

(Table 6) cont.....

Opioid	Mechanism of Action	Onset of Action	Duration of Action	Common Side Effects
Hydromorphone	Mu-opioid receptor agonist	15–30 min (oral)	4–5 hours	Respiratory depression, dizziness
Oxycodone	Mu- and kappa-opioid receptor agonist	10–15 min (oral)	3–6 hours	Dry mouth, constipation, fatigue
Fentanyl	Mu-opioid receptor agonist	5–15 min (IV)	30–60 min (IV)	Bradycardia, hypotension, chest wall rigidity
Methadone	Mu-opioid agonist + NMDA antagonist	30-45 min (oral)	8–12 hours (avg)	QT prolongation, sedation, serotonin syndrome
Buprenorphine	Partial mu-agonist, kappa antagonist	30–60 min (transdermal)	72 hours (patch)	Ceiling effect on respiratory depression

Common side effects from all opioids include constipation, sedation, nausea, tolerance, and dependence. Clinicians must balance pain control with the risk of dependence and opioid-induced hyperalgesia. The table below summarizes common side effects of opioids and their management (Table **7**).

Table 7. Opioid side effects & management.

Side Effect	Description	Management Strategies
Constipation	Very common due to decreased GI motility.	Prophylactic laxatives (*e.g.*, senna, polyethylene glycol), increased fluid intake [46].
Sedation	Often seen during initiation or dose escalation.	Dose adjustment, use of stimulant medications if needed (*e.g.*, modafinil).
Nausea	It can occur with initiation or dose increase.	Antiemetics such as ondansetron, metoclopramide [47].
Opioid Tolerance	Diminished effect over time, requiring higher doses.	Rotate opioids, use multimodal analgesia [48].
Dependence/Addiction	Physical dependence and risk of misuse, especially with long-term use.	Careful monitoring, risk assessment, and consider referral to pain or addiction specialists [49].
Opioid-Induced Hyperalgesia	Paradoxical increased sensitivity to pain due to opioid use.	Reduce opioid dose, switch agents, consider NMDA antagonists like ketamine [50].

A multimodal approach integrating these pharmacologic strategies allows for better pain control while minimizing opioid burden, improving the overall quality of life for cancer patients.

Non-Pharmacological Pain Management

Non-pharmacological approaches to cancer pain management are essential complementary components of a multimodal strategy for cancer pain management [15]. These therapies help reduce medication burden, improve the level of function, and are aimed at enhancing overall quality of life.

Physical Interventions a patient can take on include Physical Therapy and Exercise [51]. Patients who are naïve to exercise should be encouraged to start with gentle range-of-motion exercises and stretching. The goal of eventually adding strength training can alleviate musculoskeletal pain, prevent deconditioning and muscle loss, and improve mood and physical function [52]. Tailored physical therapy is especially useful in patients with limited mobility or after surgery.

Cancer patients may be referred to a pain specialist for Nerve Blocks, such as Epidural Injections, when medically indicated [53]. These interventional procedures involve the injection of local anesthetics and/or steroids near nerve roots or within the epidural space. Interventional pain is effective for focal pain syndromes, such as intractable axial back pain and radicular pain, and may offer temporary to prolonged relief [54].

Given the chronicity of cancer care, psychosocial interventions are an important aspect of long-term management [55]. Cognitive-Behavioral Therapy (CBT) helps patients reframe negative thoughts and behaviors surrounding pain [56]. CBT has demonstrated efficacy in improving coping strategies, reducing pain intensity, and enhancing overall emotional well-being [57]. Mindfulness and Relaxation Techniques, such as mindfulness meditation, guided imagery, and progressive muscle relaxation, can reduce the emotional distress associated with chronic cancer pain [58]. Furthermore, support groups and counseling should always be provided to help patients process their illness experience, manage anxiety and depression, and feel less isolated with their diagnosis. Group or individual counseling provides emotional validation and coping strategies [59].

Complementary Therapies such as acupuncture, an ancient traditional Chinese medicine technique, involve needle insertion at specific body points and may reduce cancer-related pain by modulating endorphin release and neural pathways [60]. Massage therapy has been shown to reduce pain, anxiety, and fatigue [61]. Patients should seek a licensed massage therapist (LMT) for safety and to tailor to the patient's medical status. Music therapy has been shown to improve mood, alter pain perception, and reduce physiological markers of stress in cancer patients [62].

Art therapy in supportive cancer care serves as a non-verbal outlet for expression for patients experiencing cancer pain [63]. Art therapy can involve drawing, painting, sculpting, and helping patients to explore and process complex emotions related to their illness and pain experience. Like other modalities, it can reduce anxiety, improve mood, and enhance self-esteem [64]. The act of engaging in a creative activity can help shift the focus away from the pain a patient is experiencing. A certified art therapist can help guide a patient.

These non-pharmacological therapies are most effective when integrated into a comprehensive pain management plan personalized to the patient's needs and preferences [65].

INTERVENTIONAL PAIN MANAGEMENT

Interventional pain management techniques are critical components in the multidisciplinary treatment of cancer pain [15]. When conventional pharmacologic and non-pharmacological therapies, as discussed previously, become insufficient, interventional pain procedures can offer targeted relief, reduce systemic medication use, and improve functional outcomes in patients with localized and widespread pain syndromes.

Interlaminar Epidural Steroid Injections and Selective Nerve Root Blocks

Interlaminar epidural steroid injections and selective nerve root blocks can provide coverage for axial pain and radiculopathy, reducing inflammation and pain in the epidural space [55]. These are useful in patients with cancer-related spinal stenosis or disc disease exacerbated by tumor burden or treatment effects. Nerve blocks involve the injection of local anesthetics, corticosteroids, or neurolytic agents near nerves or nerve plexuses to disrupt pain signaling.

Selective nerve root blocks can be both diagnostic and therapeutic, targeting specific nerve roots affected by tumor compression or degenerative changes. They are particularly effective in addressing radicular pain, improving both sensory symptoms and functional capacity [66].

Radiofrequency ablation (RFA) and cryoablation are used to disrupt nociceptive signaling from targeted nerves or tumor tissue. These techniques have been shown to be effective in treating focal pain from osseous metastases, peripheral nerve involvement, or resistant post-surgical pain syndromes [67]. They are commonly used to treat chronic axial spine pain.

Cancer patients may develop joint-related pain from altered biomechanics, immobility, or metastatic disease. Sacroiliac joint injections can help patients with lower back or pelvic pain due to sacroiliac dysfunction, which may arise from postural compensation, tumor invasion, or pelvic irradiation [68]. Intra-articular injections of corticosteroids in the affected joint can provide relief and restore mobility so patients can continue with their treatment plan and re-engage in physical and occupational therapy as necessary.

Sympathetic and Plexus Blocks

Celiac plexus blocks are commonly used for visceral abdominal pain, especially in patients with pancreatic or upper abdominal malignancies [69]. These blocks can significantly reduce opioid consumption and improve quality of life. Celiac plexus neurolytic blocks are a common palliative interventional technique for end-stage pancreatic cancer [70]. Neurolytic blocks involve the use of alcohol or phenol to chemically ablate the sympathetic nerve fibers transmitting nociceptive input from the pancreas and other abdominal viscera.

Other commonly performed blocks include superior hypogastric plexus blocks for pelvic malignancies and ganglion impar blocks for perineal pain secondary to rectal cancer [71].

Sympathetic nerve blocks, such as a lumbar sympathetic block or stellate ganglion block, target the autonomic nervous system and are useful in managing sympathetically maintained pain [72]. Stellate ganglion blocks have shown promise in treating cancer-related upper extremity pain and may help in cases of lymphedema secondary to malignancies such as breast cancer. Reducing sympathetic outflow can improve microcirculation and lymphatic drainage, potentially decreasing swelling and discomfort [73].

Intercostal nerve blocks have been shown to be useful for post-mastectomy pain syndrome, which often involves neuropathic pain along the chest wall following the rib cage [74]. These blocks can offer temporary but significant relief, and repeated injections or neurolysis may be considered for persistent cases and longer relief. Intercostal nerve blocks are also beneficial for pain following thoracotomies or rib metastases.

Neuromodulation: Spinal Cord Stimulation (SCS)

Neuromodulation, such as spinal cord stimulation (SCS), involves the implantation of electrodes in the epidural space to modulate pain signaling in the dorsal columns of the spinal cord [75]. The mechanism of action for SCS is partly explained by the Gate Control Theory of pain, which proposes that the stimulation of large-diameter Aβ sensory fibers can inhibit the transmission of nociceptive signals from smaller Aδ and C fibers at the spinal cord level. This "gate-control" effect occurs primarily in the substantia gelatinosa of the dorsal horn, theoretically leading to a decrease in the patient's perception of pain [76].

Additionally, SCS may influence descending inhibitory pathways and reduce central sensitization, contributing to both analgesia and improved functional capacity [77]. SCS is used in refractory cases of neuropathic cancer pain, particularly when pain involves multiple dermatomes [78]. SCS is appropriate in select cancer patients with a life expectancy sufficient to benefit from the implantation of the medical device.

Intrathecal Drug Delivery Systems

Intrathecal pumps deliver opioids, local anesthetics, or adjuvant medications (*e.g.*, clonidine, ziconotide) directly into the cerebrospinal fluid (CSF), allowing for potent analgesia with lower systemic doses [79]. The use of lower doses intrathecally is believed to lead to fewer systemic side effects of the medications as opposed to when they are taken *via* oral, intravenous, or transdermal routes.

This targeted therapy is beneficial for cancer patients with intractable pain not adequately managed by systemic therapy and can provide long-term pain relief in select cancer patients [80]. As oral opioid doses are escalated, one can develop opioid-refractory pain and respond poorly to conventional pharmacological modalities. Studies on intrathecal therapy have shown improved pain control, reduced opioid toxicity, and enhanced quality of life in appropriately selected patients [81].

Like neuromodulation, it is an invasive procedure involving the insertion of a medical device, so all patients should undergo careful multidisciplinary evaluation to assess life expectancy, functional goals, and capacity for device management. For those who meet criteria, interventional therapies can provide sustained relief in the setting of advanced cancer [82].

PAIN MANAGEMENT IN SPECIAL POPULATIONS

Populations that have unique physiological, psychological, or social considerations require a more nuanced approach to effective cancer pain management [15]. Pediatric patients, the elderly, and individuals with a history of substance use disorder will need tailored treatment strategies to ensure safety, efficacy, and overall quality of life.

Pediatric Cancer Patients

Pain in pediatric cancer patients is often under-recognized and undertreated due to multiple factors, including communication barriers, developmental differences, and provider discomfort [83]. Pediatric patients may express pain differently depending on their age, developmental stage, emotional state, and cognitive status. Pain assessment tools must be age-appropriate—for example, the FLACC scale (Face, Legs, Activity, Cry, Consolability) for infants and toddlers [84], or the Wong-Baker FACES scale [85] and Numeric Rating Scales for older children (Table **8**).

Pharmacologic treatment includes weight-based dosing for acetaminophen, NSAIDs, and opioids [86]. Opioids such as morphine remain the cornerstone for moderate to severe pain, but dosing must be carefully titrated, and side effects closely monitored. Adjuvant medications such as gabapentin, pregabalin, or antidepressants can be considered for neuropathic pain, though evidence in pediatric populations is more limited [87].

Non-pharmacological interventions, such as play therapy, distraction, guided imagery, and parental presence, play a critical role in improving a child's comfort and reducing distress [88]. Invasive techniques, including nerve blocks or epidural analgesia, may be appropriate in certain cases and should be performed by clinicians experienced in pediatric pain management [89].

Table 8. FLACC scale for pediatric pain assessment.

Category	0	1	2
Face	No expression or smile	Occasional grimace, withdrawn, disinterested	Frequent frown, clenched jaw, quivering chin
Legs	Normal position or relaxed	Uneasy, restless, tense	Kicking or legs drawn up
Activity	Normal position	Squirming, tense	Arched, rigid, or jerking
Cry	No crying	Moans or whimpers	Constant crying, screams, or sobs
Consolability	Content, relaxed	Distractible	Difficult to console

- **0** = Relaxed and comfortable
- **1–3** = Mild discomfort
- **4–6** = Moderate pain
- **7–10** = Severe pain

Elderly Cancer Patients

Elderly patients with cancer are at increased risk of undertreated pain due to age-related physiological changes, polypharmacy, cognitive impairment, and mutual fear of opioid side effects [90]. Pain assessment is also complicated by hearing or vision deficits, dementia, or altered mental status. Given these limitations, tailored pain assessment tools like the Verbal Descriptor Scale or Numeric Rating Scale, and for cognitively impaired patients, the Pain Assessment in Advanced Dementia (PAINAD) scale should be used to garner results [91].

Age-related changes in renal and hepatic function affect drug metabolism and excretion, so clinicians will start with lower initial doses and a slower titration of medication [92]. Opioids remain effective, but close monitoring for sedation, constipation, and falls is critical. Non-opioid analgesics such as acetaminophen can be first line for mild pain, while NSAIDs should be used cautiously due to cardiac, gastrointestinal, and renal side effects [93].

Adjuvants like gabapentinoids and SNRIs should be used judiciously, as they can lead to sedation and dizziness [94]. Non-pharmacologic modalities such as physical & occupational therapy, heat/cold therapy, and cognitive-behavioral techniques should be integrated when possible [95]. A comprehensive geriatric assessment can guide therapy and ensure goals of care align with functional status and life expectancy (Table **9**).

Table 9. PAINAD scale.

PAINAD Scale: Pain Assessment in Advanced Dementia			
Behavior	**0**	**1**	**2**
Breathing	Normal	Occasional labored breathing, short period of hyperventilation	Noisy labored breathing, long periods of hyperventilation, Cheyne-Stokes respirations.
Negative Vocalization	None	Occasional moan or groan, low-level speech with a negative or disapproving quality	Repeated troubled calling out, loud moaning or groaning, crying
Facial Expression	Smiling or inexpressive	Sad, frightened, frown	Facial grimacing
Body Language	Relaxed	Tense, distressed pacing, fidgeting	Rigid, fists clenched, knees pulled up, striking out, pulling away.
Consolability	No need to console	Distracted or reassured by voice or touch	Unable to console, distract, or reassure.

Patients with a History of Substance Use Disorder

Cancer pain management in patients with a history of or current substance use disorder (SUD) presents unique challenges [96]. These individuals may have higher pain thresholds, altered opioid tolerance, and are at a greater risk of misuse. Notwithstanding, their pain should not be dismissed or undertreated. Rather, a balanced approach must be set forward that addresses both adequate analgesia and addiction risk [97].

Clear documentation, close follow-up, and a multidisciplinary approach involving pain management specialists, palliative care, addiction medicine, and behavioral health providers is the ideal approach in this challenging population [98]. Long-acting opioids or patient-controlled analgesia (PCA) may be preferable to avoid peaks and troughs in serum drug levels, mitigating the risks that come with short-acting opioids.

In patients with active opioid use disorder, medications such as buprenorphine or methadone can be continued while supplementing with additional opioids for pain management, under collaborative supervision by the aforementioned clinicians [99].

Non-opioid analgesics, adjuvants, and non-pharmacological strategies should be optimized to reduce reliance on opioids [100]. Enforcement of controlled substance agreements, which may include serial urine drug testing, and clinicians relying on prescription monitoring programs can help support safe prescribing without stigmatizing the patient [101].

CHALLENGES IN PAIN MANAGEMENT

Despite significant advances in cancer pain management, there are still challenges facing optimal pain management [102]. Undertreatment, whether they be due to systemic or individual barriers, and stigma around opioid use persist. Complexities still arise in assessing and treating breakthrough pain. Long-term use of opioids for pain control can paradoxically lead to opioid-induced hyperalgesia [4]. Addressing these challenges requires a patient-centered and multidisciplinary approach. Clinicians must balance evidence-based practice with compassionate care in these unique situations.

Under-treatment of Pain: Barriers to Effective Pain Management

Globally, cancer pain remains under-recognized and undertreated [103]. Systemic factors to this include limited access to opioids, inadequate training of clinicians in the field of pain management, and time constraints in the setting of high clinical demands. Patient factors may include stoicism, concerns, and fear of dependence, addiction, and side effects [104]. Communication barriers with their healthcare providers may include cultural, socioeconomic, and language differences, which may further contribute to underreporting of pain symptoms [105].

The complexities of the opioid epidemic have led to regulatory restrictions and fear of professional scrutiny, which may deter clinicians from prescribing adequate analgesics [106]. Additionally, disparities in pain care persist, with racial and ethnic minority patients often receiving less pain control [107]. Patient and provider education, implementation of institutional protocols for standardized pain assessment, and advocacy for equitable access to pain therapies can help overcome these barriers [108].

Fear of Opioid Addiction in Cancer Patients

The opioid epidemic has increased public and clinical scrutiny of opioid prescribing, even in populations where opioids have always been medically appropriate, such as patients with cancer pain [109]. This has given rise to opiophobia—an exaggerated fear among patients, families, and providers regarding opioid use, which can lead to undertreatment [110]. While opioids carry risks of misuse, addiction is rare in cancer patients when opioids are used appropriately for pain control [111].

Given the risks, clinicians must strike a careful balance between effective analgesia and risk mitigation. Open communication about opioid goals, side effects, and monitoring strategies is essential to address fears and align expectations [16]. In selected cases, consultation with pain management or palliative care specialists may help reinforce best practices.

Breakthrough Pain: Assessment and Treatment

Breakthrough cancer pain (BTcP) is a transient increase in pain that occurs in a cancer pain patient who already has baseline pain [18]. It is typically rapid in onset, intense in severity, and may be spontaneous or triggered by an activity such as movement or dressing changes. BTcP is common, affecting up to 50–90% of patients with advanced cancer [112].

Proper assessment of BTcP includes identifying triggers, frequency, duration, and response to rescue medications [113]. Treatment generally involves short-acting opioids such as oral morphine, oxycodone, or transmucosal fentanyl formulations. The rescue opioid dose is often calculated as a fraction of 10-15% of a patient's daily opioid consumption [114]. Non-pharmacologic measures such as repositioning, heat/cold therapy, or pre-emptive dosing before activity have also been shown to be beneficial. Clinicians will need to reassess baseline medication regimens if breakthrough episodes become more frequent or poorly controlled [115].

Opioid-Induced Hyperalgesia

Opioid-induced hyperalgesia (OIH) is a paradoxical condition in which increasing opioid doses lead to heightened pain sensitivity rather than relief [116]. It is characterized by diffuse, non-localized pain and can be difficult to distinguish from tolerance or disease progression.

The mechanism of OIH is not fully understood but may involve central sensitization, excitatory neurotransmitter upregulation, and activation of N-methyl-D-aspartate (NMDA) receptors [117]. Management strategies include reducing or rotating opioids, using NMDA antagonists such as ketamine, and incorporating adjuvant medications [118]. Awareness of OIH is important to prevent inappropriate opioid escalation and to guide rational, evidence-based multidisciplinary pain management.

MULTIDISCIPLINARY APPROACH TO CANCER PAIN

Cancer pain management involves a multidisciplinary approach coordinated by healthcare professionals, patients, and their families□15□. Pain in cancer patients is often multifactorial—arising from tumor burden, treatment-related side effects, psychological distress, and comorbid conditions. A collaborative care model improves pain outcomes, minimizes lapses in care, and ensures comprehensive support throughout the continuum of a patient's course of treatment [119].

Role of Oncologists, Palliative Care Specialists, and Pain Specialists

Oncologists are the gatekeepers for patients with cancer-related pain [120]. They play a central role in identifying pain patterns, initiating first-line analgesic treatments, and referring patients to appropriate services when standard regimens are no longer sufficient.

Palliative care specialists bring an advanced care planning approach to symptom management. Their expertise includes pharmacologic optimization as well as addressing psychological and emotional needs [121]. Early integration of palliative care has been shown to improve quality of life, reduce symptom burden, and even extend survival rates [122].

Pain medicine specialists provide advanced skills in interventional procedures and multimodal strategies [123]. Cancer pain patients can also rely on radiation oncologists, surgical oncologists, psychologists, pharmacists, physical therapists, and social workers, with each specialty offering a unique approach to pain management.

Effective communication among specialties ensures efficient multidisciplinary care [124]. It is also important to establish clear communication about goals of care, especially in patients with advanced disease or shifting prognoses [125].

Incorporating Family and Caregivers in the Management Plan

Incorporating family members and caregivers plays a critical role in providing emotional support, recognizing changes in pain, advocating for the patient, and assisting with adherence [126]. Their involvement improves practical aspects of pain control and emotional well-being.

Education of caregivers should include training on pain assessment tools, medication schedules, side effect management, and escalation protocols [127]. Support for caregivers *via* counseling, respite services, and caregiver support groups mitigates caregiver burden [128].

Ethical and Legal Considerations

Pain management in cancer care involves the intricacies of ethics, medicine, and public policy [129]. Clinicians have the duty of providing compassionate and effective pain relief while also safeguarding against potential misuse, diversion, and adverse outcomes. With the opioid epidemic being under public scrutiny, healthcare providers are forced to navigate a complex landscape of ethical obligations and legal regulations while providing clinical care [121].

Balancing Pain Relief with Concerns of Opioid Misuse

The primary ethical principle guiding cancer pain management is beneficence where clinicians are acting to promote the well-being of their patients to relieve suffering [130]. Opioids remain the mainstay of moderate to severe pain control for cancer patients. However, the rising incidence of opioid misuse and addiction in the general population has led to opiophobia among providers and patients alike [131]. Concerns over dependence, regulatory surveillance, and liability may result in undertreatment of legitimate cancer pain.

Clinicians must balance these concerns by applying risk mitigation strategies without compromising effective pain control [132]. This includes using controlled substance agreements and regular reevaluations of functional capacity and goals of care. The use of online prescription monitoring programs has also helped reduce the risks of misuse and diversion [133]. It is important to note that the risk of addiction is low in cancer patients when opioids are prescribed appropriately [134]. Concerns over misuse should not override the need to treat pain compassionately.

Decision-Making in End-of-Life Care

In end-of-life care, the ethical goal of pain management shifts toward comfort-based and palliative care [135]. Decisions around analgesia should prioritize the patient's expressed goals, desires, and values while respecting their autonomy. Opioid dosing at end-of-life care may be escalated more rapidly to relieve suffering, even while theoretically risking a closer onset of death.

The doctrine of double effect is an ethical principle where an action can be morally justified even if it has positive and negative consequences [136]. The intent of symptom relief by opioid escalation can lead to a life-shortening result, but such actions are considered ethically and legally permissible.

Legal Regulations Surrounding Opioid Prescribing

Clinicians should also remain apprised of federal and state-level laws regulating opioid prescribing [137]. In the U.S., the Controlled Substances Act classifies opioids based on potential for misuse and mandates secure documentation, recordkeeping, and prescription practices. States may have additional requirements such as mandatory use of prescription drug monitoring programs (PDMPs) every few months, limits on initial prescription durations to 5 days, and continuing medical education (CME) mandates for opioid prescribers [138].

There are exemptions for patients with cancer, palliative, and hospice care. Recognizing these exceptions is important to prevent inappropriate restriction of access to necessary medications due to fear of legal repercussions [139].

FUTURE DIRECTIONS IN CANCER PAIN MANAGEMENT

Oncology is always advancing; thus, the approaches to managing cancer-related pain are also evolving [15]. Traditional pain management strategies have centered around pharmacologic and interventional modalities. The future may entail more precise and individualized therapies. Emerging technologies in gene therapy, immunotherapy, and molecular medicine are paving the way for a more tailored and effective approach to pain relief [140].

Emerging Therapies

Gene therapy represents a novel frontier in cancer pain management [141]. Experimental models have studied the use of viral vectors to deliver genes that encode for anti-inflammatory cytokines, opioid peptides, or ion channel modulators directly into the nervous system [142]. In some of these preclinical studies, intrathecal delivery of genes encoding enkephalins or endomorphins has shown analgesic effects. These novel methods aim to provide long-term tailored pain relief without systemic side effects. Gene therapy is still in investigational phases, but it holds promise for patients with chronic cancer pain.

Immunotherapy may also secondarily influence pain. CAR-T cell therapies alter the tumor microenvironment, potentially reducing inflammation, peritumoral edema, and neuropathic pain caused by tumor invasion [143]. However, there is still much work to be done here as immunotherapy can also cause pain syndromes, such as immune-mediated neuropathies [144].

Personalized Pain Management Based on Genomics

Advances in genomics and precision medicine may soon allow clinicians to predict individual pain susceptibility, response to medications, and risk of side effects [145]. It is known that certain genetic polymorphisms can affect drug metabolism enzymes such as CYP2D6 and CYP3A4 [146]. Approximately 5–10% of Caucasian patients are poor metabolizers of codeine due to CYP2D6 mutations and may benefit from alternative opioids [147]. Opioid receptors such as OPRM1 or inflammatory cytokines (*e.g.*, IL-6, TNF-α) can influence how a patient experiences and responds to pain treatments.

In the future, pain management regimens may be personalized based on genomic profiles, which can potentially increase efficacy while minimizing toxicity [148]. Pharmacogenomic testing could identify patients at risk of opioid-induced neurotoxicity or hyperalgesia, expediting early adoption of non-opioid or interventional approaches [149]. As these technologies become more accessible and cost-effective, personalized pain management may become the clinical standard of care of the future.

CONCLUSION

Cancer pain remains a challenging area for patients and clinicians alike. Cancer pain management is multifaceted and involves studying its underlying mechanisms, coming up with assessment strategies, and creating pharmacologic and non-pharmacologic treatments.

A multidisciplinary patient-centered approach is essential for optimal pain management. Individualized treatment plans should incorporate the patient's clinical status, goals of care, physical and psychological well-being, and social support system. Whether using standard analgesics, interventional procedures, or emerging genomic tools, pain management should be tailored to the unique needs of each patient. Advances in gene therapy, immunotherapy, and pharmacogenomics hold promise for the future.

Clinicians will need to maintain commitment to continued education and ethical practice. Research will continue to close gaps in knowledge, develop novel treatments, and improve outcomes. Equipping clinicians with evidence-based tools and maintaining open communication among providers, patients, and caregivers will ensure that pain relief remains a priority for all individuals living with cancer.

REFERENCES

[1] Fallon M. Neurological aspects of cancer pain. Br J Anaesth 2013; 111(1): 105-11. [http://dx.doi.org/10.1093/bja/aet208] [PMID: 23794652]

[2] Caraceni A, Portenoy RK. An international survey of cancer pain characteristics and syndromes. Pain 1999; 82(3): 263-74. [http://dx.doi.org/10.1016/S0304-3959(99)00073-1] [PMID: 10488677]

[3] Mantyh PW. Cancer pain and its impact on diagnosis, survival and quality of life. Nat Rev Neurosci 2006; 7(10): 797-809. [http://dx.doi.org/10.1038/nrn1914] [PMID: 16988655]

[4] Mercadante S. Malignant bone pain: pathophysiology and treatment. Pain 1997; 69(1): 1-18. [http://dx.doi.org/10.1016/S0304-3959(96)03267-8] [PMID: 9060007]

[5] Smith HS. Visceral pain: the ins and outs, the ups and downs. Pain Physician 2012; 15(2): E183-91.

[6] Paice JA. Mechanisms and management of neuropathic pain in cancer. J Support Oncol 2003; 1(2): 107-20. [PMID: 15352654]

[7] Bennett MI, Rayment C, Hjermstad M, Aass N, Caraceni A, Kaasa S. Prevalence and aetiology of neuropathic pain in cancer patients: A systematic review. Pain 2012; 153(2): 359-65. [http://dx.doi.org/10.1016/j.pain.2011.10.028] [PMID: 22115921]

[8] Bruera E, Portenoy RK. Cancer Pain: Assessment and Management. Cambridge University Press 2003. [http://dx.doi.org/10.1017/CBO9780511550096]

[9] Coleman RE. Metastatic bone disease: clinical features, pathophysiology and treatment strategies. Cancer Treat Rev 2001; 27(3): 165-76. [http://dx.doi.org/10.1053/ctrv.2000.0210] [PMID: 11417967]

[10] Deandrea S, Montanari M, Moja L, Apolone G. Prevalence of undertreatment in cancer pain. A review of published literature. Ann Oncol 2008; 19(12): 1985-91. [http://dx.doi.org/10.1093/annonc/mdn419] [PMID: 18632721]

[11] Clarke JL, Perez HR, Jacks LM, Panageas KS, DeAngelis LM. Leptomeningeal metastases in the MRI era. Neurology 2010; 74(18): 1449-54. [http://dx.doi.org/10.1212/WNL.0b013e3181dc1a69] [PMID: 20439847]

[12] Cavaletti G, Marmiroli P. Chemotherapy-induced peripheral neurotoxicity. Nat Rev Neurol 2010; 6(1 2): 657-66. [http://dx.doi.org/10.1038/nrneurol.2010.160] [PMID: 21060341]

[13] Staff NP, Grisold A, Grisold W, Windebank AJ. Chemotherapy-induced peripheral neuropathy: A current review. Ann Neurol 2017; 81(6): 772-81. [http://dx.doi.org/10.1002/ana.24951] [PMID: 28486769]

[14] Chow E, Wong R, Hruby G, *et al.* Management of side effects of palliative radiation therapy. Curr Probl Cancer 2009; 33(5): 272-310.

[15] Paice JA, Ferrell B. The management of cancer pain. CA Cancer J Clin 2011; 61(3): 157-82. [http://dx.doi.org/10.3322/caac.20112] [PMID: 21543825]

[16] Caraceni A, Hanks G, Kaasa S, *et al.* Use of opioid analgesics in the treatment of cancer pain: evidence-based recommendations from the EAPC. Lancet Oncol 2012; 13(2): e58-68. [http://dx.doi.org/10.1016/S1470-2045(12)70040-2] [PMID: 22300860]

[17] Wiffen PJ, Wee B, Derry S, Bell RF, Moore RA. Opioids for cancer pain - an overview of Cochrane reviews. Cochrane Database Syst Rev 2017; 7(7): CD012592. [PMID: 28683172]

[18] Zeppetella G. Breakthrough pain in cancer. Br J Anaesth 1999; 83(1): 109-12.

[19] Mystakidou K, Tsilika E, Parpa E, *et al.* Pain assessment in advanced cancer: patient self-report vs. systematic evaluation. J Pain Symptom Manage 2004; 27(6): 523-30. [PMID: 15165650]

[20] Cleeland CS. Measurement of pain by subjective report. In: Chapman CR, Loeser JD, Eds. Advances in Pain Research and Therapy. New York: Raven Press 1989; Vol. 12: pp. 391-403.

[21] Dworkin RH, Turk DC, Farrar JT, *et al.* Core outcome measures for chronic pain clinical trials: IMMPACT recommendations. Pain 2005; 113(1): 9-19. [http://dx.doi.org/10.1016/j.pain.2004.09.012] [PMID: 15621359]

[22] Downie WW, Leatham PA, Rhind VM, Wright V, Branco JA, Anderson JA. Studies with pain rating scales. Ann Rheum Dis 1978; 37(4): 378-81. [http://dx.doi.org/10.1136/ard.37.4.378] [PMID: 686873]

[23] Cleeland CS, Ryan KM. Pain assessment: global use of the Brief Pain Inventory. Ann Acad Med Singap 1994; 23(2): 129-38. [PMID: 8080219]

[24] Melzack R. The McGill Pain Questionnaire: Major properties and scoring methods. Pain 1975; 1(3): 277-99. [http://dx.doi.org/10.1016/0304-3959(75)90044-5] [PMID: 1235985]

[25] Turk DC, Monarch ES. Biopsychosocial perspective on chronic pain. In: Gatchel RJ, Turk DC, Eds. Psychological Approaches to Pain Management. 2nd ed. New York: Guilford Press 2002; pp. 3-29.

[26] Kroenke K, Spitzer RL, Williams JBW. The PHQ-9. J Gen Intern Med 2001; 16(9): 606-13. [http://dx.doi.org/10.1046/j.1525-1497.2001.016009606.x] [PMID: 11556941]

[27] Gatchel RJ, Peng YB, Peters ML, Fuchs PN, Turk DC. The biopsychosocial approach to chronic pain: Scientific advances and future directions. Psychol Bull 2007; 133(4): 581-624. [http://dx.doi.org/10.1037/0033-2909.133.4.581] [PMID: 17592957]

[28] Lutz S, Berk L, Chang E, *et al.* Palliative radiotherapy for bone metastases: an ASTRO evidence-based guideline. Int J Radiat Oncol Biol Phys 2011; 79(4): 965-76. [http://dx.doi.org/10.1016/j.ijrobp.2010.11.026] [PMID: 21277118]

[29] Even-Sapir E, Metser U, Mishani E, Lievshitz G, Lerman H, Leibovitch I. The detection of bone metastases in patients with high-risk prostate cancer: 99mTc-MDP Planar bone scintigraphy, single- and multi-field-of-view SPECT, 18F-fluoride PET, and 18F-fluoride PET/CT. J Nucl Med 2006; 47(2): 287-97. [PMID: 16455635]

[30] Tuma J. Bone scanning in oncology. AJR Am J Roentgenol 1995; 165(5): 1137-47. [PMID: 7717220]

[31] Alberti P, Rossi E, Cornblath DR, *et al.* Chemotherapy-induced peripheral neurotoxicity: classification, diagnosis, and prevention. Nat Rev Neurol 2022; 18(1): 71-80.

[32] de Wit R, van Dam F, Loonstra S, *et al.* The Amsterdam Pain Management Index compared to eight frequently used outcome measures to evaluate the adequacy of pain treatment in cancer patients with chronic pain. Pain 2001; 91(3): 339-49. [http://dx.doi.org/10.1016/S0304-3959(00)00455-3] [PMID: 11275392]

[33] Pergolizzi JV, Raffa RB. The WHO pain ladder: do we need another step? Pract Pain Manag 2014; 14 (1)

[34] McNicol ED, Strassels SA, Goudas LC, Lau J, Carr DB. NSAIDs or paracetamol for cancer pain. Cochrane Database Syst Rev 2005; 1: CD005180.
[PMID: 15654708]

[35] Hardy J, Zeppetella G, Porta-Sales J. Pain control with low-dose oral opioids in cancer patients with renal failure. Support Care Cancer 2010; 18(5): 613-7.
[PMID: 20352266]

[36] Finnerup NB, Kuner R, Jensen TS. Neuropathic pain: from mechanisms to treatment. Physiol Rev. 2021; 101(1): 259-321.
[http://dx.doi.org/10.1152/physrev.00040.2019] [PMID: 32926021]

[37] Smith EM, Pang H, Cirrincione C, *et al.* Effect of duloxetine on chemotherapy-induced painful peripheral neuropathy. JAMA 2013; 309(13): 1359-67.
[http://dx.doi.org/10.1001/jama.2013.2813] [PMID: 23549581]

[38] Backonja M, Beydoun A, Edwards KR, *et al.* Gabapentin for the symptomatic treatment of painful neuropathy in patients with diabetes mellitus: a randomized controlled trial. JAMA 1998; 280(21): 1831-6.
[http://dx.doi.org/10.1001/jama.280.21.1831] [PMID: 9846777]

[39] Lunn MP, Hughes RA, Wiffen PJ. Duloxetine for treating painful neuropathy or chronic pain. Cochrane Database Syst Rev 2009; 4(4): CD007115.
[PMID: 19821395]

[40] Vecht CJ, Haaxma-Reiche H, van Putten WL, *et al.* Initial bolus of corticosteroids in metastatic spinal cord compression? A randomised trial. Neurology 1989; 39(9): 1255-7.
[http://dx.doi.org/10.1212/WNL.39.9.1255] [PMID: 2771077]

[41] Shakespeare DT, Boggild M, Young C. Anti-spasticity agents for multiple sclerosis. Cochrane Database Syst Rev 2003; 4(4): CD001332.
[PMID: 14583932]

[42] Häuser W, Petzke F, Fitzcharles MA. Efficacy, tolerability and safety of cannabinoids for chronic pain. Pain 2018; 159(12): 2438-49.

[43] Bruera E, Kim HN. Cancer Pain. JAMA 2003; 290(18): 2476-9.
[http://dx.doi.org/10.1001/jama.290.18.2476] [PMID: 14612485]

[44] Fallon M, Cherny N, Hanks G, Kaasa S. Opioid therapy: guidelines for daily practice. J Clin Oncol 2001; 19(9): 2542-54.
[PMID: 11331334]

[45] Knotkova H, Fine PG, Portenoy RK. Opioid rotation: the science and the limitations of the equianalgesic dose table. J Pain Symptom Manage 2009; 38(3): 426-39.
[http://dx.doi.org/10.1016/j.jpainsymman.2009.06.001] [PMID: 19735903]

[46] McPherson ML. Demystifying Opioid Conversion Calculations. 2nd ed., Bethesda: ASHP 2018.
[http://dx.doi.org/10.37573/9781585284306]

[47] Sykes NP. The relationship between opioid use and laxative use in terminally ill cancer patients. Palliat Med 1998; 12(5): 375-82.
[http://dx.doi.org/10.1191/026921698674125048] [PMID: 9924600]

[48] Bruera E, MacEachern T, Ripamonti C. The management of nausea and vomiting in cancer patients. Cancer Treat Rev 1989; 16(1): 49-65.
[PMID: 2471590]

[49] Mercadante S. Opioid rotation for cancer pain. Cancer 1999; 86(9): 1856-66.
[http://dx.doi.org/10.1002/(SICI)1097-0142(19991101)86:9<1856::AID-CNCR30>3.0.CO;2-G]

[PMID: 10547561]

[50] Paice JA, Portenoy R. Opioid therapy in patients with cancer. J Clin Oncol 2014; 32(16): 1721-6. [http://dx.doi.org/10.1200/JCO.2013.52.5196] [PMID: 24799468]

[51] Angst MS, Clark JD. Opioid-induced Hyperalgesia. Anesthesiology 2006; 104(3): 570-87. [http://dx.doi.org/10.1097/00000542-200603000-00025] [PMID: 16508405]

[52] Schmitz KH, Campbell AM, Stuiver MM, *et al.* Exercise is medicine in oncology: Engaging clinicians to help patients move through cancer. CA Cancer J Clin 2019; 69(6): 468-84. [http://dx.doi.org/10.3322/caac.21579] [PMID: 31617590]

[53] Courneya KS, Friedenreich CM. Physical activity and cancer control. Semin Oncol Nurs 2007; 23(4): 242-52. [http://dx.doi.org/10.1016/j.soncn.2007.08.002] [PMID: 18022052]

[54] Deer TR, Krames E, Mekhail N, *et al.* The appropriate use of neurostimulation: new and evolving neurostimulation therapies and applicable treatment for chronic pain and selected disease states. Neuromodulation 2014; 17(6): 599-615. [http://dx.doi.org/10.1111/ner.12204] [PMID: 25112892]

[55] Manchikanti L, Singh V, Cash KA, *et al.* A comparative effectiveness evaluation of percutaneous adhesiolysis and epidural steroid injections in managing lumbar post-surgery syndrome: a randomized, equivalence controlled trial. Pain Physician 2014; 17(6): E705-16. [PMID: 19935992]

[56] Syrjala KL, Jensen MP, Mendoza ME, Yi JC, Fisher HM, Keefe FJ. Psychological and behavioral approaches to cancer pain management. J Clin Oncol 2014; 32(16): 1703-11. [http://dx.doi.org/10.1200/JCO.2013.54.4825] [PMID: 24799497]

[57] Keefe FJ, Abernethy AP, C Campbell L. Psychological approaches to understanding and treating disease-related pain. Annu Rev Psychol 2005; 56: 601-30. [http://dx.doi.org/10.1146/annurev.psych.56.091103.070302] [PMID: 15709948]

[58] Ehde DM, Dillworth TM, Turner JA. Cognitive-behavioral therapy for individuals with chronic pain: Efficacy, innovations, and directions for research. Am Psychol 2014; 69(2): 153-66. [http://dx.doi.org/10.1037/a0035747] [PMID: 24547801]

[59] Garland SN, Tamagawa R, Todd SC, Speca M, Carlson LE. Increased mindfulness is related to improved stress and mood following participation in a mindfulness-based stress reduction program in individuals with cancer. Integr Cancer Ther 2013; 12(1): 31-40. [http://dx.doi.org/10.1177/1534735412442370] [PMID: 22505593]

[60] Uitterhoeve RJ, Bensing JM, Grol RP, Demulder PHM, Van Achterberg T. The effect of communication skills training on patient outcomes in cancer care: a systematic review of the literature. Eur J Cancer Care (Engl) 2010; 19(4): 442-57. [http://dx.doi.org/10.1111/j.1365-2354.2009.01082.x] [PMID: 20030702]

[61] Garcia MK, McQuade J, Haddad R, *et al.* Systematic review of acupuncture in cancer care: a synthesis of the evidence. J Clin Oncol 2013; 31(7): 952-60. [http://dx.doi.org/10.1200/JCO.2012.43.5818] [PMID: 23341529]

[62] Jane SW, Wilkie DJ, Gallucci BB, Beaton RD, Huang HY. Effects of a full-body massage on pain intensity, anxiety, and physiological relaxation in Taiwanese patients with metastatic bone pain: a randomized controlled trial. Pain 2011; 152(10): 2432-42. [http://dx.doi.org/10.1016/j.pain.2011.06.021] [PMID: 21802850]

[63] Bradt J, Dileo C, Grocke D, Magill L. Music interventions for mechanically ventilated patients. Cochrane Database Syst Rev 2010; 12(12): CD006902. [PMID: 21154376]

[64] Geue K, Goetze H, Buttstaedt M, Kleinert E, Richter D, Singer S. An overview of art therapy interventions for cancer patients and the results of research. Complement Ther Med 2010; 18(3-4):

160-70.
[http://dx.doi.org/10.1016/j.ctim.2010.04.001] [PMID: 20688262]

[65] Wood MJM, Molassiotis A, Payne S. What research evidence is there for the use of art therapy in the management of symptoms in adults with cancer? A systematic review. Psychooncology 2011; 20(2): 135-45.
[http://dx.doi.org/10.1002/pon.1722] [PMID: 20878827]

[66] Syrjala KL, Jensen MP. Nonpharmacologic management of cancer pain. J Clin Oncol 2013; 31(16): 1936-41.

[67] Manchikanti L, Boswell MV, Datta S, *et al.* Comprehensive review of therapeutic interventions in managing chronic spinal pain. Pain Physician 2009; 4(12): E123-98.
[http://dx.doi.org/10.36076/ppj.2009/12/E123] [PMID: 19668281]

[68] Kim PS, Kim BH, Lee JW, *et al.* Selective nerve root blocks for cancer pain. Korean J Pain 2017; 30(2): 67-74.
[http://dx.doi.org/10.3344/kjp.2019.32.2.67] [PMID: 31091504]

[69] Notaro JR, Gelman MI. Radiofrequency ablation for the treatment of pain associated with metastatic cancer. Curr Pain Headache Rep 2016; 20(7): 47.
[PMID: 27278441]

[70] DePalma MJ, Ketchum JM, Saullo TR. Etiology of chronic low back pain in patients having undergone lumbar fusion. Pain Med 2011; 12(5): 732-9.
[http://dx.doi.org/10.1111/j.1526-4637.2011.01098.x] [PMID: 21481166]

[71] Nagels W, Pease N, Bekkering G, Cools F, Dobbels P. Celiac plexus neurolysis for abdominal cancer pain: a systematic review. Pain Med 2013; 14(8): 1140-63.
[http://dx.doi.org/10.1111/pme.12176] [PMID: 23802777]

[72] Staats PS, Hekmat H, Sauter P, Lillemoe KD. The effects of alcohol celiac plexus block, pain, and quality of life in patients with pancreatic cancer. Pain Med 2001; 2(1): 28-34.
[http://dx.doi.org/10.1046/j.1526-4637.2001.002001028.x] [PMID: 15102315]

[73] Amr YM. Effect of early intervention with superior hypogastric plexus block in cancer pelvic pain. Pain Physician 2010; 13(2): 119-24.

[74] Huntoon MA. Lumbar sympathetic block. Tech Reg Anesth Pain Manage 2002; 6(2): 77-82.

[75] Narouze S, Vydyanathan A, Kapural L, Sessler DI, Mekhail N. Ultrasound-guided stellate ganglion block: description of technique and efficacy of block. Pain Physician 2007; 10(6): 757-62.
[PMID: 17987098]

[76] Shah UJ, Shah GU. Efficacy of intercostal nerve block in relieving pain in post thoracotomy patients. Indian J Anaesth 2010; 54(2): 135-8.

[77] North RB, Kidd DH, Farrokhi F, Piantadosi SA. Spinal cord stimulation versus repeated lumbosacral spine surgery for chronic pain: a randomized, controlled trial. Neurosurgery 2005; 56(1): 98-107.
[http://dx.doi.org/10.1227/01.NEU.0000144839.65524.E0] [PMID: 15617591]

[78] Melzack R, Wall PD. Pain mechanisms: a new theory. Science 1965; 150(3699): 971-9.
[http://dx.doi.org/10.1126/science.150.3699.971] [PMID: 5320816]

[79] Harvey SC, Hassenbusch SJ 3rd, Kerns RD. Intrathecal drug delivery systems in the management of chronic pain: a review of efficacy, complications, and cost-effectiveness. Pain Med. 2000; 1(4): 310-330.
[http://dx.doi.org/10.1046/j.1526-4637.2000.00042.x] [PMID: 11725117]

[80] Kumar K, Hunter G, Demeria D. Spinal cord stimulation in treatment of chronic benign pain: challenges in treatment planning and present status, a 22-year experience. Neurosurgery 2006; 58(3): 481-96.
[http://dx.doi.org/10.1227/01.NEU.0000192162.99567.96] [PMID: 16528188]

[81] Smith TJ, Staats PS, Deer T, *et al.* Randomized clinical trial of an implantable drug delivery system compared with comprehensive medical management for refractory cancer pain: impact on pain, drug-related toxicity, and survival. J Clin Oncol 2002; 20(19): 4040-9. [http://dx.doi.org/10.1200/JCO.2002.02.118] [PMID: 12351602]

[82] Hassenbusch SJ, Portenoy RK, Cousins M, Buchser E. Polyanalgesic Consensus Conference 2000. J Pain Symptom Manage 2001; 21(1): 47-53.

[83] Deer TR, Krames ES, Hassenbusch SJ, *et al.* Polyanalgesic Consensus Conference 2007: recommendations for the management of pain by intrathecal drug delivery. Neuromodulation 2007; 10(4): 300-28. [http://dx.doi.org/10.1111/j.1525-1403.2007.00128.x] [PMID: 22150890]

[84] Pope JE, Deer TR, Falowski S, *et al.* Multidisciplinary consensus on best practices for intrathecal drug delivery. Neuromodulation 2017; 20(2): 96-132. [PMID: 28042904]

[85] Friedrichsdorf SJ, Postier A, Eull D, *et al.* Pain outcomes in a US children's hospital: a prospective cross-sectional survey. Hosp Pediatr 2015; 5(1): 18-26. [http://dx.doi.org/10.1542/hpeds.2014-0084] [PMID: 25554755]

[86] Merkel SI, Voepel-Lewis T, Shayevitz JR, Malviya S. The FLACC: a behavioral scale for scoring postoperative pain in young children. Pediatr Nurs 1997; 23(3): 293-7. [PMID: 9220806]

[87] Wong DL, Baker CM. Pain in children: comparison of assessment scales. Pediatr Nurs 1988; 14(1): 9-17. [PMID: 3344163]

[88] Anghelescu DL, Burgoyne LL, Faughnan LG, Mandrell BN. Pediatric cancer pain management. Cancer Contr 2015; 22(4): 451-65.

[89] Gilchrist L. Chemotherapy-induced peripheral neuropathy in pediatric cancer patients. Semin Pediatr Neurol 2012; 19(1): 9-17. [http://dx.doi.org/10.1016/j.spen.2012.02.011] [PMID: 22641071]

[90] Fortier MA, Chou J, Maurer EL, Kain ZN. Acute and postoperative pain in children. Pediatr Clin North Am 2013; 60(5): 1083-101. [PMID: 24093897]

[91] Zernikow B, Wamsler C, Michel E, *et al.* Pediatric cancer pain management using WHO analgesic guidelines. Pain 2005; 117(1-2): 126-34.

[92] Hadjistavropoulos T, Herr K, Turk DC, *et al.* An interdisciplinary expert consensus statement on assessment of pain in older persons. Clin J Pain 2007; 23(1) (Suppl. 1): S1-S43. [http://dx.doi.org/10.1097/AJP.0b013e31802be869] [PMID: 17179836]

[93] Warden V, Hurley AC, Volicer L. Development and psychometric evaluation of the Pain Assessment in Advanced Dementia (PAINAD) scale. J Am Med Dir Assoc 2003; 4(1): 9-15. [http://dx.doi.org/10.1097/01.JAM.0000043422.31640.F7] [PMID: 12807591]

[94] Schofield P. The assessment of pain in older people: UK national guidelines. Age Ageing 2018; 47 (Suppl. 1): i1-i22. [http://dx.doi.org/10.1093/ageing/afx192] [PMID: 29579142]

[95] Reid MC, Eccleston C, Pillemer K. Management of chronic pain in older adults. BMJ 2015; 350(feb13 2): h532. [http://dx.doi.org/10.1136/bmj.h532] [PMID: 25680884]

[96] LeBlanc TW, Smith JM, Currow DC. Symptom burden in older patients with advanced cancer: a population-based study. J Am Geriatr Soc 2015; 63(8): 1607-14.

[97] Ferrell BA. Pain evaluation and management in the nursing home. Ann Intern Med 1995; 123(9): 681-

7.
[http://dx.doi.org/10.7326/0003-4819-123-9-199511010-00007] [PMID: 7574224]

[98] Passik SD, Weinreb HJ. Managing chronic nonmalignant pain: Overcoming obstacles to the use of opioids. Adv Ther 2000; 17(2): 70-83.
[http://dx.doi.org/10.1007/BF02854840] [PMID: 11010058]

[99] Pergolizzi J, Böger RH, Budd K, *et al.* Opioid use for moderate to severe chronic non-cancer pain: consensus statement. Pain Pract 2008; 8(5): 287-313.
[http://dx.doi.org/10.1111/j.1533-2500.2008.00204.x] [PMID: 18503626]

[100] Mehta A, Chan LS. Understanding of the concept of "total pain". J Hosp Palliat Nurs 2008; 10(1): 26-32.
[http://dx.doi.org/10.1097/01.NJH.0000306714.50539.1a]

[101] Alford DP, Compton P, Samet JH. Acute pain management for patients receiving maintenance methadone or buprenorphine therapy. Ann Intern Med 2006; 144(2): 127-34.
[http://dx.doi.org/10.7326/0003-4819-144-2-200601170-00010] [PMID: 16418412]

[102] Vowles KE, McEntee ML, Julnes PS, Frohe T, Ney JP, van der Goes DN. Rates of opioid misuse, abuse, and addiction in chronic pain. Pain 2015; 156(4): 569-76.
[http://dx.doi.org/10.1097/01.j.pain.0000460357.01998.f1] [PMID: 25785523]

[103] Starrels JL, Becker WC, Alford DP, Kapoor A, Williams AR, Turner BJ. Systematic review: treatment agreements and urine drug testing to reduce opioid misuse in patients with chronic pain. Ann Intern Med 2010; 152(11): 712-20.
[http://dx.doi.org/10.7326/0003-4819-152-11-201006010-00004] [PMID: 20513829]

[104] Breivik H, Cherny N, Collett B, *et al.* Cancer-related pain: a pan- European survey of prevalence, treatment, and patient attitudes. Ann Oncol. 2009; 20(8): 1420–1433.
[PMID: 19395383]

[105] Kimberlin C, Brushwood D, Allen W, Radson E, Wilson D. Cancer patient and caregiver experiences: communication and pain management issues. J Pain Symptom Manage. 2004 Dec; 28(6): 566-78.
[http://dx.doi.org/10.1016/j.jpainsymman.2004.03.005] [PMID: 15589081]

[106] Green CR, Anderson KO, Baker TA, *et al.* The unequal burden of pain: confronting racial and ethnic disparities in pain. Pain Med 2003; 4(3): 277-94.
[http://dx.doi.org/10.1046/j.1526-4637.2003.03034.x] [PMID: 12974827]

[107] Meghani SH, Byun E, Gallagher RM. Time to take stock: a meta-analysis and systematic review of analgesic treatment disparities for pain in the United States. Pain Med 2012; 13(2): 150-74.
[http://dx.doi.org/10.1111/j.1526-4637.2011.01310.x] [PMID: 22239747]

[108] Volkow ND, McLellan TA. Curtailing diversion and abuse of opioid analgesics without jeopardizing pain treatment. JAMA 2011; 305(13): 1346-7.
[http://dx.doi.org/10.1001/jama.2011.369] [PMID: 21467287]

[109] Anderson KO, Green CR, Payne R. Racial and ethnic disparities in pain: causes and consequences of unequal care. J Pain 2009; 10(12): 1187-204.
[http://dx.doi.org/10.1016/j.jpain.2009.10.002] [PMID: 19944378]

[110] Paice JA. Cancer pain management: strategies for safe and effective opioid prescribing. J Natl Compr Canc Netw 2010; 8(9): 1081-9.
[PMID: 27226517]

[111] Vissers KCP, Besse K, Hans G, Devulder J, Morlion B. Opioid rotation in the management of chronic pain: where is the evidence? Pain Pract 2010; 10(2): 85-93.
[http://dx.doi.org/10.1111/j.1533-2500.2009.00335.x] [PMID: 20070552]

[112] Oldenmenger WH, Sillevis Smitt PAE, van Dooren S, Stoter G, van der Rijt CCD. A systematic review on barriers hindering adequate cancer pain management and interventions to reduce them: A critical appraisal. Eur J Cancer 2009; 45(8): 1370-80.

[http://dx.doi.org/10.1016/j.ejca.2009.01.007] [PMID: 19201599]

[113] Fallon M. Opioid analgesia for cancer pain. Curr Opin Support Palliat Care 2013; 7(1): 8-14. [PMID: 23196380]

[114] Portenoy RK, Lesage P. Management of cancer pain. Lancet 1999; 353(9165): 1695-1700. [PMID: 10371416]

[115] Portenoy RK, Hagen NA. Breakthrough pain: definition, prevalence and characteristics. Pain 1990; 41(3): 273-81. [http://dx.doi.org/10.1016/0304-3959(90)90004-W] [PMID: 1697056]

[116] Davies AN, Dickman A, Reid C, Stevens AM, Zeppetella G. The management of cancer-related breakthrough pain: Recommendations of a task group of the Science Committee of the Association for Palliative Medicine of Great Britain and Ireland. Eur J Pain 2009; 13(4): 331-8. [http://dx.doi.org/10.1016/j.ejpain.2008.06.014] [PMID: 18707904]

[117] Mercadante S. Pharmacotherapy for breakthrough cancer pain. Drugs 2012; 72(2): 181-90. [http://dx.doi.org/10.2165/11597260-000000000-00000] [PMID: 22233484]

[118] Mao J. Opioid-induced abnormal pain sensitivity: implications in clinical opioid therapy. Pain 2002; 100(3): 213-7. [http://dx.doi.org/10.1016/S0304-3959(02)00422-0] [PMID: 12467992]

[119] Dobscha SK, Corson K, Perrin NA, *et al.* Collaborative care for chronic pain in primary care: a cluster randomized trial. JAMA. 2009 Mar 25; 301(12): 1242–1252.

[120] Lee MO, Silverman SM, Hansen H, Patel VB, Manchikanti L. A comprehensive review of opioid-induced hyperalgesia. Pain Physician 2011; 3(14): 145-61. [http://dx.doi.org/10.36076/ppj.2011/14/145] [PMID: 21412369]

[121] Bruera E, Paice JA. Cancer pain management: safe and effective use of opioids. Am Soc Clin Oncol Educ Book 2015; 35(35): e593-9. [http://dx.doi.org/10.14694/EdBook_AM.2015.35.e593] [PMID: 25993228]

[122] Ripamonti CI, Santini D, Maranzano E, Berti M, Roila F. Management of cancer pain: ESMO Clinical Practice Guidelines. Ann Oncol 2012; 23 (Suppl. 7): vii139-54. [http://dx.doi.org/10.1093/annonc/mds233] [PMID: 22997447]

[123] Temel JS, Greer JA, Muzikansky A, *et al.* Early palliative care for patients with metastatic non-smal--cell lung cancer. N Engl J Med 2010; 363(8): 733-42. [http://dx.doi.org/10.1056/NEJMoa1000678] [PMID: 20818875]

[124] Zimmermann C, Swami N, Krzyzanowska M, *et al.* Early palliative care for patients with advanced cancer: a cluster-randomised controlled trial. Lancet 2014; 383(9930): 1721-30. [http://dx.doi.org/10.1016/S0140-6736(13)62416-2] [PMID: 24559581]

[125] Epstein AS, Volandes AE. The Magic of Conversation — Patient-Centered Communication in Cancer. JAMA Oncol. 2020; 6(6): 892–893. [http://dx.doi.org/10.1001/jamaoncol.2020.1256] [PMID: 32492028]

[126] Oldenmenger WH, Sillevis Smitt PAE, van Dooren S, Stoter G, van der Rijt CCD. A systematic review on barriers hindering adequate cancer pain management and interventions to reduce them: A critical appraisal. Eur J Cancer 2009; 45(8): 1370-80. [http://dx.doi.org/10.1016/j.ejca.2009.01.007] [PMID: 19201599]

[127] Hui D, Bruera E. Integrating palliative care into the trajectory of cancer care. Nat Rev Clin Oncol 2016; 13(3): 159-71. [http://dx.doi.org/10.1038/nrclinonc.2015.201] [PMID: 26598947]

[128] Sun V, Grant M, McMullen CK, *et al.* Surviving colorectal cancer: long-term, persistent ostomy-specific concerns and adaptations. J Wound Ostomy Continence Nurs 2013; 40(1): 61-72. [http://dx.doi.org/10.1097/WON.0b013e3182750143] [PMID: 23222968]

[129] Hudson PL, Remedios C, Thomas K. A systematic review of psychosocial interventions for family carers of palliative care patients. BMC Palliat Care 2010; 9(1): 17. [http://dx.doi.org/10.1186/1472-684X-9-17] [PMID: 20687960]

[130] Dionne-Odom JN, Azuero A, Lyons KD, *et al.* Benefits of early versus delayed palliative care to informal family caregivers of patients with advanced cancer. J Clin Oncol 2015; 33(13): 1446-52. [http://dx.doi.org/10.1200/JCO.2014.58.7824] [PMID: 25800762]

[131] Harsanyi H, Cuthbert C, Schulte F. The stigma surrounding opioid use as a barrier to cancer-pain management: an overview of experiences with fear, shame, and poorly controlled pain in the context of advanced cancer. Curr Oncol. 2023 Jun 17; 30(6): 5835–5848. [http://dx.doi.org/10.3390/curroncol30060437] [PMID: 37366920]

[132] Beauchamp TL, Childress JF. Principles of Biomedical Ethics. 7th ed., New York: Oxford University Press 2012.

[133] Volkow ND, McLellan AT. Opioid abuse in chronic pain—misconceptions and mitigation strategies. N Engl J Med 2016; 374(13): 1253-63. [http://dx.doi.org/10.1056/NEJMra1507771] [PMID: 27028915]

[134] Manchikanti L, Helm S II, Fellows B, *et al.* Opioid Epidemic in the United States. Pain Physician 2012; 3S(15) (Suppl.): ES9-ES38. [http://dx.doi.org/10.36076/ppj.2012/15/ES9] [PMID: 22786464]

[135] Patrick SW, Fry CE, Jones TF, Buntin MB. Implementation of prescription drug monitoring programs associated with reductions in opioid-related death rates. Health Aff (Millwood) 2016; 35(7): 1324-32. [http://dx.doi.org/10.1377/hlthaff.2015.1496] [PMID: 27335101]

[136] Fishman SM. Responsible Opioid Prescribing: A Physician's Guide. 2nd ed., Washington, DC: Waterford Life Sciences 2012.

[137] Cherny NI, Portenoy RK. Sedation in the management of refractory symptoms: guidelines for evaluation and treatment. J Palliat Care 1994; 10(2): 31-8. [http://dx.doi.org/10.1177/082585979401000207] [PMID: 8089815]

[138] Sulmasy DP. Double effect principle. In: Post SG, Ed. Encyclopedia of Bioethics. 3rd ed. New York: Macmillan Reference 2004; pp. 709-13.

[139] Practitioner's Manual: An Informational Outline of the Controlled Substances Act. Washington, DC: US Department of Justice 2006.

[140] Model policy for the use of controlled substances for the treatment of pain. J Pain Palliat Care Pharmacother 2005; 19(2): 73-8. [http://dx.doi.org/10.1080/J354v19n02_14] [PMID: 16061467]

[141] Opioid Policy Principles for People with Cancer, a History of Cancer, and Survivors. Washington, DC 2017.

[142] Lotan D, Fenig E, Bejar J, Berkenstadt H. New directions in cancer pain management: The future is personalized. Isr Med Assoc J 2020; 22(7): 450-4. [PMID: 33236576]

[143] Fink DJ. Gene therapy for pain: a perspective. Pain Med 2013; 14(4): 505-6.

[144] Fink DJ, Wechuck J, Mata M, *et al.* Gene therapy for pain: Results of a phase I clinical trial. Ann Neurol 2011; 70(2): 207-12. [http://dx.doi.org/10.1002/ana.22446] [PMID: 21796661]

[145] Majzner RG, Mackall CL. Tumor antigen escape from CAR T-cell therapy. Cancer Discov 2018; 8(1 0): 1219-26. [http://dx.doi.org/10.1158/2159-8290.CD-18-0442] [PMID: 30135176]

[146] Bennett CL, Jiang R, Alpaugh RK, *et al.* Immunotherapy-induced neuropathies: current knowledge

and future perspectives. Curr Oncol Rep 2020; 22(5): 46.
[PMID: 32296952]

[147] Nishizawa D, Ikeda K. Pharmacogenomics of opioid pain sensitivity. Drug Metab Pharmacokinet 2014; 29(1): 12-7.
[PMID: 24284432]

[148] Klepstad P, Rakvag TT, Kaasa S, *et al.* The 118 A>G polymorphism in the human mu-opioid receptor gene influences pain perception and morphine requirements in cancer patients. Pain 2004; 109(3): 415-9.

[149] Gasche Y, Daali Y, Fathi M, *et al.* Codeine intoxication associated with ultrarapid CYP2D6 metabolism. N Engl J Med 2004; 351(27): 2827-31.
[http://dx.doi.org/10.1056/NEJMoa041888] [PMID: 15625333]

SUBJECT INDEX

A

B

C

D

E

F

G

H

I

K

L

M

Q

R

S

T

U

V

W

www.ingramcontent.com/pod-product-compliance
Ingram Content Group UK Ltd.
Pitfield, Milton Keynes, MK11 3LW, UK
UKHW060011051026
15591UKWH00002B/150
* 9 7 9 8 8 9 8 8 1 3 7 4 1 *